D1736907

THE SOMATIZING DISORDERS

ILLNESS AS A WAY OF LIFE

THE
SOMATIZING
DISORDERS
ILLNESS AS A WAY OF LIFE

Charles V. Ford, M.D.
Vanderbilt University School of Medicine
Nashville

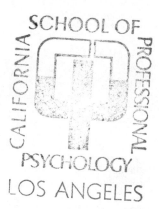

ELSEVIER BIOMEDICAL
New York · Amsterdam · Oxford

Elsevier Science Publishing Co., Inc.
52 Vanderbilt Avenue, New York, New York 10017

Sole distributors outside the United States and Canada:
Elsevier Science Publishers B. V.
P.O. Box 211, 1000 AE Amsterdam, The Netherlands

Library of Congress Cataloging in Publication Data
Ford, Charles V.
    The somatizing disorders.

    Includes bibliographical references and index.
    1. Medicine, Psychosomatic. 2. Sick—Psychology. 3. Physician and patient.
    I. Title. [DNLM: 1. Factitious disorders. 2. Somatoform disorders. WM 90
    F699s]
RC49.F67   1983   616.08   82-13947
ISBN 0-444-00752-0

Manufactured in the United States of America

Dedicated to the memory of my father
Clifford Ford, 1910–1981

CONTENTS

ACKNOWLEDGMENTS

The assistance of several faculty members of the Department of Psychiatry, Vanderbilt University, who critically reviewed portions of the manuscript and offered valuable suggestions, is greatly appreciated. They are Virginia Abernethy, Professor (anthropology); Edward Arnold, Assistant Professor; Mark Kelly, Assistant Professor (medical psychology); and Perry Nicassio, Assistant Professor (medical psychology).

I am also indebted to Selena Cunningham, my secretary, and to Evelyn Ford, my wife, for their efforts in preparing the manuscript for publication.

1

INTRODUCTION AND OVERVIEW

Health is accorded a positive value in Western society, yet paradoxically many persons choose illness as a way of life. This choice is usually, but not always, unconsciously determined, and the patient will state that health is preferable and indeed repetitively seek medical care.

THE CONCEPT OF SOMATIZATION

Somatization is a process by which the body (the soma) is used for psychological purposes or for personal gain. Any one symptom or constellation of symptoms may concurrently serve more than one function, including issues related to intrapsychic conflicts, interpersonal relationships, and social or environmental problems.

Examples of the psychological uses of somatization include (1) displacement of unpleasant affects (emotions) into a physical symptom, e.g., preoccupation with bowel dysfunction in place of experiencing the underlying depression; (2) the use of the symptom to communicate, via symbolic means, an idea or emotion, e.g., hysterical paraplegia to symbolize and communicate feelings of helplessness; (3) the alleviation of guilt through suffering, e.g., a pain syndrome experienced after the death of someone who was ambivalently regarded.

Examples of personal gains obtained by somatization include (1) the capacity to manipulate interpersonal relationships, e.g., "not tonight dear, I have a headache"; (2) the intention to obtain release from duties and responsibilities, e.g., absence at place of employment or excuse for not completing housework; (3) financial gain, e.g., disability payments or compensation for pain after a "whiplash" injury; (4) the seeking of attention or a closer relationship or sympathy from another person; e.g., the concern and worry elicited in response to skin lesions surreptitiously self-induced.

Interpersonal and psychic gains from somatization are not distinct from those observed in the psychological uses of genuine organic illness. It is not at all infrequent for persons with diseases of unquestioned organic etiology to capitalize upon their illness to serve a variety of needs. However, there are some individuals who repetitively use their bodies as a means of handling life stresses. Persons who use physical symptoms as a lifestyle have somatoform disorders such as hypochondriasis.

THE FREQUENCY OF SOMATIZATION

If the process of somatization were comparatively rare, it would be of intellectual interest but of little impact upon medical practice and medical economics. Quite the contrary is true. Despite the fact that only a miniscule portion of the medical curriculum is devoted to the diagnosis and treatment of somatizing disorders, patients with these symptoms occupy a significantly large proportion of the practicing physician's time.

Several investigations from different geographical locations suggest a remarkably high frequency of patient visits to a physician at which time no evidence of disease can be found. Studying consecutive patients in an English medical clinic Culpan and Davies (1960) found that only 43% had organic disease alone, 13% had organic disease and psychological problems, 6% had no diagnosis, and 38% had no disease and only psychological problems. When the same investigators studied patients at a surgical clinic, the figures were weighted in favor of organic disease: 66% of the patients had organic disease only, 16% had both organic disease and psychiatric symptoms, 13% had no diagnosis, and 5% had only psychological symptoms.

A review of the charts of 692 outpatients of the medical clinic at Mount Sinai Hospital, Chicago, Ill., disclosed that only 37.4% had organic disease alone, 39.6% had a diagnosis of a functional disorder (e.g., depression or psychogenic back pain), and a diagnosis of a functional disorder was implied in 23.1% (Hilkevitch, 1965).

An analysis of 1000 consecutive visits to a California health maintenance organization (HMO) disclosed that 11.6% of all persons fit into a category called the "worried well." The patients who comprised the "worried well" group were not well defined, but presumably they were persons concerned about symptoms but with no evidence of disease. Visits by "well" patients for purposes such as refills of birth control prescriptions constituted 56.8% of all patient visits. Therefore, of patients who were symptomatic, 26.9% had no evidence of disease (Garfield et al., 1976).

It is not only outpatients who utilize medical services for nonmedical disease. Multiple studies have demonstrated that women with "hysteria" are at least twice as likely as other women to have had surgical operations (Bibb and Guze, 1972; Cohen et al., 1953; DeVaul and Faillace, 1980). There is no evidence to indicate that the hysterics have more organic disease requiring a greater extent of surgical intervention than other women. Patients with other somatoform disorders, such as chronic pain syndromes, are also prone to an increased rate of hospitalizations and surgical operations (Swanson and Maruta, 1980).

Illness is not randomly distributed among persons in the population. Hinkle and Wolff (1958) studied four distinct population groups and found that for each group approximately 50% of all illness episodes were accounted for by only 25% of the population. Illnesses tended to occur in clusters, and it was estimated that at least one third of all the illnesses were influenced to some degree by the attempts of the individual to adapt to events and situations encountered. People with a high frequency of illness were viewed as having more illness because of their continuing inability to make an adequate adjustment to their milieu.

A detailed investigation (Hinkle et al., 1956) of one highly selected and stable group (male telephone company employees) indicated that over a 20-year period 10% of the men experienced 34% of the total sickness disability (days off work), while the healthiest 10% of the men experienced only 1% of the sickness disability. The data did not fit a random distribution pattern and could not be accounted for by a few men suffering extended major illnesses.

The finding that illness does not occur in random distribution has also been confirmed in studies of military populations where there is a consistent finding that a relatively small proportion of naval personnel account for a disproportionately large proportion of all visits to sick bay (see Chapter 3.).

That a relatively few persons experience a disproportionately large number of illnesses suggests that either these people are unusually prone to disease processes *or* that this group consists of persons who repetitively somatize. It cannot be denied that some people, by chance or constitution, appear to suffer more disease than others. However, it is probable that a large proportion, probably the majority, of those people who overutilize medical services are somatizers.

THE SOCIOECONOMIC IMPACT OF SOMATIZATION

Medical care is an increasing portion of the gross national product of the United States. At the present time the annual costs for medical care exceed $200 billion (U.S. Bureau of the Census, 1980). If one were to assume that 10% of all medical care (not including psychiatric treatment) is provided to persons with no organic disease, then the total cost would be $20 billion per annum. This figure does not even include disability payments or time lost from work. Somatization is a large industry!

Viewed differently, if the 25% of the people who use 50% of the medical services provided were to reduce their medical care utilization to the same average rate as the rest of the populace, then overall medical services would be reduced by 25%! Obviously such a reduction is an unrealistic goal. The point is that a large portion of medical care services are directed toward persons without disease and/or are overutilized by some persons who may or may not have evidence of disease. These services are offered in a fashion consistent with the disease model; but because these patients do not have organic disease it is not unreasonable to propose that the treatment they receive is not very effective.

American medicine has increasingly become tied to technology. Feats such as organ transplantation and computerized imagery of the brain are now taken for granted. Associated with this new technical virtuosity has been the accelerating cost of medical care and disquieting evidence of dissatisfaction with the medical profession (Boyle and Morriss, 1979). There are also sobering hints that less technically sophisticated treatment approaches may have an equally good outcome (Kane et al., 1974; Mather et al., 1971). It would seem reasonable that increased attention to the relatively neglected somatizing disorders and to the doctor–patient relationship would be cost effective and help to ameliorate the growing dissatisfaction with the medical profession. Despite the seeming logic of this proposal, physicians appear to be hesitant to alter the manner in which they practice medicine.

PHYSICIANS AND SOMATIZING BEHAVIOR

Illness as a way of life for the somatizing patient is, when viewed from the opposite perspective, also a way of life for the physician. Instead of *being sick* the physician devotes his life to the *care of the sick*; there is daily contact with all aspects of illness. Despite having chosen a life based upon caring for the sick, many physicians are disillusioned and resent the dependency of their regressed patients. Patients who do not play by the rules (e.g., have a disease that can be diagnosed and treated by the use of scientific principles) are especially resented. It often comes as a surprise to learn that some patients do not seem to want to get well and that others may even have self-induced disease. The fresh enthusiasm of the young medical student is lost in the resulting resentment, and patients are referred to (out of their presence) by the use of defamatory slang. The physician's behavior changes and direct interpersonal contacts with patients are minimized. It would be absurd to blame somatizing disorders for all problems physicians have with their patients. Yet, considering the high frequency with which the average physician comes into contact with these patients, and a general lack of skills in their management, these interactions are inevitably frustrating and lead to decreased satisfaction in the practice of medicine.

A STRATEGY TO INVESTIGATE SOMATIZATION: A READER'S GUIDE

This book proposes to study systematically the various forms of somatizing behavior. However, because somatization does not occur as a process isolated from the rest of medical practice, it is first necessary to review our current ideas about normal illness behavior before going on to study *abnormal illness behavior*. Therefore, the first part of this book focuses upon basic understandings of how people become identified as patients, the sick role, and normal psychological responses to acute and chronic diseases.

With this perspective of normal illness behavior in mind, the second portion of the book reviews in detail each of the major somatoform disorders. These include hysteria, hypochondriasis, malingering, factitious disease, Munchausen syndrome, chronic pain syndrome, and disability syndromes. Each of these topics are explored in regard to phenomenology, theoretical constructs, and suggested therapeutic strategies and techniques.

In this book the so-called "psychosomatic" diseases will not be considered as somatizing disorders. Current etiologic views of these chronic diseases (e.g., asthma, ulcerative colitis, rheumatoid arthritis) tend toward seeing them as multidetermined disorders with constitutional, environmental, and psychological issues all playing a role in their symptomatic expression. Previous views that the "psychosomatic" diseases may be a symbolic expression of a specific conflict have been discarded by most investigators working in this area of medicine. Although the classic psychosomatic diseases may be somewhat more sensitive to psychological issues than other diseases, the difference is quantitative rather than qualitative. All disease processes appear to be influenced by psychosocial stressors, and, in a reciprocal fashion, the psychological state of the patient is influenced by the disease (Leigh and Reiser, 1977).

The third portion of this book is centered on the doctor–patient relationship. This relationship is regarded as a primary issue both in understanding the etiology of somatizing behavior and as a primary treatment modality. A comprehensive knowledge of the doctor–patient relationship requires an investigation of both sides of this interpersonal dyad. Therefore the "other side" of the relationship, the characteristics of the physicians, is also investigated in Chapter 12.

The last chapter synthesizes the various themes presented throughout the book. The abnormal illness behavior displayed in somatizing disorders is related to illness behavior associated with organic disease. Features that are common to, or that differentiate, the various somatizing disorders are reviewed. The unique relationships between patients who experience illness as a way of life and their physicians are explored. Finally, general strategies for diagnosis and treatment of the various somatizing disorders are suggested.

Each chapter has been constructed so that it can be read as a separate unit. However, some cross-indexing has been necessary to reduce redundancy.

REFERENCES

Bibb, R.C., and Guze, S.B. 1972. Hysteria in a psychiatric hospital. Am J Psychiatry 129:224–228.

Boyle, J., and Morriss, J. 1979. The crisis in medicine: Models, myths and metaphors. Et Cetera 36:269–274.

Cohen, M.E., Robins, E., Purtell, J.J., Altmann, M.W., and Reid, D.E. 1953. Excessive surgery in hysteria. JAMA 151:977–986.

Culpan, R., and Davies, B. 1960. Psychiatric illness at a medical and a surgical outpatient clinic. Compr Psychiatry 1:228–235.

DeVaul, R.A., and Faillace, L.A. 1980. Surgery-proneness: A review and clinical assessment. Psychosomatics 21:295–299.

Garfield, S.R., Collen, M.G., Feldman, R., Soghikian, K., Richart, R.H., and Duncan, J.H. 1976. Evaluation of an ambulatory medical-care delivery system. N Engl J Med 294:426–431.

Hilkevitch, A. 1965. Psychiatric disturbance in outpatients of a general medical outpatient clinic. Int J Neuropsychiatry 1:372–375.

Hinkle, L.E., and Wolff, H.G. 1958. Etiologic investigations of the relationships between illness, life experiencies and the social environment. Ann Intern Med 49:1373–1388.

Hinkle, L.E., Pinsky, R.H., Bross, I.D.J., and Plummer, N. 1956. The distribution of sickness liability in a homogeneous group of "healthy adult men." Am J Hyg 64:220–242.

Kane, R., Leymaster, C., Olsen, D., Wolley, F.R. and Fisher, 1974. Manipulating the patient: A comparison of the effectiveness of physicians and chiropractice care. Lancet 1333–1336.

Leigh, H., and Reiser, M.F. 1977. Major trends in psychosomatic medicine: The psychiatrist's evolving role in medicine. Ann Intern Med 87:233–239.

Mather, H.G., Pearson, N.G., Read, K.L.W., Shaw, D.B., Steed, G.R., Thorne, M.G., Geurrier, C.J., Erant, C.D., McHugh, P.M., Chowdhury, N.R., Jafarg, M.H., and Wallace, T.S. 1971. Acute myocardial infarction: Home and hospital treatment. Br Med J 3:334–338.

Swanson, D.W., and Maruta, T. 1980. Patients complaining of extreme pain. Mayo Clin Proc 55:563–566.

United States Bureau of the Census. 1980. Statistical Abstract of the United States (101st ed.). Washington, D.C.: U.S. Government Printing Office.

2

DISEASE, ILLNESS, AND HEALTH

The process by which a person becomes sick and is identified as a patient involves interactions of biologic, psychological, environmental, and social factors. People vary as to their propensity to become sick; and when ill, all people do not behave in the same manner.

ILLNESS BEHAVIOR

As an introduction, let us examine the following real life scenario. The various elements are illustrative of different aspects of illness behavior.

A group of physicians on rounds enter a hospital room and greet the first patient, a white-haired woman in her late 60s. The patient immediately accosts the attending physician with the statement that she feels fine and that she sees no reason to be in the hospital. On questioning she relates that she has always been in good health and has never been hospitalized other than for childbirth. She states that she had come to the hospital reluctantly, and only after insistent urging by her children, after she had experienced a transient episode of crushing chest pain. She initially demands to be discharged but then relents to the persuasion of her physicians to remain until certain laboratory tests have been completed.

Moving on to the next bed the medical team finds another woman of approximately the same age. This woman is a "familiar face" immediately recognized because of several prior hospital admissions for poorly defined symptoms. She immediately begins a litany of physical complaints. It is necessary to interrupt her history to discover that the immediate reason for this hospital admission was, similar to the first patient, an episode of transient chest pain. Intermixed with the woman's report of multiple physical symptoms are complaints about the hospital food and the care she has received; she angrily reports that a nurse took 35 minutes to answer her bell the previous night. When a tactful suggestion concerning discharge is made she immediately becomes more accommodating and suggests that perhaps "a few more tests" are in order before she leaves the hospital. As the physicians attempt to leave her bedside she clutches the sleeve of one, moans, extends her arm, and asks that he inspect the "painful" site of a venipuncture.

Later, out in the hall, the discussion, with the laboratory results now available, indicates that the first woman has elevated enzymes, indicative of a small myocardial infarct. The physicians express both concern and admiration for the "crusty old lady." For the second woman all laboratory findings are again within normal limits. The physicians' discussion revolves around the need for dynamite to get the "old turkey" out of the hospital.

What has been observed is two patients of similar age and symptoms displaying remarkably different *illness behavior*. It is important to note that the illness behavior elicited very different emotional responses and attitudes from the physicians.

Illness behavior is a term suggested by Mechanic (1962) to describe the various types of behavior that persons may have in regard to their perceptions of bodily symptoms and their evaluation of symptoms, as well as the various courses of action that they may take (or not take) as a consequence. Some examples are as follows: Is an abdominal pain interpreted as "indigestion" or as a symptom of disease? Does the person as a consequence of a symptom perceive himself to be "sick" and behave accordingly (e.g., going to bed), or is the symptom interpreted as merely an annoying ache or pain associated with the process of aging? Does the symptom elicit a decision that the person should consult a physician for further evaluation?

DISEASE, ILLNESS, AND HEALTH

At this point it is important to differentiate between illness and disease. These terms (along with "sickness," a nonspecific term incorporating elements of both disease and illness) are often used interchangeably by the lay public and many physicians. However, such nonspecific use of the terms blurs important distinctions, which allow one to conceptualize the role that illness behavior plays in the presentation of symptoms by a patient to a physician.

Disease refers to objective anatomic deformations and pathophysiologic conditions. These changes can be objectively demonstrated or inferred (although sophisticated diagnostic equipment may be required) and may be caused by such varied etiologic factors as degenerative processes, trauma, toxins, and infectious agents.

The study of disease has been the almost exclusive focus of the bioscientific medical model which has increasingly predominated modern medicine (Boyle and Morriss, 1979; Engel, 1977; Kleinman et al., 1978). This has been particularly true in the United States since the Flexner report of 1910. At that time medical schools were rated primarily by the degree to which they utilized scientific principles in their educational programs (Engel, 1973). This emphasis on the scientific aspects of medical care has led to immense therapeutic and technologic advances in the treatment of disease states. Paradoxically these technologic advances have received the awe and admiration of the general public but have not been associated with increased respect for the medical profession. To the contrary, there is evidence that the general populace has become more disenchanted with physicians (Boyle and Morriss, 1979; Kleinman et al., 1978). It is entirely possible, and probable, that patients are less satisfied with physicians because, in their preoccupation with disease, physicians have neglected the fact that disease is only one aspect of illness. But it is usually the condition of illness that brings a person to a physician.

Illness refers to " ... experiences of disvalued changes in states of being and in social function" (Eisenberg, 1977). Therefore illness takes into account the personal nature of suffering, alienation from usual gratifying activities, and the decreased capacity to participate in society (Apple, 1960; Herzlich, 1973). Illness has a subjective quality and the many personal aspects unique to each individual.

From the above definitions and concepts of disease and illness, it is readily seen that disease and illness often accompany one another. A middle-aged man with an acute myocardial infarction has objective evidence of a disease state; in addition he experiences illness because of his personal subjective distress and his inability to participate in his usual activities.

Although it is often assumed that a person's symptoms and consequent behavior will parallel the degree of disease, this is often not the situation. Divergence may occur in either direction. There may be extensive disease with little suggestion of illness or there may be little or no evidence of disease, despite which the person experiences disabling illness. Some clinical examples will clarify this point.

A 55-year-old contractor was sitting in his pickup truck at a construction site when it was hit by another vehicle. When seen at a local emergency room there was no evidence of injury, except for very minor contusions. He was seen in psychiatric consultation 18 months later at the insistence of his insurance company. The patient had, at that time, already sought consultation with a total of 35 different physicians and/or medical centers for subjective complaints of unilateral pain and swelling. No objective evidence of a disease process had been demonstrated in any of the 35 separate consultations. The patient was transported from one medical center to another, lying supine in the back of a station wagon driven by his wife. He was unable to work and ceased almost all of his relationships with other persons. It is important to note that the patient had been an extremely hard worker since childhood. In recent years he had spent all of his "spare time" caring for a sick relative with a disabling chronic disease (see Humpty Dumpty syndrome, Chapter 6).

In contrast to the above is the case history of a 50-year-old college professor. This man suffered from chronic lymphoma and, during the 6 months preceding a psychiatric evaluation, was hospitalized briefly with herpes zoster and later for an iridectomy for treatment of acute narrow angle glaucoma. Despite this medical history the patient described himself as "healthy." Despite evidence of significant disease and the inevitable transient setbacks, the patient continued to teach his classes, had good relationships with his grown children, and maintained a warm relationship, including sexual activity, with his wife. Therefore this man had not become chronically "ill" and regarded himself as "healthy."

Health is a word or concept most people take for granted. Health is usually defined as an absence of illness or disease, which connotes a passive quality to the idea of health. Because the layman may not know how to interpret symptoms accurately, particularly if they are not disabling, the perception of health may continue in the presence of considerable disease. In general one's perception of health is closely allied with the ability to carry out normal day-to-day activities, and only when there is interference with these activities does the feeling of being ill arise. Therefore for many people, if not most, health is the opposite of illness rather than of disease.

There is, however, another way of looking at health: as an active homeostatic process. With this theoretical construct health is seen as an active process of maintaining a disease-free state. Thus one can view a whole range of activities and attitudes as constituting "health behavior" (Kasl and Cobb, 1966). Health behavior is complementary to, rather than the opposite of, illness behavior. An active participation in maintaining health may include a variety of behaviors, such as being careful about diet and weight, participation in exercise programs, and the avoidance of toxins, including tobacco smoke. Other active behaviors for health maintenance include using seat belts in automobiles, obtaining proper immunizations, and learning effectively to manage and cope with life stresses (Knowles, 1977). Consistent with this view of actively maintaining health would be the acquisition of knowledge about basic physiology and common disease states, such as the early warning symptoms of cancer.

THE PROCESS OF DISEASE AND ILLNESS

There is a general tendency for the lay public to think of disease (and illness) as a stochastic process. That is to say that a disease "hits" randomly, afflicting unfortunate victims. After the perception of a symptom the victim (patient) seeks assistance from a physician with the hope of being restored to his/her previously healthy state.

Although some aspects of the above formulation may have partial validity, the actual process of disease and illness is far more complicated. This process involves the interaction of multiple variables reflecting biologic, psychological, and environmental (including social) factors. As is demonstrated later in this chapter, even a disease process so apparently simple as a bacterial infection is influenced by personal factors.

An outline of some of the interacting factors relative to disease and illness is provided by Figure 1. Even this relatively detailed schema does not include all possible variables and interactions.

The initial step in the disease process is the influence of a pathogen. The pathogenic influence may be a toxin, degenerative process, infectious agent, etc. This pathogenic influence is modified by the body defenses, such as immunologic processes, fibroblast response, and other homeostatic mechanims. If the defensive mechanisms are inadequate to immediately restore the body to its normal state symptoms may develop. (Symptoms are defined as a sensation of bodily or psychological states which are perceived as out of the

FIGURE 1. A schematic view of the process of illness and disease (not all possible relationships are shown).

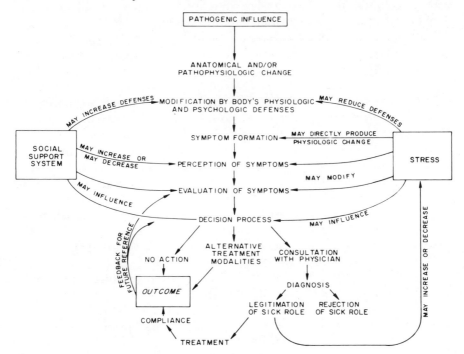

ordinary and may be interpreted as abnormal.) Psychological mechanisms such as denial may block the perception of symptoms, or anxiety may intensify the perception of symptoms. Symptoms may also arise directly from psychological reactions, such as the physiologic concomitants of emotional states.

Once the symptom has been perceived, a process of evaluation follows. The symptom may be discounted and interpreted as a normal physiologic process, or, on the contrary, it may be interpreted as possibly indicative of serious disease. The person's evaluation process is influenced by variables, including previous experience, cultural orientation, and general knowledge about medicine and physiology (Fabrega, 1973, 1974).

A decision follows from evaluation of a symptom. The person must evaluate variables such as available resources (Is a physician available? How much will it cost?) in relationship to personal belief systems (religious beliefs or cultural determinants such as belief in voodoo) in deciding whether to seek further assistance and of what type. Many, perhaps most, persons will not seek medical care at this point but will instead decide to take no action, to self-remedy, or to seek an alternative treatment system such as consultation with a Christian Science practitioner or informal discussion with a pharmacist.

Symptoms and brief periods of illness are very common and usually do not result in medical consultation. Mechanic (1975) has stated that the most common reason for seeing a physician is the common cold, but most people with a cold do not seek medical attention! Studies of subjects who maintained health logs or diaries indicate that most illness episodes (75–95%) do not result in physician consultation (Demers et al., 1980; Roghmann and Haggerty, 1973; White et al., 1961). Yet many of these illness episodes (or symptoms) would be regarded by a physician as potentially serious (Berg and LoGerfo, 1979).

When a decision is made to seek medical consultation, an important question is why did the person decide to see a doctor at that particular time? Often symptoms have been present for weeks or months before the physician is consulted. Psychosocial stress has been posited as an important influence determining when a symptom may elicit a physician consultation (Tessler et al., 1976; Zola, 1973). McWhinney (1972) suggests that there are a number of reasons that determine why and when a patient seeks medical care. Among these are that (1) the symptoms have become intolerable in terms of pain, discomfort, or disability; (2) the symptoms have caused anxiety and the patient fears their consequences; and (3) the symptoms are actually a mask for a problem in living.

A person becomes a "patient" at the time medical consultation has been sought. Eisenberg (1980) has observed that the transition to patienthood (and from patienthood back to person) represent social decision points rather than boundaries determined by shifting biologic parameters. It is the process of illness, not disease, that determines a person's efforts to seek help.

The physician evaluates the patient through the medical interpretation of the symptom, by physical findings of examination, and by a variety of diagnostic aides (i.e., blood studies, x-rays). The diagnosis is established, often modified by the physician's personal belief system and psychological characteristics and after "negotiation" with the patient (Balint, 1957). The diagnosis (and treatment) to be accepted by the patient, must be compatible with his/her personal belief system and cultural orientation. For example, patients holding certain folk medicine views " . . . may change physicians if they are told that they have both high blood (pressure) and low blood (anemia). In folk nosology these are obviously exclusive so the physician making such diagnoses is thought a "fool" (Snow, 1974).

The physician's diagnosis may be that there is no disease (or illness) present. However, more frequently a disease is diagnosed and consequently this legitimizes the "sick role." (The sick role is such an important element in the concept of illness that the following chapter is devoted to that topic.) Following the establishment of a diagnosis the physician then "prescribes" a treatment program, which the patient may follow to a variable extent. Studies of patients' compliance suggest that the patients often cooperate with prescribed therapeutic interventions far less frequently than their physicians realize (Blackwell, 1973).

Increased stress, as reflected by a larger number of life changes, also occurs after an illness experience (Rahe and Arthur, 1968). Presumably this increased stress reflects the effect of the illness upon the person's life. The illness can also serve to decrease stress. Patients having regional enteritis were reported to have exacerbations of their diseases at times when they felt that they were struggling with insoluble conflicts. Often, responses of the social environment to their illnesses provided solutions to their problems (Ford et al., 1969).

A number of experiences along this pathway described will provide new knowledge for the patient and will be utilized during future illness episodes (Fabrega, 1973, 1974). For example, a patient may be less likely to seek medical care in the future if prior medical treatment was ineffective or if it increased personal suffering.

DISEASE, ILLNESS, AND THE RELATIONSHIP TO STRESS AND SOCIAL SUPPORT

During the last two decades there has been considerable emphasis on the role of stress preceding disease states. Early work emphasized the importance of loss and feelings of helplessness (Engel, 1967; Schmale, 1958) and later the concept of stress as a consequence of life change was elaborated. In an effort to measure and to standardize the extent of stress experienced by a person the idea of life change units (LCUs) was developed by Holmes and Rahe (1967). A wide variety of events occur in a person's life which elicit responses. These life events may be positive or negative and the degree to which an individual responds to any one type of event is highly dependent upon personal characteristics of that individual. A specific type of life event may have different meanings to different persons. Coping mechanisms and the presence or absence of social support (see below) may significantly modify the degree of stress to the individual. A wide variety of diseases have been demonstrated to have an onset, or symptomatic expression, statistically correlated with increased life change units in their victims. These include such diverse disorders as myocardial infarction (Rahe et al., 1974), sickle cell disease (Leavell and Ford, 1982), and diabetes (Grant et al., 1974). Although these correlations are statistically significant, they account for a relatively small degree of the variance, and this suggests that there are other important variables in the disease–illness process (Rahe and Arthur, 1978). It is a gross oversimplification to view stress as a direct etiologic factor in the development of disease or in the elaboration of patterns of illness behavior. Keeping this caveat in mind, however, psychosocial stress remains a very important concept and, in a generic manner, does influence the disease–illness process at several points (see Figure 1). These may be summarized as follows:

1. Stress, both of a physical or psychological nature, may modify the body's defenses and thereby increase susceptibility to pathogenic influences. For example, immunosuppression has been shown to be reduced in high-stress situations (Solomon et al., 1974).
2. Stress, by inducing emotional responses, may therefore lead to various physiologic changes associated with different emotional states. An example would be increased muscular tension associated with increased responsibility at work (Holmes and Wolff, 1952).
3. The feeling that one is stressed may intensify the perception of concurrently existing physical symptoms (Ford et al., 1976).
4. The sensation of being stressed may lead one to evaluate a perceived symptom differently than if one were in a nonstressed state (Mechanic, 1972).
5. Stress may influence the decision-making process in terms of what course of action to take in regard to a physical symptom. People who feel stressed are in general more likely to seek medical attention than those who are not (Tessler et al., 1976).
6. Illness (the sick role) itself may serve to reduce the stress that an individual experiences (Ford et al., 1969).

Although the association of stress antecedent to the development of illness has received much publicity, including featured articles in the Sunday tabloids, the personal assets of the patient in modifying the effects of stress are probably of equal importance. Social support appears to be an important factor that exerts a favorable effect in the process of disease and illness (Cobb, 1976; Eisenberg, 1979). Eisenberg has succinctly described this role in an editorial entitled, "A friend, not an apple, a day will keep the doctor away" (Eisenberg, 1979).

The statistical evidence for the power of social support in modifying illness is as impressive as that for the power of psychosocial stress in initiating illness. Nuckolls and colleagues (1972) computed the incidence of pregnancy complications in various groups of women using psychosocial stress and the women's personal assets as variables. Psychosocial stress was measured using the Homes–Rahe Schedule of Recent Events, and the estimate of the women's personal assets placed emphasis upon their social support systems. This well-designed prospective study disclosed that a high incidence of pregnancy complications was associated with high stress and low social support. In the absence of stress there was no significant relationship between social support and pregnancy complications.

An excellent epidemiologic investigation found that persons who lacked social and community ties had an increased mortality rate (Berkman and Syme, 1979). Factors included in the social network were marriage, contacts with close friends and relatives, church membership, and informal and formal group associations. The finding of increased mortality for the more socially isolated subjects persisted even when age, smoking history, health practices, alcohol consumption, use of health services, socioeconomic status, and health problems were taken into account. The evidence, therefore, was the lack of social support rather than some other confounding variable that increased the mortality rate. The findings were impressive in that the quatrile of subjects who were least socially connected, when compared to the quatrile who were most socially connected, had an increased mortality risk of 2.3 for men and 2.8 for women over the nine-year study.

The degree to which social contacts can influence health is impressive. Using the simple characteristic of frequency of church attendance it has been shown that frequent-church-attending white males had statistically lower blood pressure when they were compared to infrequent attenders. This beneficial effect persisted even when factors such as age, obesity, cigarette smoking, and socioeconomic status were taken into account. It appeared that factors such as the provision of interpersonal relationships and such difficult to define entities as "maintenance of hope" provided the beneficial effect (Graham et al., 1978).

From the preceding brief review of the effects of stress and social support it becomes readily apparent that the process of both disease and illness are intimately connected with the life situation and life events in any individual. The nonspecificity of "stress" and "social support" should not lead to the interpretation that attention to these details is nonscientific. Quite the contrary! The logical conclusion is that these are important variables that must be considered by the *scientific* physician. Failure to control for all known variables is nonscientific! Yet, many physicians trained within the biomedical model pride themselves upon their scientific approach and decide that the personal, social, and psychological aspects of patient care, which are not easily quantified, are irrelevant to their practice of medicine.

All patients present themselves to physicians as part and parcel of some aspect of illness behavior. This behavior is generated as a consequence of changes in their usual life activities. Such changes may be, but are not necessarily, initiated by a disease process. The patient comes to the physician not so much because of disease but because there is the perception or fear of illness. To quote Cassell (1976), *"Doctors do not treat disease; they treat patients who have diseases* .... A patient is a person with both an illness and a disease; the patient is made better to the extent that both the illness and the disease are made better."

Illustrative Case History

The following case history demonstrates how separate the processes of illness and disease can be in the same patient and how the patient may use a disease in the service of reducing the illness.

A 62-year-old disabled widowed motel maid was hospitalized 6 times within a period of 14 months. The indications for these hospitalizations, paid for by Medicare and Medicaid, were episodes of uncontrolled hypertension. Poor compliance with medications was suspected but was not proven until the most recent hospitalization when a nurse found medications, which had been ordered for the patient, in a waste basket. Psychiatric consultation was requested at that time.

The patient was cooperative with the consulting psychiatrist and offered the history that she was depressed and often did not understand "why I do things." By depression the patient meant that she was lonely and isolated, living in a housing project, and felt frightened to leave her apartment. In addition finances were a struggle as her disability payments totaled only $200.00 per month. She explained, with a smile on her face, how nice the food was at the hospital and about the good care that she received from the nurses. She admitted that at home she frequently did not take her antihypertensive medications because there was no one to "coax" her to do so.

Psychological testing was obtained and indicated an IQ of 75, passive-dependent and compulsive personality characteristics, and mild depression. There was no suggestion of psychosis.

The psychiatric consultant was not impressed that the patient displayed any symptoms of a major depression. Instead, she appeared to have a "simple" quality and to be manipulating the health care system in a fairly open manner in an effort to cope with the unhappy life. The consultant's recommendations revolved around efforts for social agencies to provide more interpersonal support in an effort to reduce her need to use hospitals for that purpose.

This case illustrates a situation where a person had both a disease (hypertension) and an illness (disability). Neither were directly causal to the other, but paradoxically the patient used her disease, and perpetuated the disease, in an effort to reduce her illness. Because the illness was ignored the good care that the patient received in treatment for her disease failed to be effective.

ILLUSTRATIONS OF DISEASE AND ILLNESS

To further explore certain aspects of the intermingling of illness behavior, life events, and disease processes I have chosen three medical "disorders." They are (1) streptococcal pharyngitis ("strep throat"), an example of a disease with a highly specific pathogen; (2) reactive hypoglycemia—a frequently diagnosed condition which may or may not be indicative of a disease process; and (3) medical student illness, a syndrome without physiologic or pathologic changes, which is a fascinating type of illness behavior probably initiated by stress.

Streptococcal Pharyngitis

Streptococcal pharyngitis (strep throat) is a common acute infectious disease with a known pathogen. If the acute disease is not treated some victims will develop chronic manifestations of rheumatic heart disease or glomerulonephritis, both believed to be related to autoimmunologic processes.

A one-year prospective study (Meyer and Haggerty, 1962) involving 100 subjects in 16 lower-middle-class families demonstrated that there was no relationship between streptococcal illness episodes and the number or type of streptococci present as measured by frequent cultures from throat swabs! Thus, despite the presence of a known pathogenic organism, factors other than the presence of the organism were more important in determining the onset of disease. The significant factors were age (2- to 5-year-olds were more susceptible), season (illness episodes were slightly more common in late winter and spring), and closeness of contact with an infected person (illness episodes were twice as frequent when sleeping in the same room as an infected person). No relationships were found when the number of illness episodes was computed for the sex of the patient, presence or absence of tonsils, allergic history, changes in weather, type of housing, or family size.

Of major importance was the finding that about one quarter of the streptococcal acquisitions and illnesses followed acute family crises; these infections were about four times as likely to be preceded as to be followed by acute stress. Parents were able to predict which child was most likely to become sick in 11 out of the 16 families. Another factor relating stress to the potential severity of subsequent disease was that antistreptolysin increases were seen in only 21% of the patients in the low-stress families as compared to 47% of the patients in the moderate-high-stress families. (Statistically significant at the $p = .01$ level.)

From this study it would appear that several factors other than the pathogen itself play a part in determining which persons may become sick with a well-defined infectious disease. Among these factors, and possibly the most important, are the influences of family crises and chronic stress.

Reactive Hypoglycemia

Reactive hypoglycemia has become popularly known through several books written for the lay public. It has been implicated as the etiology for such diverse conditions as alcoholism and rheumatoid arthritis.

The physiologic rationale for reactive hypoglycemia is that when blood glucose falls below normal levels homeostatic mechanisms are activated to return the concentration of blood glucose to normal. This is particularly likely to occur approximately 2 hours following the ingestion of a high carbohydrate meal. The sequence of events is as follows: elevated blood glucose initiates the release of insulin, which if it "overshoots," acts to decrease the concentration of blood glucose below normal levels. This hypoglycemia then causes the release of growth hormone, cortisol, glucagon, and epinephrine. The effect of the epinephrine, possibly associated with mild transient cerebral hypoglycemia, may result in transient neurologic symptoms such as headache, tremor, and light-headedness, and may be perceived by the patient as an abnormal state. Other nonspecific symptoms often associated with reactive hypoglycemia include emotional lability, depression, fatigue, depression, difficulty in thinking, nausea, and visual disturbances. These symptoms are very similar to some psychiatric disorders, particularly anxiety neuroses or an agitated depression.

Hypoglycemia may be a symptom of severe underlying disease such as an insulinoma or early diabetes mellitus. However, low blood glucose levels (below 50 mg) occur frequently in normal asymptomatic individuals (Burns et al., 1965). Therefore a single laboratory finding of low blood glucose is not of much diagnostic significance (Permutt, 1979).

An investigation (Ford et al., 1976) of individuals who had been previously diagnosed as having "reactive hypoglycemia" disclosed that approximately one third of the group had evidence of an underlying disease, usually prodromal diabetes mellitus. There was no evidence of any disease process in the other two thirds of the group. Irrespective of the presence or absence of underlying disease there was no difference in either the number or the nature of the presenting symptoms between the two groups! On careful examination it was evident that there was frequently an ongoing life crisis, often reflecting a sexual conflict, which had engendered the nonspecific symptoms. These symptoms had led to medical attention. The focus upon the symptoms, with the assistance of an inaccurate medical diagnosis, served, at least temporarily, to help cope with the acute stress (Ford, 1977).

An illustrative example is that of a middle-aged woman who, conflicted about her sexual relationship with her husband, used symptoms referrable to "hypoglycemia" to identify herself as sick and therefore to avoid sexual activity.

Medical Student Disease

"Medical student disease" is a well-known and fascinating phenomenon. It is estimated that 70–80% (Woods et al., 1966) of all medical students at some time during their medical school education become convinced or fearful that they have a disease. The disease "chosen" may be one that is currently being studied (such as in pathology) or that of a patient for whom the student is caring. Symptom choice appears to be influenced by "a variety of accidental, historical and learning factors in which the mechanisms of identification play a major role" (Hunter et al., 1964). Rather than just being a syndrome of the sophomore year, it has been found to occur with equal frequency through the four years of training (Woods et al., 1966). The student with "medical student disease" frequently seeks medical consultation with faculty or peers and not infrequently seeks laboratory or x-ray examinations in order to further evaluate the possibility of diagnosis. Another type of typical student behavior is to study the disease intensely in order to learn more about it. Hunter and coworkers differentiated "medical student's disease" from true hypochondria, and, although they noted that it may be associated with personal stress, they did not regard the syndrome as having much psychiatric significance. However, Woods and colleagues found that medical student disease often occurred during periods of general emotional turmoil in the personal and academic lives of the students whom they studied. Conflicts about concerns over personal and mental health and sexuality were common. These authors also found that the occurrence of medical student disease was associated with a tendency toward greater psychopathology as evidenced by MMPI (Minnesota Multiphasic Personality Inventory) scores. They recommended that the presence of the syndrome may be a signal of emotional disturbance and an indication of a need for psychiatric assistance.

Mechanic (1972) has pointed to medical student disease as an example of how stress and the acquisition of new knowledge may interact. Random bodily events (e.g., extrasystoles), or physiologic concomitants of emotional states related to stress, are evaluated differently as the student obtains previously unknown information about specific disease processes. These symptoms may then be mistakenly *attributed* to a pathologic entity. Factors important to the special situation of the medical student include the stressful nature of medical school and experiences with persons who have suffered life-threatening diseases. As a consequence the student often develops an increased sense of vulnerability.

Interpretation and Implications

The three disorders described above were chosen from a large number of possibilities because they serve to illustrate important steps in the process of disease and illness.

With streptococcal infections there is no question as to the presence of a real, potentially life-threatening disease process. Yet, even with this well-defined disease, personal crises and stressful social situations influence both the initiation and long-term course of the disease.

The myriad of nonspecific symptoms associated with hypoglycemia may reflect a disease process such as early diabetes mellitus, a normal physiologic state, a psychiatric syndrome such as anxiety neurosis, or merely a current life stress. The nature of the symptoms alone does not differentiate between these three diagnostic possibilities. The patient who perceives symptoms typical of the hypoglycemia syndrome may respond to these symptoms with a variety of illness behaviors reflecting personality characteristics, concurrent life events, emotional states, and how the symptoms might be utilized to cope with stress or conflict.

Medical student illness is an example of how the acquisition of limited new knowledge (incorporated within the disease model) associated with acute personal stress and feelings of personal vulnerability may lead to illness behavior because of the misperception of a disease state.

From these disorders it can be seen that stress can influence the process of disease and/or the perception of illness. The symptoms that a patient experiences may elicit a wide range of different interpretations. Evaluating the patient from the narrow perspective of the disease model may lead to inappropriate or inadequate treatment.

SUMMARY

The loss of *health* and a person's subjective experience of suffering and social disability is termed *illness*, while objective pathophysiologic changes are termed *disease* processes. Illness and disease are not correlated on a one-to-one basis. The action, or lack of action, that a person takes in response to a symptom is called *illness behavior*. Illness behavior is determined by the individual's personality characteristics, past experiences, current life events (stress), and the presence or absence of social support. The extent of illness that a person experiences in response to a disease, and whether or not he/

she becomes identified as a patient, are largely determined by factors unrelated to the disease process. To quote Zola (1973), "Rather than being a narrow and limited concept, health and illness are on the contrary empirically quite elastic. In short it is not merely that health and illness has sociological aspects, for it has many aspects, but really that there is a sense in which health and illness *are* social phenomena."

Contemporary Western culture usually interprets illness in terms of the disease model promulgated by bioscientific medicine. Because of pervasive confusion concerning the difference between disease and illness the person who has a propensity to use the body for psychological purposes or for personal gain (somatization) will frequently be inappropriately identified as diseased. Some persons may also find that cultural attitudes toward sick persons and the benefits afforded to them provide a way to cope with life problems. As a consequence many people who are not diseased, or whose disease is minimally related to their perceived disability, may either seek or be assigned to the sick role.

REFERENCES

Apple, D. 1960. How laymen define illness. J. Health Hum Behav 1:219–225.

Balint, M. 1957. *The Doctor, His Patient and the Illness.* New York: International Universities Press.

Berg, A.O., and LoGerfo, J.P. 1979. Potential effect of self-care algonithms on the number of physician visits. N Engl J Med 300:535–537.

Berkman, L.F., and Syme, S.L. 1979. Social networks, host resistance and mortality: A nine year followup of Alameda County residents. Am J Epidem 109:186–204.

Blackwell, B. 1973. Patient compliance. N Engl J Med 289:249–252.

Boyle, J., and Morriss, J. 1979. The crisis in medicine: Models, myths and metaphors. Et Cetera 36:269–274.

Burns, T.W., Bregant, R. VanPeenan, H.J., and Hood, T.E. 1965. Observations on blood glucose concentrations of human subjects during continuous sampling. Diabetes 14:186–193.

Cassell, E.J. 1976. *The Healer's Art.* Philadelphia, Pa.: Lippincott, pp 47–83.

Cobb, S. 1976. Social support as a moderator of life stress. Psychosom Med 38:300–314.

Demers, R.Y., Altamore, R., Mustin, H., Kleinman, A., and Leonardi, D. 1980. An exploration of the dimensions of illness behavior. J Fam Pract 11:1085–1092.

Eisenberg, L. 1977. Disease and illness: Distinctions between professional and popular ideas of sickness. Cult Med Psychiatry 1:9–23.

Eisenberg, L. 1979. A friend, not an apple, a day will help keep the doctor away. Am J Med 66:551–553.

Eisenberg, L. 1980. What makes persons "patients" and patients "well"? Am J Med 69:277–286.

Engel, G.L. 1967. A psychological setting of somatic disease: The 'giving up–given up' complex. Proc Roy Soc Med 60:533–535.

Engel, G.L. 1973. Enduring attributes of medicine relevant for the education of the physician. Ann Int Med 78:587–593.

Engel, G.L. 1977. The need for a new medical model: A challenge for biomedicine. Science 196:129–136.

Fabrega, H. 1973. Toward a model of illness behavior. Medical Care 11:470–484.

Fabrega, H. 1974. *Disease and Social Behavior.* Cambridge, Mass.: MIT Press, Chap. 6.

Ford, C.V. 1977. Hypoglycemia, hysteria, and sexual function. Med Aspects Human Sexuality 11:63–72.

Ford, C.V., Bray, G.A., and Swerdloff, R.S. 1976. A psychiatric study of patients referred with a diagnosis of hypoglycemia. Am J Psychiatry 133:290–294.

Ford, C.V., Glober, G.A., and Castelnuovo-Tedesco, P. 1969. A psychiatric study of patients with regional enteritis. JAMA 208:311–315.

Graham, T.W., Kaplan, B.H., Loroni-Huntley, J.C., et al. 1978. Frequency of church attendance and blood pressure elevation. J Behav Med 1:37–42.

Grant, I., Kyle, G.C., Teichman, A., and Mendels, J. 1974. Recent life events and diabetes in adults. Psychosom Med 36:121–128.

Herzlich, C. 1973. *Health and Illness: A Social Psychological Analysis.* New York: Academic Press.

Holmes, T.H., and Rahe, R.H. 1967. The social readjustment rating scale. J Psychosom Res 11:213–218.

Holmes, T.H., and Wolff, H.G. 1952. Life situations, emotions and backache. Psychosom Med 14:18–33.

Hunter, R.C.A., Lohrenz, J.G., and Schwartzman, A.E. 1964. Nosophobia and hypochondriasis in medical students. J Nerv Ment Dis 139:147–152.

Kasl, S.V., and Cobb, S. 1966. Health behavior, illness behavior and sick role behavior. Arch Environ Health 12:246–266.

Kleinman, A., Eisenberg, L., and Good, B. 1978. Culture illness and care. Clinical lessons from anthropologic and cross cultural research. Ann Intern Med 88:251–258.

Knowles, J.H. 1977. The responsibility of the individual. In *Doing Better and Feeling Worse: Health in the United States.* Knowles, J.H., ed. New York: Norton, pp 57–80.

Leavell, S.R., and Ford, C.V. 1982. Sickle cell disease: Psychiatric features and the relationship of symptoms to stress. Presented at the Annual Meeting of the American Academy of Psychosomatic Medicine, Chicago, Ill. November 21.

McWhinney, I.R. 1972. Beyond diagnosis. N Engl J Med 287:384–387.

Mechanic, D. 1972. The concept of illness behavior. J. Chronic Dis 15:189–194.

Mechanic, D. 1972. Social psychologic factors affecting the presentation of bodily complaints. N Engl J Med 286:1133–1139.

Mechanic, D. 1975. Sociocultural and social-psychological factors affecting personal responses to psychological disorder. J Health Soc Behav 16:393–404.

Meyer, R.J., and Haggerty, R.J. 1962. Streptococcal infections in families: Factors altering individual susceptibility. Pediatrics 29:539–549.

Nuckolls, K.B., Cassel, J., and Kaplan, B.H. 1972. Psychosocial assets, life crisis and the prognosis of pregnancy. Am J Epidemiol 95:431–441.

Permutt, M.A. 1979. Is it really hypoglycemia? If so, what should you do? Resident Staff Physician 25(August):25–41.

Rahe, R.H., and Arthur, R.J. 1968. Life-change patterns surrounding illness experience. J Psychosom Res 11:341–345.

Rahe, R.H., and Arthur, R.J. 1978. Life change and illness studies: Past history and future directions. J Hum Stress 4:3–15.

Rahe, R.H., Romo, M., Bennett, L., and Siltanen, P. 1974. Recent life changes, myocardial infarction and abrupt coronary death. Studies in Helsinki. Arch Int Med 133:221–228.

Roghmann, K.J., and Haggerty, R.J. 1973. Daily stress, illness and use of health sources in young families. Pediatr Res 7:520–526.

Schmale, A.H. 1958. Relationship of separation and depression to disease. I. A report on a hospitalized medical population. Psychosom Med 20:259–277.

Snow, L. 1974. Folk medical beliefs and their implications for care of patients. Ann Intern Med 81:82–96.

Solomon, G.F., Amkraut, A.A., and Kasper, P. 1974. Immunity, emotions and stress. Psychother Psychosom 23:209–217.

Tessler, R., Mechanic, D., and Dimond, M. 1976. The effect of psychological distress on physician utilization: A prospective study. J Health Soc Behav 17:353–364.

White, K.L., Williams, T.L., and Breenberg, B.G. 1961. The ecology of medical care. N Engl J Med 265:885–892.

Woods, S.M., Natterson, J., and Silverman, J. 1966. Medical students disease: Hypochondriasis in medical education. J Med Educ 41:785–790.

Zola, I.K. 1973. Pathways to the doctor—From person to patient. Soc Sci Med 7:677–689.

3

THE SICK ROLE

During the past three decades there has been rapid growth and significant contributions in a new field of study, *medical sociology*. This field critically explores the social aspects of medical care, including factors influencing medical utilization, patterns of medical practice, and alternate treatment modalities such as chiropractic.

A major topic of research in medical sociology has been the *sick role*, a concept initially proposed by Parsons (1951). The term "role" as used by sociologists defines an individual's relationship to society in regard to a number of rights and obligations that are assumed a priori because of one's occupation, social status, or personal circumstances (Twaddle, 1972). A person can simultaneously occupy several roles, although usually behavior will be consistent with only one role at a time. Examples include the roles of parent, law enforcement officer, and husband. Each is associated with certain obligations and rights which may be defined by law or, more usually, just by general societal expectations.

The sick role as described by Parsons is viewed as having a deviant status from the rest of society; to be sick is to be different. Associated with this deviant position are two major rights and two major obligations. The first right is that the sick person is released from the normal and usual social obligations of society, for example, attending school or work. The second right is that the sick person is absolved from blame for his condition; he cannot be expected to get well merely by will power and he must be cared for by others. In regard to the obligations, the sick person is expected to want to get well, to seek competent technical help, and to cooperate with such help in an effort to get well.

Parson's definitions of the sick role were not derived from research data but were initially put forth as heuristic postulates. These seminal postulates have subsequently elicited an immense quantity of research designed to investigate various aspects of how people behave in regard to illness. In general this research has validated Parsons' original description in that most people in society accept, to a greater or lesser degree, each of the stated rights and obligations. However, a variety of socioeconomic, cultural, and demographic factors influence the degree to which any one individual would endorse the descriptions of each of these rights and obligations (Arluke et al., 1979; Segall, 1976a). For example, Anglo-Saxon Protestants are more likely to object to the idea that dependency should accompany the sick role (Segall, 1976b). The Parsonian concept of the sick role model appears to fit best when one is dealing with an acute disabling illness for which a known cure is available, such as an infectious illness. The model has severe limitations when the illness is chronic or of less well-determined etiology such as psychiatric disorders (see below). The concept of a unitary sick role has been challenged, and instead it has been suggested that there are a variety of sick roles (Gordon, 1966; Segall, 1976a; Twaddle, 1969).

Considerations of the sick role have led to fruitful research in describing different types of illness behavior and the characteristics of people most likely to exhibit those behaviors. The concept of the sick role is especially important in the consideration of the somatizing disorders because most of the time the apparent goal (either conscious or unconscious) is to obtain the status of a sick person.

To facilitate organization, a number of different factors that influence entry into or out of the sick role are outlined. However, it must be kept in mind that any one individual may simultaneously fit into more than one category.

FACTORS INFLUENCING ENTRY INTO THE SICK ROLE

Age, Sex, and Socioeconomic Status

When persons of various ages are questioned about criteria that legitimize assumption of the sick role there is a direct correlation between age and perceived legitimacy. That is to say, the older one is the more one feels entitled to assume the sick role (Petroni, 1969a). The relationship of sex to legitimacy of the sick role is less clear. It has been suggested that women have more right to assume the sick role than men because they have fewer conflicting role responsibilities (Mechanic, 1965), but the data of Petroni (1969a) suggest no differences between the sexes.

Studies of the effect of socioeconomic status (SES) upon the tendency to adopt or reject the sick role are confounded by a number of variables. Among these is the fact that disease appears to be more prevalent in the lower socioeconomic classes, and this is concretely demonstrated by a shorter life expectancy for those groups (Antonovsky, 1972). Chronic illnesses such as peptic ulcer and hypertension have also been shown to be more prevalent among poorer people (Schwab et al., 1974).

Although a greater tendency among lower SES persons to accept the sick role might be logically expected (Kadushin, 1964), the limited data available are not consistent with that expectation. McBroom (1970) found no substantial differences among different social classes. Contrary to the expectation that persons of the lower social classes might be more ready to seek the sick role status, McBroom's study of applicants for social security disability benefits found "... a tendency for higher status persons to see themselves as more limited than those of lower status on both functional and social dimensions." There was no evidence to indicate that lower status persons tended to overreport their symptoms.

Many variables operate when one attempts to evaluate illness behavior in different social classes. Petroni (1969c) found that family size is one such variable. His findings indicated that family size was inversely related to both illness frequency and doctor visits in lower SES families but not in the middle class. One interpretation of this finding is that illness (including a visit to a physician) may have a greater adverse financial impact upon a large lower class family.

Cultural Factors

Attitudes toward being sick and the implications of illness vary among different cultural (ethnic) groups.

Two groups compared more frequently than others are Jewish people and Anglo-Saxon Protestants. Mechanic and Volkart (1961) found that Jewish college students (particularly those of higher SES) were more likely to engage in illness behavior than their white Protestant classmates. Such behavior included a greater tendency to visit physicians, to take medications, and to be absent from classes when ill. Mechanic (1963) interpreted this behavior as consistent with the high value that Jewish culture places upon health and particularly upon "healthy-looking" children (Zborowski, 1958). That such a cultural value may serve the group as a survival factor is shown by the fact that Jews have the lowest infant mortality rates, even in lower class immigrants (Anderson, 1958). Twaddle (1969) also found that Jews were more oriented toward the use of physicians than other groups studied. In this study Protestants were more resistant to seeing physicians and more likely to use extended nonphysician referral networks. Segall (1976b) in a study of sick role attitudes, found differences between Jewish and Protestant women to be statistically nonsignificant. However, there was a trend for Jewish women to be more willing to adopt the sick role. Protestant women were more likely to be uncertain concerning their feelings. It appeared that the white Protestant women were primarily objecting to the dependency that accompanies adoption of the sick role. They were as willing as the Jewish patients to accept other dimensions of the sick role.

Self-Reliance

Self-reliance, the feeling that one should handle one's own problems, has been shown to be a factor in reducing willingness to adopt the sick role (Phillips, 1965). However, this value interacts with others, including education (positive correlation with seeking health care) and a high value on health. People who are most likely to seek health care are those persons with low self-reliance who place a high value on health.

Psychosocial Stress

Personal stress appears to be one of the important variables in determining one's inclination to adopt the sick role. In an oft-quoted study of university students Mechanic and Volkart (1961) measured stress (as defined by nervousness and loneliness) and the tendency to adopt the sick role (as measured by tendency to seek medical evaluation in hypothetical situations). When the results of this questionnaire study were correlated with the number of visits to the university's student health center it was found that both increased stress and the tendency to adopt the sick role were correlated with the number of visits. Of the two the latter was the more powerful variable.

Thurlow (1971) investigated individual employees and found that a person's perception of the variability of his or her environment was significantly related to the number of his/her subsequent illnesses.

A very well-controlled and statistically sophisticated prospective study of enrollees in a prepaid health plan demonstrated that distress was one of the most important factors affecting the use of physician services. Tessler and coworkers (1976) concluded that distress has a direct causal role in initiating contacts with physicians; social and psychological problems act as triggers for physician utilization. This effect was not caused by higher levels of disease among the distressed.

Social Support

The quality of one's social support appears to influence the tendency to adopt the sick role. For example, it has been found that low social support (living alone) leads to increased medical utilization and is a more important variable in initiating visits to a physician than is actual health status (Blake et al., 1980).

Investigating the relationship between the sick role and the attitudes of spouses, Petroni (1969b) found that wives were more instrumental in influencing illness behavior in their husbands than vice versa.

The Sick Role as Coping Behavior

Because the traditional sick role (the Parsonian model) exempts the occupant of the role from usual social obligations, there are some obvious inherent potential benefits. The sick role may be used by the person to rationalize personal failures or inadequacies, particularly of a characterologic nature, or the need to accept welfare by using the explanation that one cannot be blamed for illness nor expected to perform at the same level as a healthy person (Cole and Lejeune, 1972). In some societies the physician may act as a gatekeeper, determining the distribution of certain sparce commodities. Thus Shuval and colleagues (1973) have noted that in Israel, a significant proportion of a physician's time may be spent in providing certificates. These certificates (legitimizing the sick role) are used to excuse absences from work, to obtain housing privileges, and so forth. As a consequence of this activity, the physician serves a social function in helping people cope with failure.

RELINQUISHING THE SICK ROLE

The foregoing discussion has focused upon factors that may predispose or facilitate a more ready entry into the sick role. Another perspective is looking at those factors that may be associated with a person's capacity to relinquish the sick role after a serious illness. We shall look at some factors influencing recovery from heart disease because cardiac dysfunction is universally accepted as implying serious disease and therefore legitimizing the sick role.

Brown and Rawlinson (1975), in a study of behavior following open heart surgery, found that those persons who were more reluctant to assume the sick role before open heart surgery were also more eager to exit from it. To the contrary, those persons who had become more confirmed in their sick role attitudes before surgery found it more difficult to surrender the sick role following surgery. Surprisingly, factors such as the complexity of the operation, time on the heart pump, or the presence of other health problems failed to correlate with the patient's tendency to relinquish the sick role. Demographic factors related to illness behavior after surgery suggested that men and younger persons tended to abandon the sick role after surgery to a greater extent than women and older patients. Patients who were less depressed, who reported fewer physical or psychological symptoms on the Cornell Medical Index, and who were "repressors" in coping style also tended to more readily relinquish the sick role.

Gundle and coworkers (1980) investigated factors related to psychosocial outcome after coronary bypass surgery. Patients studied were mostly of lower SES. Despite a good physiologic result from surgery most of the subjects were found to be functioning poorly; 87% were unemployed, and 57% were sexually impaired. The most significant factor related to postoperative functioning was that of the duration of symptoms prior to the operation. A duration of symptoms over 8 months was associated with a significantly poorer adjustment after surgery, irrespective of the success of the operation. The investigators reported that those patients who had prolonged symptoms (particularly those who also had limited education and income) commonly evidenced a damaged self-concept which was reinforced, rather than repaired, by the experience of surgery.

The above findings were largely consistent with earlier work by Garrity (1973), who found that, after the first myocardial infarction, a man was more likely to return to work if he pereived his health as being good. This perception of health (not necessarily reflective of the objective findings of the physician) was related to the man's perception of his health before the myocardial infarction. Other factors associated with an increased probability of return to work were higher socioeconomic status and the personality characteristic of being more "fatalistic." The number of hours worked during a week after a myocardial infarction was related to the number of hours a week man worked prior to his heart attack and were inversely correlated with how worried the man perceived his family to be.

The importance of the attitudes of spouses and other family members about relinquishing the sick role has been noted by Bursten and D'Esopo (1965). These authors reported three cases where the patient's rehabilitation was impaired via "double messages" to the patient from relatives in regard to getting well. In one case the patient's wife obviously enjoyed her new importance in her family and business roles caused by her husband's illness, and she subtly encouraged him to remain in the sick role.

THE SICK ROLE AND THE NATURE OF THE ILLNESS

As mentioned above the sick role as described by Parsons best fits societal expectations when the illness is acute and visibly disabling and when a specific known cure is available.

There is less willingness to afford the benefits of the sick role if the illness is judged to be the fault of the sick person (Phillips, 1965). A specific example is that alcoholics are generally not regarded as legitimate incumbents of the sick role benefits (Chalfant and Kurtz, 1971). There is also reluctance to regard persons with psychiatric or psychosocial problems as legitimate occupants of the sick role (Blackwell, 1967).

Chronic diseases present special problems for consideration of the sick role. A complete recovery cannot be anticipated and because patients with those diseases are often ambulatory their capacity for other roles may be partial rather than total (Kassebaum and Baumann, 1965). For example, a chronically ill person may be able to attend some social activities yet have severe limitations for employment. The incongruity with usual expectations of the sick role has been highlighted by Callahan and colleagues (1966). They note that the chronically ill person may experience conflict between efforts to be more independent to meet societal demands, yet be expected to be dependent in response to the needs of the health care team. Along similar lines, Eardley (1977) comments that the Parsonian model is referrable to comparatively few modern illnesses. She noted that chronic illness is much more common than acute disease, and that total dependence upon the physician may prove to be counterproductive in rehabilitation. She suggests that a teacher–student relationship may be more appropriate for many illnesses than the authoritarian model conceptualized in the Parsonian model.

AN EPIDEMIOLOGIC STUDY OF ILLNESS REPORTING AND THE SICK ROLE

Military populations in many ways approximate ideal groups for epidemiologic study. A military unit is composed of a fairly homogeneous group of individuals in terms of sex, age, education, and health status. Those individuals with notable health problems have been previously eliminated by the screening process of induction physical examinations. Other factors important for epidemiologic studies are that the subjects experience very similar environmental conditions, including food and water. Illness reporting is channeled through a single agency where records of all illnesses, even minor, are maintained. The authoritarian nature of the military also facilitates 100% cooperation among prospective subjects!

All of the above advantages for an ecologic study are even more true for a naval ship. The crew experiences very similar climatic changes, exposure to infectious illnesses, stresses from combat operations, and so forth.

Noting the above advantages for epidemiologic research, a U.S. Naval research team undertook a series of investigations of illness reporting by the crews of several U.S. Navy ships (Doll et al., 1969; Rahe et al., 1970; Rubin et al., 1969a, 1969b, 1971a, 1971b, 1972). The investigations took place during the time of the Viet Nam War, and the crews were studied during their ships' deployments to the Mediterranean or to Southeast Asia.

The methodology employed was similar, although not necessarily identical, for all ships that included an attack carrier, a battleship, and several cruisers. Information obtained at the time of deployment included demographic and personal history data, determination of recent life changes, and a Health Opinion Survey. Illness rates and their timing (e.g., combat periods) were computed by a review of medical records which noted each visit made by a crew member to sick bay. It was notable that, with one exception (the battleship where all illness rates tended to be unusually high), relatively few crew members accounted for a high percentage of all illness episodes. This finding was most marked for the group of naval aviators where 12.4% of the men had 46.7% of all reported illnesses and 25.6% of the men accounted for 74.3% reported illness. Another finding, which tended to be constant across the different ships, was that younger, less-experienced men had a higher frequency of reported illness. Not surprisingly those men who worked in hostile environments and/or performed hazardous or physically demanding tasks also reported more illness. Decreased job satisfaction was also associated with increased rates of illness. Illness rates were higher in those individuals who had prospectively indicated a greater preoccupation with their health as suggested by their responses on the Health Opinion Survey.

A consistent finding of the naval study was differences between races in illness reporting. Blacks had higher rates of illness than did whites and Filipinos were lower than either whites or blacks. This finding appeared to be related to cultural factors rather than to demographic variables such as younger age or more arduous duty. In fact, it was noted that, on the average, blacks reported a higher degree of job satisfaction than whites.

The relationship between stress and illness rates was notable. Illness became more frequent at times of combat duty than during periods of time spent in port. The amount of stress as estimated by life change units (LCUs) on the Schedule of Recent Events that an individual had experienced in the 6 months prior to deployment of the ship was also significantly rated to the frequency of illness during the period of deployment. An increased total of LCUs was associated with increased illness rates. The predictive value of LCUs as determined by the Schedule of Recent Events was greatest for the older and better-educated crew members. This finding was not unexpected because the test had been standardized, using well-educated middle-class subjects. A revised scoring technique was used to estimate life stress in enlisted personnel, and this different scoring system proved to be of more predictive power than that derived from civilian subjects. Interestingly it appears that issues related to conflict (legal difficulties or fighting with one's wife) appears to be more predictive of illness in the enlisted men than were issues related to loss. This may reflect the possibility that conflict for these younger men was a more frequently occurring event than was loss.

In summary, the findings of this very well-designed epidemiologic study confirmed previous reports with civilian subjects. A small percentage of the men accounted for a disproportionate number of the illness episodes. Illness reporting was most common in those individuals who were under the greatest stress, both current and during the preceding 6 months, and those who were judged to have the fewest coping skills. In general job satisfaction was inversely correlated with the rate of illness.

THE SICK ROLE AND SOMATIZATION

Consideration of the concept of the sick role leads us to postulate that somatization may be motivated (either consciously or unconsciously) by the desire to seek those privileges afforded to the sick person by society. These privileges include a release from obligations such as work, school, military duty, or fulfilling one's role as a homemaker, spouse, or parent.

A review of those characteristics which appear to predispose to someone's adoption of the sick role indicates that the sick role is more attractive when (1) it is more culturally acceptable; (2) the social support system is perceived to be inadequate; (3) the individual feels under psychosocial stress; (4) the sick role resolves personal and social problems; (5) the individual is less self-reliant; and (6) coping skills are decreased.

It is suggested that the sick role can be used to solve certain problems in living *but* that society does not accept emotional disorders or difficulties in coping with life problems to be an acceptable entry into the sick role. However, the stress that the patient experiences can be translated into a somatic complaint. Thus a homemaker feeling overburdened by the responsibility of small children may complain of a backache and be afforded the sick role, thereby achieving transient relief from her responsibilities.

SUMMARY

The Parsonian concept of the sick role has stimulated widely varied and productive research of sociological issues in medicine. With this further investigation, it is apparent that the sick role is not a simple and well-defined entity but instead serves as a useful unifying general principle with which to examine certain aspects of illness behavior. The sick role not only describes, but to some extent determines some expectations of the sick person's behavior; there are prevalent attitudes that a person should not be afforded full benefits of the sick role when he/she is responsible for the illness suffered.

Examination of society's attitudes toward the sick role offers at least one of the possible motivations of somatizing behavior. Present societal–cultural concepts of illness are highly influenced by the disease model. Therefore a person who suffers from emotional or social disability (which may be considered to be one's own fault) must translate the illness into one which is socially acceptable. Thus an inadequacy that is socially unacceptable, when transformed into a somatic symptom and defined as a disease, becomes an acceptable means of entry into the sick role.

REFERENCES

Anderson, O. 1958. Infant mortality and social and cultural factors: Historical trends and currents patterns. In *Patients, Physicians and Illness*. Jaco, E.G., ed. Glencoe, Ill.: Free Press, pp 12–24.

Antonovsky, A. 1972. Social class, life expectancy and overall mortality. In *Patients, Physicians and Illness*, 2nd ed. Jaco, E.G., ed. New York: Free Press.

Arluke, A., Kennedy, L., and Kessler, R.C. 1979. Reexamining the sick role concept: An empirical assessment. J Health Soc Behav 20:30–36.

Blackwell, B.L. 1967. Upper middle class and adult expectations about entering the sick role for physical and psychiatric dysfunctions. J Health Soc Behav 8:83–95.

Blake, R.L., Roberts, C., Mackey, T., and Hosokawa, M. 1980. Social supports and utilization of medical care. J Family Prac 11:810–812.

Brown, J.S., and Rawlinson, M. 1975. Relinquishing the sick role following open heart surgery. J Health Soc Behav 16:12–27.

Bursten, B., and D'Esopo, R. 1965. The obligation to remain sick. Arch Gen Psychiat 12:402–407.

Callahan, E.M., Carroll, S., Revier, P., Gilhooly, E., and Dunn, D. 1966. The "sick role" in chronic illness: Some reactions. J Chron Dis 19:883–897.

Chalfant, H.O., and Kurtz, R.A. 1971. Alcoholics and the sick role: Assessments by social workers. J Health Soc Behav 12:66–72.

Cole, S., and Lejeune, R. 1972. Illness and the legitimation of failure. Am Soc Rev 37:347–356.

Doll, R.E., Rubin, R.T., and Gunderson, E.K.C. 1969. Life stress and illness patterns in the U.S. Navy II: Demographic variables and illness onset in an attack carrier crew. Arch Environ Health 19:748–752.

Eardley, A. 1977. The sick role and its relevance to doctors and patients. Practitioner 219:385–390.

Garrity, T.F. 1973. Vocational adjustment after first myocardial infarction: Comparative assessment of several variables suggested in the literature. Soc Sci Med 7:705–717.

Gordon, G. 1966. *Role Theory and Illness: A Sociology Perspective*. New Haven, Conn.: Yale College and University Press.

Gundle, M.J., Reeves, B.R., Tate, S., Raft, D., and McLauria, L.P. 1980. Psychosocial outcome after coronary artery surgery. Am J Psychiatry 137:1591–1594.

Kadushin, C. 1964. Social class and the experience of ill health. Sociological Inquiry 34:67–80.

Kassebaum, G.G., and Baumann, B.O. 1965. Dimensions of the sick role in chronic illness. J Health Hum Behav 6:16–27.

McBroom, W.H. 1970. Illness, illness behavior and socioeconomic status. J Health Soc Behav 11:319–326.

Mechanic, D. 1963. Religion, religiosity and illness behavior: The special case of the Jews. Hum Organ Clgh Bull 22:202–208.

Mechanic, D. 1965. Perception of parental response to illness: A research note. J Health and Human Behav 6:253–257.

Mechanic, D., and Volkart, E.H. 1961 Stress, illness behavior and the sick role. Am Soc Rev 26:51–58.

Parsons, T. 1951. Social structure and dynamic process: The case of modern medical practice. In *The Social System*. New York: Free Press, pp 428–479.

Petroni, F.A. 1969a. The influence of age, sex and chronicity in perceived legitimacy to the sick role. Sociology Soc Res 53:180–193.

Petroni, F.A. 1969b. Significant others and illness behavior: A much neglected sick role contingency. Sociological Q 10:32–41.

Petroni, F.A. 1969c. Social class, family size and the sick role. J Marriage Family 31:728–735.

Phillips, D.L. 1965. Self reliance and the inclination to adopt the sick role. Soc Forces 43:555–563.

Rahe, R.H., Gunderson, E.K.E., and Arthur, R.J. 1970. Demographic and psychosocial factors in acute illness reporting. J Chron Dis 23:245–255.

Rubin, R.T., Gunderson, E.K.E., and Doll, R.E. 1969a. Life stress and illness patterns in the U.S. Navy I. Environmental variables and illness onset in an attack carrier's crew. Arch Environ Health 19:740–747.

Rubin, R.T., Gunderson, E.K.E., and Arthur, R.J. 1969b. Life stress and illness patterns in the U.S. Navy III: Prior life change and illness onset in an attack carrier's crew. Arch Environ Health 19:753–757.

Rubin, R.T., Gunderson, E.K.E., and Arthur, R.J. 1971a. Life stress and illness patterns in the U.S. Navy IV: Environmental and demographic variables in relation to illness onset in a battleship's crew. J Psychosom Res 15:277–288.

Rubin, R.T., Gunderson, E.K.E., and Arthur, R.J. 1971b. Life stress and illness patterns in the U.S. Navy V: Prior life change and illness onset in a battleship's crew. J Psychosom Res 15:89–94.

Rubin, R.T., Gunderson, E.K.E., and Arthur, R.J. 1972. Life stress and illness patterns in the U.S. Navy VI: Environmental, demographic and prior life change variables in relation to illness onset in naval aviators during a combat cruise. Psychosom Med 34:533–547.

Schwab, J.J., Fennell, F.B., and Warheit, G.J. 1974. The epidemiology of psychosomatic disorders. Psychosomatics 15:88–93.

Segall, A. 1976a. The sick role concept: Understanding illness behavior. J Health Soc Behav 17:163–170.

Segall, A. 1976b. Socio-cultural variation in sick role behavioral expectations. Soc Sci Med 10:47–51.

Shuval, J.T., Antonovsky, A., and Davies, A.M. 1973. Illness: A mechanism for coping with failure. Soc Sci Med 7:259–265.

Tessler, R., Mechanic, D., and Dimond, M. 1976. The effect of psychological distress on physician utilization: A prospective study. J Health Soc Behav 17:353–364.

Thurlow, H.J. 1971. Illness in relation to life situation and sick role tendency. J Psychosom Res 15:73–88.

Twaddle, A.C. 1969. Health decisions and sick role variations: An exploration. J Health Soc Behav 10:105–115.

Twaddle, A.C. 1972. The concepts of sick role and illness behavior. In *Advances in Psychosomatic Medicine, vol. 8, Psychosocial Aspects of Physical Illness.* Lipowski, Z.J., ed. Basel: Karger, pp 162–179.

Zboroswki, M. 1958. Cultural components in response to pain. In *Patients, Physicians and Illness.* Jaco, E.G., ed. Glencoe, Ill. Free Press, pp 256–268.

4

PSYCHOLOGICAL RESPONSES TO
ACUTE AND CHRONIC DISEASE

The preceding two chapters have focused upon the process of disease and illness and the sociological aspects of being sick, including factors which influence the utilization of medical services. Disease also has a very personal aspect, in its meaning to the individual, in the reality of how it influences one's life, in the intrapsychic perception of distress, and in the initiation of a variety of coping mechanisms as the person attempts to readjust his/her life.

Before proceeding to the somatizing disorders, which represent abnormal illness behavior, it is useful to have some concepts of what constitutes "normal" illness behavior and response to disease in order that the two types of behavior can be compared. A number of different clinicians have described the psychological processes in response to disease, and the following brief review incorporates the ideas of both prior reports and my own clinical experience.

DISEASE AS A THREAT

The emergence of a disease process threatens the usual "steady state" of a person's life. Different types of threats have been described by Engel (1962), Kiely (1972), and Strain and Grossman (1975). These include the following:

1. The threat to one's sense of self. Being sick is being different so there is a challenge to one's core identity as a healthy person who performs certain activities and has responsibilities. Included in this threat is the fear of loss of life itself, and therefore one's very existence, or the state of "being," is also brought into question.
2. The threat of injury to the body, the loss of bodily functions such as

bowel and bladder control or even the loss of body parts. This type of anxiety falls into the category of "castration anxiety."

3. The threat that one's state of being diseased and otherwise damaged will make one less respected and/or loved. For example, certain diseases carry with them a stigma that persists even when the disease is asymptomatic. With these diseases the patient's identity is to some extent defined by the disease, e.g., a person with a seizure disorder is known as an epileptic.
4. The threat of possible loss of interpersonal relationships through separation (such as hospitalization or loss of mobility) from friends and relatives. This type of anxiety falls into the general category of "separation anxiety."
5. The threat the dysfunction will be permanent and result in the loss of usual gratifying activities, including the ability to express biological drives such as sexual activity.

THE PERSONAL MEANING OF ILLNESS

Faced with limitations imposed by the state of being sick, and threatened by further implications of having a disease state, the sick person must engage in the cognitive activity of searching for a personal meaning of the illness (Lazarus, 1974). The various meanings that illness may have for an individual have been categorized by Lipowski (1969) as follows:

1. The illness may be viewed as a challenge—an obstacle which must be overcome, e.g., the trials of Job.
2. The illness may be seen as an enemy which threatens to destroy the person.
3. The illness may be interpreted as a punishment for past transgressions, often of a sexual nature. For example, one patient offered the opinion that his medically related impotence was punishment for adolescent masturbation.
4. The illness may be interpreted as evidence of an inherent weakness in the person.
5. The illness may be interpreted as a relief. It may be welcomed as a reprieve from societal expectations, demands, or responsibilities. A concrete example would be a disease which would exempt a young man from military conscription.
6. Illness may be a strategy to cope with the demands of life. Examples would include the use of illness to obtain disability benefits or to excuse one from the sexual requests of a spouse.
7. Illness and disease may be interpreted as an irreparable loss or damage. For example, an adolescent with diabetes may see himself/herself as inferior and anticipate an impaired life.

8. Illness may be interpreted as a positive value. In this line of reasoning the illness state is regarded as helping a person have a greater sense of the meaning of life or of a greater appreciation of esthetic values.

PERSONAL FACTORS INFLUENCING THE THREAT AND MEANING OF ILLNESS

The preceding list of threats and individual interpretations of disease is not exhaustive, and any one individual may construct a meaning of his/her individual illness which incorporates more than one element. The specific meaning and the perceived degree of threat is determined by a number of personal factors such as previous life experiences, and current life situations (Verwoerdt, 1972). Among these personal factors are age and sex.

The age at which a person develops a disease may be associated with certain developmental tasks and therefore determine some aspects of the emotional reaction. For example, the young child who has recently mastered basic bodily functions such as bowel and bladder control may react with shame and regression with the emergence of a disease which threatens those hard-won developmental skills. An adolescent who is struggling with the conflict of independence–dependence in relationship to his or her parents may not acknowledge the existence of a disease (e.g., diabetes) which might threaten the capacity for independence. Adolescents are also extremely sensitive to any disease process that may affect physical appearance. Any defect or difference from other members of the peer group tends to be magnified in its perception by the adolescent.

Young men, particularly those with family responsibilities, react intensely to any threat to their earning power and to their capacity to see themselves as providers. Mothers of small children often respond with a feeling of guilt that their diseases may interfere with their capacity to care for their children. Older patients often react to disease with intense anxiety fearing that it may signal a decline leading to death, or that it may interfere with their capacity to remain independent. Disease may also be equated in the elderly with the idea of being forced to give up independence and to have to live in a nursing home.

As a broad generalization men tend to react comparatively more adversely to disabilities which interfere with physical activity and women tend to react more adversely to disease processes which interfere with physical appearance and attractiveness (Simon, 1971).

PSYCHOLOGICAL REACTIONS TO DISEASE

Several psychological reactions to the process of disease have been noted so consistently with a wide variety of patients that these reactions should be considered to fall within a broad definition of normal responses (Abram,

1972; Verwoerdt, 1972). However, if any of these responses is exaggerated in extent or unduly prolonged in duration then the response may be considered atypical or pathological. These normal responses include the following.

Denial

The person with a disease attempts to hide from himself that he may be sick, or the implications of having certain symptoms.

"Denial" is often used as a very general term incorporating at one end of a continuum the conscious suppression of unpleasant thoughts to, at the other end of the continuum a psychotic distortion of reality. Most people with a disease process engage in efforts to rationalize symptoms or to direct thinking away from the potential seriousness of their disease. For example, a woman may delay seeking medical advice in regard to a small hard breast mass with the rationalization that it is just a bit of fibrosis. At times the degree of denial can reach psychotic proportions. I have personally seen an elderly spinster who was brought to the hospital with a cabbage-sized necrotic exophytic vulvar carcinoma.

In its more usual and normal function denial serves to protect the emotional state of the patient, to help provide a sense of continuity with the "healthy state" and to promote an optimistic view of the future. "Normal" denial should not interfere with the rational decision process of obtaining and complying with medical care but rather serve to protect the psyche from unacceptable and disabling emotional distress.

Regression

The state of being sick almost inevitably leads to some degree of psychological regression; that is to say that the person functions at a psychologically less-mature level. The degree of regression varies; it can be represented by merely a more intensely inner-directed preoccupation with the self and bodily function or, at the other extreme, it may be demonstrated by overt childlike behavior complete with urinary incontinence.

Disease itself, and often potentiated by the process of hospitalization, appears to promote a lower level of psychological functioning and more specifically an increased dependency upon other people. Reality factors may demand this increased reliance on other people; a man weak with a ravaging infectious disease may require someone to feed him. But in addition frequently there are also increased demands upon others for attention, decision making, and minor self-care activities usually assumed by the patient. Most people, including relatives and health care personnel, tend to respond instinctively to the sick person and accede to these demands as an acceptable part of being sick.

Unfortunately the procedures of some hospitals and the attitudes of some health care personnel facilitate regression. Personal belongings, including shoes, may be removed; the patient may be treated as a child in reference to bedtime and even spoken to in the voice tones usually reserved for small children, "Now is the time for our bath."

Anxiety and Fear

Anxiety is a ubiquitous and, when not disabling, a normal and necessary part of human development and psychological functioning. Anxiety can be viewed as an alerting function that warns of danger from internal psychic processes. From a physiologic standpoint fear is similar to anxiety but usually fear refers to an alerting function of perceived external danger. Both anxiety and fear are prominent in disease. There are external, reality validated events of which to be fearful and there is also the continual input of fantasy, inappropriate guilt and self-critical attitudes which generate anxiety. Fear and anxiety alert the sick person to the possibility and anticipation of experiencing loss. Examples of these losses are loss of comfort, bodily part or function, and interpersonal relationships. Because the sick person has already experienced a loss of some extent, the anxiety of anticipating further loss is not unreasonable.

Grief

Grief is the normal emotion experienced when one has experienced a loss. The loss of health, body function, or body part must be acknowledged in the psychological experience of a person. Grief includes features of anger, preoccupation with the lost object, feelings of guilt and self-recrimination, a disruption of the usual patterns of behavior and thinking, a depressed mood and the need to work through (or mourn) the loss (Lindemann, 1944). Some elements of the grief process may be more prominent in some patients than in others but many of the various psychological reactions noted in sick persons (e.g., guilt or anger) represent aspects of necessary grief work. Patients may rage against the gods for the injustice of their having been inflicted with disease, or they may be preoccupied with guilt from feelings of responsibility for their disease.

The grief associated with disease must be distinguished from a major depression. With grief a depressed mood is common, but the lowered mood is not ever-present nor persistent for the long periods of time which characterize a major depression. The latter is characterized by a more persistent depressed mood and is associated with changes in vegetative functions such as sleep, appetite, and bowel function. In the normal situation the grief associated with physical illness is worked through, and the sick person comes to a new acceptance of himself, often reflecting some alterations in such important issues as body image.

Personality Change with Chronic Illness: A Prospective Study

Prospective investigations to determine an individual's changes in response to a chronic illness are difficult because of the time and expense required. One such study, which utilized the Cattell Sixteen Personality Questionnaire has been reported (Barton and Cattell, 1972). Over 500 New Zealand high school seniors took the test and then repeated it 5 years later. Those subjects who had experienced a chronic illness during the interim were compared to subjects who reported no chronic illness.

Findings indicated that the chronic illness group differed from the healthy group when results obtained from the original test were compared. They scored lower on qualities of ego strength and emotional maturity and had traits reflecting greater sensitivity, dependency, and overprotectedness.

Five years later the chronic illness group had test scores indicating a failure to progress in the qualities of ego strength and emotional stability. They appeared to be more dependent and sensitive and in addition had become more insecure, tense, apprehensive, self-reproaching, and troubled.

Results from a single self-report questionnaire type of study must be interpreted cautiously. However, the findings from this objective investigation are compatible with clinical observations. Regression, guilt and anxiety all increased in these young subjects who had experienced a chronic illness.

COPING WITH DISEASE

Concurrent with perceptions of a change in health, the threats of further losses, and the search for the meaning of illness are the efforts made by the sick person to adapt to the new and potentially dangerous situation. Adaptive tasks include learning how to deal with pain, developing adequate interpersonal relationships with health care staff, preparing for an uncertain future, and preserving a reasonable balance and a satisfactory self-image (Moos and Tsu, 1977). Coping processes can be defined as functions whose aim is to reduce, deflect, or eliminate anticipated harm (Kiely, 1972).

The concept of coping can be divided into two major categories: coping style (reflecting an individual's long-standing characteristic mode of coping with stress) and coping tactics or techniques.

Coping Style

Coping style has a close relationship with the personality pattern because a "personality" is determined by the "characteristic" techniques that an individual uses to deal with his/her everyday life situations. However, in regard to physical illness, one's prior experiences with disease, either personal or with close relatives, may be also incorporated in the coping style utilized when one becomes sick.

Lipowski (1970) identified two major cognitive coping styles related to bodily disease or injury: minimization and vigilant focusing. Minimization refers to a style characterized by a tendency to ignore, deny, or rationalize the input of information concerning one's illness and its consequences. These persons often use repression, denial, "forgetting," and a fuzzy impression-istic type of cognitive style as habitual modes of coping, and many of them can be diagnostically described as having hysterical personalities (Kiely, 1972).

The other major coping style in regard to illness is that of "vigilant focusing." This mode of coping is most commonly seen in obsessional, alert, anxiety-prone, intellectualizing individuals. They must know what is happening to them, and why, and try consistently to obtain as much information as possible from physicians or other sources in order to make sense of their experience.

Lipowski (1970) also described three behavioral coping styles (as opposed to cognitive coping style); they are "tackling," an active approach toward problems; "capitulating," a passive and withdrawing behavior in response to disease; and "avoiding," a behavioral style characterized by behavioral attempts to deny and get away from the exigencies of illness.

Coping Techniques

Coping tactics or techniques refer to more specific psychological mechan-isms or behaviors used to adapt to the presence of disease. Lazarus (1974), who emphasized that the person's cognitive appraisal of stress determines the degree of perceived threat, distinguishes two types of coping techniques: direct actions taken by a patient to alter his environment and palliative activities, which are in turn divided into intrapsychic processes such as denial and somatically oriented devices such as drugs or alcohol.

In reality, the behavioral and intrapsychic processes are not so separate as implied by definitions. It is also important to note that, while the ego defense mechanisms can all be considered to be coping mechanisms, the various tactics used in coping go far beyond those intrapsychic processes. A few examples of the numerous coping tactics used in disease states follow.

Suppression

Suppression is a psychological mechanism by which the person voluntarily excludes material from consciousness. This is often accomplished by focusing attention in another direction. Thus a sick person, rather than dwelling upon symptoms and limitations, may become interested in a book or watching television. The material being suppressed is always voluntarily available to the person, and attention can be redirected to the disease process when it is prudent to do so.

Displacement

In the psychological process known as displacement psychic energy is "displaced" from the area of worry and anxiety to another less conflicted area. For example, a man with symptoms of bronchogenic carcinoma of the lung may, instead, focus his complaints to a physician around a relatively innocuous disorder such as hemorrhoids.

Overcompensation

Using the technique of overcompensation, a person may attempt to deny the effects of a physical defect by efforts and behavior which would negate the disability. The lay literature is replete with accounts of athletes who overcame physical defects to become outstanding in their chosen sport.

Mastery

The person who employs mastery often concurrently uses *intellectualization*. There is an attempt to master a disease by learning as much about it as possible and also acquiring those techniques required for care of the disease. For example, someone with end-stage renal disease may learn everything possible about management of uremia and be an active participant in a home hemodialysis program.

Acceptance and Substitution

Acceptance and substitution is a mature coping mechanism, and the afflicted person learns to accept the limitations of illness and then substitutes and obtains pleasure from new activities. An example is the permanently disabled athlete who "learns" how to enjoy spectator sports as a fan.

PSYCHOLOGICAL RESPONSES IN ILLUSTRATIVE DISEASES

Diabetes Mellitus

Diabetes mellitus is a common chronic disease, which may have its onset at various ages. Because most symptoms can be controlled through the patient's compliance with medical care (although there are many progressive complications such as blindness and premature death) it serves as an excellent example to illustrate chronic disease and illness behavior.

Psychological factors associated with diabetes have been the subject of numerous articles in the medical literature. Recent critical reviews of this literature (Greydanus and Hoffman, 1979; Hauser and Pollets, 1979) suggest that there is little consistent evidence to support theories that psychological factors are etiologic in diabetes, that there is a particular personality associated with diabetes, or that there is a notable increase in the incidence of psychiatric illness in patients who have diabetes. There does appear to be more substantial evidence (although not all investigators are unanimous in this finding) that diabetics suffer from lower self-esteem and may have more depressive symptoms than control subjects.

There is general consensus that the onset of diabetes in adolescence is frequently associated with multiple emotional problems, including disturbances in body image, low self-esteem, and acting-out behavior. The struggles that adolescents typically experience with parents as they resolve normal conflicts about dependecy–independency may, with the diabetic adolescent, be acted out over issues such as diet, urine checks, and medical clinic visits. A delay in the normal progression of ego development in the diabetic adolescent has been reported (Hauser and Pollets, 1979).

The physician can be of therapeutic use to the adolescent by helping him/her assume responsibility and self-care for the disease and thereby achieve a sense of mastery over a disease that often leaves the victim with a feeling of helplessness. Failure to take the developmental needs of the adolescent into account may result in repetitive episodes of ketoacidosis or hypoglycemia.

Pregnancy is a time in a diabetic woman's life when emotional issues may be exaggerated. Complications of pregnancy are increased by the presence of diabetes, and the diabetic woman may have more intense conflicts about issues of femininity, dependency, and anger during pregnancy. These conflicts may be handled by massive psychological denial, which tends to make medical care more difficult (Leeman, 1970).

The symptoms of diabetes have been shown to be sensitive to psychosocial stress (Grant et al., 1974). There is evidence that an increased number of life events is correlated with indices of poorer medical control such as glycosuria and frequent changes in the dosage of insulin (Bradley, 1979). Still further, there is an apparent correlation between loss and depression and episodes of ketoacidotic coma (Rosen and Lidz, 1949; Slawson, 1963). This manifestation of poor medical control can clearly be the result of behavior influenced by both conscious and unconscious motivation.

The following clinical history of a diabetic woman illustrates many of the psychological issues of chronic illness in general and of diabetes mellitus in particular.

A 33-year-old married mother of two children was seen for psychiatric evaluation and treatment after an episode of ketoacidotic coma. The referring internist had noted that she appeared "depressed" and had recommended to her that she seek treatment. The patient was cooperative to the suggestion of psychotherapy, and she indicated to the psychiatrist that she had chronic marital problems related to her husband's apparent disinterest and unpredictable behavior.

Past history indicated that the patient was healthy until 14 years of age when she inexplicably became amenorrheic. This was associated with depression, anxiety, and the fear that her primary goal in life, to become a mother, could not be achieved. Subsequently developing symptoms of weight loss and polyuria led to a diagnosis of diabetes. Treatment with insulin reversed all symptoms, including resumption of her normal menstrual cycle. However, her parents, both successful professionals, fought viciously over which of the two was responsible for her illness. The father, who was more passive than the mother, eventually capitulated and symbolically assumed blame by the ritualistic presentation to the patient of a year's supply of insulin syringes each year on her birthday!

The patient, who was very physically attractive, began to date her future husband while both were teenagers. He abused her by insults and by openly flaunting relationships with other girls. However, when he proposed marriage she eagerly accepted, feeling grateful that he would accept "damaged merchandise." Because of her diabetes she had given up hope that anyone would ever be interested in her. She became pregnant early in the marriage, and when her husband failed to be attentive she neglected control of her diabetes, which resulted in a prolonged hospitalization. The product of the pregnancy was a slightly deformed child (clubfoot), and the patient had severe guilt feelings for her behavior during her pregnancy. A second pregnancy was uneventful. The marriage continued, apparently stable but unrewarding. The patient's husband continued his detached relationship with her, and she in turn was sexually withholding and frequently neglected housework because she "didn't feel well." Interspersed were several episodes of severe ketoacidosis. She continued to take insulin but refused to test her urine.

Psychotherapy initially focused upon the patient's complaints about her husband, but the patient progressively gained insight about her low self-esteem, lack of assertiveness, and how she used passive-aggressive techniques in an attempt to deal with her husband. After 3 years of therapy she "confessed" that each episode of ketoacidosis (including the hospitalization for coma) had resulted from her failure to give herself insulin because of anger at her husband.

As a result of psychotherapy, all episodes of ketoacidosis ceased and (perhaps paradoxically) the relationship with her husband improved as she became more assertive. Psychotherapy was successfully discontinued after 5 years, although some passive-aggressive characterologic features persisted. The patient's attitudes toward her disease and her capacity for management of the diabetes had improved immensely.

Dwarfism

The preceding discussion might mislead one to believe that disease inevitably produces devastating psychological consequences in the afflicted person. Fortunately this is not true, and many persons, including those with severe chronic diseases, learn to adjust their lives in a manner which maintains psychological health.

Dwarfs are a group of people who have severe underlying disease and a markedly different appearance from other people. Although one might anticipate a high frequency of psychopathology in this group, such is not the case; the large majority of these people have made a good adjustment to life.

There are two major types of dwarfism, achondroplastic and hypopituitary. The latter is often associated with other hormonal deficiencies in addition to inadequate growth hormone. Achondroplasia is a hereditary disorder of cartilage, which has the symptomatic expression of very short stature with a normal trunk. The face is affected at times, resulting in a grotesque appearance because of changes in the nose and frontal bossing. Complications such as hip degeneration or instability of the back often occur later in life.

Despite the obvious differences in physical appearance and complications of a medical nature, a psychiatric study of 16 adult dwarfs failed to demonstrate more psychopathology in this group than would have been expected by chance (Brust and Ford, 1976). Rather, it was discovered that the dwarfs had effectively used a variety of coping mechanisms, which resulted in their having a high degree of psychological well-being and confident self-identities. They engendered respect in the investigators for their capacity to deal with adversity. Stresses associated with a markedly short stature were reported, and there were histories of childhood neuropathic traits. However, by adulthood most of these subjects had learned that the important issue in life was how to relate to others. Therefore they had mastered the ability to set others at ease and had developed a pleasant interpersonal style. One finding was that male dwarfs were less well adjusted than females, possibly reflecting societal attitudes; it is anticipated that women are normally of shorter stature.

The important point is that a chronic disease which results in an obviously different body shape than other people does not automatically lead to a psychological disorder. An extrapolation is that when psychological disorders occur in other chronic diseases it would be a mistake to assume immediately that they are a result of the disease process.

Summary and Conclusions

The emergence of a serious disease is regarded as a severe threat to the usual normal state of an individual. This threat (which is modified by the cognitive apparatus) results in psychological distress which can best be described as a grief response. Transient regression to a more immature and dependent level of psychological functioning is very common.

Most individuals are able to employ coping mechanisms which allow for psychological reconstitution at different levels of functioning. Maladaptive efforts at coping may lead to long-term adjustment problems and psychiatric syndromes. However, the persistence of psychiatric symptoms should not be automatically attributed to the existence of organic disease because many persons with severe chronic disease have no evidence of psychiatric illness. A review of the psychological factors associated with diabetes mellitus indicates that there may be an interplay of abnormal illness behavior and genuine organic disease. From a clinical viewpoint there is often no sharp differentiation between the somatizing disorders and an organic disease process.

REFERENCES

Abram, H.S. 1972. The psychology of chronic illness. J Chronic Dis 25:659–664.

Barton, K., and Cattell, R.B. 1972. Personality before and after a chronic illness. J Clin Psychol 28:464–467.

Bradley, C. 1979. Life events and the control of diabetes mellitus. J Psychosom Res 23:159–162.

Brust, J.S., and Ford, C.V. 1976. Psychiatric aspects of dwarfism. Am J Psychiatry 133:160–164.

Engel, G.L. 1962. *Psychological Development in Health and Disease.* Philadelphia, Pa.: Saunders.

Grant, I., Kyle, G.C., Teichman, A., and Mendels, J. 1974. Recent life events and diabetes in adults. Psychosom Med 36:121–128.

Greydanus, D.E., and Hoffman, A.D. 1979. Psychological factors in diabetes mellitus. Am J Dis Child 133:1061–1066.

Hauser, S.T., and Pollets, D. 1979. Psychological aspects of diabetes mellitus: A critical review. Diabetes Care 2:227–232

Kiely, W.F. 1972. Coping with severe illness. In *Advances in Psychosomatic Medicine 8: Psychosocial Aspects of Physical Illness.* Lipowski, Z.J., ed. Basel: Karger, pp 105–118.

Lazarus, R.S. 1974. Psychological stress and coping in adaptation and illness. Int J Psychiatry Med 5:321–333.

Leeman, P. 1970. Dependency, anger and denial in pregnant diabetic women: A group approach. Psychiatr Q 44:1–12.

Lindemann, E. 1944. Symptomatology and management of acute grief. Am J Psychiatry 101:141–148.

Lipowski, Z.J. 1969. Psychosocial aspects of disease. Ann Int Med 71:1197–1206.

Lipowski, Z.J. 1970. Physical illness, the individual and the coping process. Psychiatry Med 1:91–102.

Moos, R.H., and Tsu, V.D. 1977. The crisis of physical illness: An overview. In *Coping with Physical Illness.* Moos, R.H., ed. New York: Plenum.

Rosen, H., and Lidz, T. 1949. Emotional factors in the precipitation of recurrent diabetic acidosis. Psychosom Med 16:211–215.

Simon, J.I. 1971. Emotional aspects of physical disability. Am J Occup Ther 25:408–410.

Slawson, P.F. 1963. Emotional factors in repetitive diabetic acidosis. Psychosomatics 4:344–352

Strain, J.J., and Grossman, S. 1975. Psychological reactions to medical illness and hospitalization. In *Psychological Care of the Medically Ill.* New York: Appleton-Century-Crofts, pp. 23–36.

Verwoerdt, A. 1972. Psychopathological responses to the stress of physical illness. In *Advances in Psychosomatic Medicine 8: Psychosocial Aspects of Physical Illness.* Lipowski, Z.J., ed. Basel: Karger, pp 119–141.

5

HYSTERIA

The fascinating history of hysteria as told by Veith (1965) dates back at least to 1900 B.C. when Egyptian papyri described diseases attributed to displacement or wandering of the uterus. Treatment techniques employed by Egyptian physicians included applying a variety of fragrant and aromatic substances to the women's pudenda in an effort to attract the uterus back into its "normal" anatomic position.

The term hysteria dates from the time of the *Corpus Hippocraticum* and is derived from the Greek word *hustera*, meaning uterus. "Elderly virgins as well as widows, including those who had had children, were thought to be particularly vulnerable to hysterical afflictions caused by irregular menses; marriage was recommended to them as the speediest way of achieving a cure" (Veith, 1965). Thus an association with both menstrual disorders and sexual issues has been present in the story of hysteria for at least 2500 years.

During the Middle Ages, hysteria was often confused with demonic possession. Diagnostic studies were performed by various means of torture such as the use of hot irons to determine areas of anesthesia, and therapeutic interventions were largely limited to eradicating the demons by burning the "patient" at the stake!

In the mid-19th century, Briquet, through careful study of more than 400 hysterics, determined that the disorder was related to the brain rather than to physical pathology of the female genitalia. He proposed that unfavorable environmental events acted upon the affective part of the brain in predisposed individuals (Mai and Merskey, 1981). Charcot accepted these formulations of Briquet's and believed that the hysteric was predisposed by heredity. He proposed that a traumatic event led to an idea, and the idea caused a "functional" or "dynamic" lesion in the brain (Havens, 1966). Freud visited Charcot in Paris for a period of six months in the late 19th century. Freud was profoundly influenced by the great French neurologist, and when he returned to Vienna his work with hysterics led to the concept of repression and subsequent formulations of psychoanalytic theory.

HYSTERIA: THE CONFUSING TERMINOLOGY

With the passage of time, the concept of hysteria has evolved into multiple meanings, and the term has progressively lost any specific diagnostic meaning (Hyler and Spitzer, 1978). There are at least six major uses of the word "hysteria." Clarification of these various meanings of hysteria is necessary in order to facilitate understanding of the terms as they are used in this book and by others.

There various uses of "hysteria" include (hysterical) conversion reaction; hysterical personality; hysteria as a form of repetitive somatizing behavior (also known as somatization disorder or Briquet's syndrome); as a contagious group process, e.g., a "hysterical" crowd; as a pejorative term in either men or women, e.g., "He is nothing but a hysteric"; and to connote a specific constellation in psychoanalytic theory, e.g., the use of the term to refer to a woman who has unresolved conflicts which originated during the oedipal stage of psychosexual development.

This chapter addresses only three of the aforementioned categories. Hysterical (histronic) personality will be briefly discussed with an emphasis upon description and diagnostic criteria. Although the hysterical personality is not per se a somatizing disorder, this personality description is often used when various aspects of somatiation are discussed. Conversion reactions (or "disorders") are included here because of their traditional association with hysteria. In fact, earlier terminology usually included the entire phrase "hysterical conversion reaction." Conversion reactions do represent an important form of somatizing behavior, but as discussed below they are by no means synonymous with, and often occur independently of, other "hysterical" phenomenon. Finally, Briquet's syndrome (or somatization disorder) is included because it is a well-defined disorder of repetitive somatizing behavior which incorporates many earlier concepts of hysteria.

THE HYSTERICAL PERSONALITY

Descriptions of the hysterical personality vary, and the definition of the disorder as well as of its etiology has been the subject of a number of psychoanalytically oriented articles (Blinder, 1966; Easser and Lesser, 1965; Halleck, 1967; Hollender, 1971; Lazare, 1971; Marmor, 1953). There is consensus that there is a wide spectrum in the phenomenology of the hysterical personality, and there appears to be increasing acceptance of the policy of labeling those at the more pathologic end of the continuum as "borderline" personalities. However, it must be stressed that borderline personality does not consist exclusively of patients with hysteroid features. The hysterial personality as described by Chodoff and Lyons (1958) is characterized by "...persons who are vain and egocentric, who display labile and excitable but shallow affectivity, whose dramatic attention-seeking and histrionic behavior may go to the extremes of lying and even pseudologic phantastica, who are very conscious of sex, sexually provacative yet frigid, and who are dependently demanding in interpersonal situations." These persons use to a great extent the ego defense mechanisms of repression, displacement, isolation, and projection.

Psychodynamic explanations for the hysterical personality have varied. Earlier hypotheses put emphasis upon conflicts in the "oedipal" stage of psychosexual development. More recently the important paper of Marmor (1953), which stressed fixations at the oral stage of psychosexual development, has found wide acceptance. A further elaboration of this formulation is that the hysterical woman's efforts to maintain relationships with men, often in a coquettish or sexually provocative manner, are actually motivated by attempts to use these men as substitute mothers (Hollender, 1971). The hysteric is motivated by similar needs (unconscious) for mothering in the repetitive seeking of medical attention from physicians (Halleck, 1967). Recently Chodoff (1982) has proposed that the hysterical personality is a caricature of femininity which develops under the influence of cultural forces, particularly male domination. He suggests that machoism may be the male equivalent of the hysterical personality in women and that there should be a corresponding diagnostic niche for the "macho" personality disorder.

The observations of Shapiro (1965), who has described the "hysterical style," provide a different and useful way of looking at the hysterical personality. Shapiro describes a hysterical cognitive style that typifies the manner by which these people process information. Hysterical cognition is viewed as global and impressionistic, relatively diffuse, and lacking in sharpness and fine detail. There is distractibility with the train of thought easily interrupted by transient influences. The hysterical person tends to cognitively respond quickly and to be susceptible to that which is immediately impressive. From the above qualities are derived the frequently described hysterical characteristics: suggestibility, romance and fantasy to fill in for a factually depleted inner world, judgments which are quick and labile, and an emotionality which is superficial but not deeply experienced.

The term "hysterical personality" has been criticized on the basis that it is not descriptive of the disorder, and the Diagnostic and Statistical Manual (DSM) III (1980) of the American Psychiatric Association now uses the term "histronic personality." The DSM III diagnostic criteria (see Table 1) for "histronic personality" are not significantly different from the description by Chodoff and Lyons (1958) of the "hysterical personality," except for less emphasis on sexual issues.

TABLE 1. DSM III Diagnostic Criteria for Histrionic Personality Disorder

The following are characteristic of the individual's current and long-term functioning, are not limited to episodes of illness, and cause either significant impairment in social or occupational functioning or subjective distress.

A. Behavior that is overly dramatic, reactive, and intensely expressed, as indicated by at least three of the following:
   1. Self-dramatization, e.g., exaggerated expression of emotions
   2. incessant drawing of attention to oneself
   3. craving for activity and excitement
   4. overreaction to minor events
   5. irrational, angry outbursts or tantrums

B. Characteristic disturbances in interpersonal relationships as indicated by at least two of the following:
   1. perceived by others as shallow and lacking genuineness, even if superficially warm and charming
   2. egocentric, self-indulgent, and inconsiderate of others
   3. vain and demanding
   4. dependent, helpless, constantly seeking reassurance
   5. prone to manipulative suicidal threats, gestures, or attempts

American Psychiatric Association, *Diagnostic and Statistical Manual of Mental Disorders,* Third Edition, p 315, Washington, D.C., APA 1980. Reprinted by permission.

CONVERSION REACTIONS

Conversion phenomena are defined as symbolic representations of psychical conflict in terms of motor or sensory manifestations (Campbell, 1981). Recognized since antiquity, these are manifested in a wide variety of symptomatic presentations (Engel, 1970). Examples include pseudoseizures, "hysterical mutism" and tunnel vision. Conversion phenomena differ from malingering in that the patient does not have conscious control over the symptom, and they differ from psychophysiologic reactions in that there is no demonstrable anatomic or pathophysiologic abnormality (except as a secondary response such as disuse atrophy).

One often hears comments made to the effect that conversion reactions were a product of Victorian culture and no longer exist because of greater medical and psychological sophistication. The available data, however, do not bear this out (Lewis and Berman, 1965; Stephens and Kamp, 1962). It appears that the more grossly nonphysiologic and dramatic symptoms occur in patients from less well-educated backgrounds, and that more sophisticated persons have more complex symptoms which often closely simulate known medical diseases (Stephens and Kamp, 1962; Ziegler et al., 1960). Thus dramatic conversion reactions such as "hysterical" gait disorders occur more frequently in culturally deprived areas such as Appalachia (Weinstein et al., 1969), and university centers tend to see patients who frequently present with pain syndromes (Ziegler et al., 1960). In fact, Engel (1970) has expressed the opinion that pain is the most common conversion symptom seen today.

Conversion in Children

Conversion reactions occur in children and appear to be fairly common. One report (Maloney, 1980) indicated that 16.7% of pediatric patients seen in psychiatric consultation were diagnosed as having a conversion reaction, and another report (Proctor, 1958) indicated a frequency of 13% diagnosed as such in a consecutive unselected series of child psychiatric patients. Interestingly, the sex distribution of conversion disorders in children is almost equal (Maloney, 1980; Proctor, 1958), and it has been hypothesized that "hysteria" is more common in boys than in adult men because dependency and passitivity are not socially condoned in men. In the series reported by Maloney (1980), of those children who were diagnosed as having a conversion reaction, 97% came from a family with a recent stress, 77% came from a family with communication problems, and 58% of the patients had an unresolved grief reaction. In addition, 90% of these children had a depressed parent.

The symptoms of most children with conversion reactions remit within a relatively short period of time, with or without psychotherapy. However, whether or not symptoms remit, it has been recommended that the children should be engaged in psychotherapy which is aimed at alteration of the underlying psychopathology. Without treatment, it is likely that the child will again become symptomatic in the future.

Conversion in Adults

Most, but by no means all, adult patients with conversion reactions are women, and the average age is about 40 years. Contrary to popular belief, all males with conversion are not compensation cases (Ziegler et al., 1960). The personalities of patients with conversion disorders are frequently described as immature or dependent, and a singificant number are the only child or the youngest of their sibships. Many conversion reaction patients have a hysterical personality, but this is by no means universal. The concurrence of conversion reaction and hysterical personality was 9% in one series (Stephens and Kamp, 1962), noted to be less than half the group in another series (Ziegler et al., 1960), and over half the group in still another study (Lewis and Berman, 1965).

Etiologic Theories of Conversion

Theories of the etiology of conversion phenomena revolve around three major themes: neurophysiologic, behavioral, and psychoanalytic explanations (Jones, 1980). The various etiologic explanations are not mutually exclusive because a mixture of factors may be operative for any one patient or different factors in different patients.

Neurophysiologic theories suggest that there is an inherent defect or weakness in certain brain functions. Ludwig (1972) proposed a theoretical model of hysteria which suggested that the disorder is basically a dysfunction of attention and recent memory due to corticofugal inhibition of afferent stimulation. A recent detailed neuropsychological investigation (utilizing the Reitan Battery) of hysterics yielded findings that these patients, when compared to various other control groups, including normals, exhibited bifrontal cerebral impairment and globally a greater dysfunction of the nondominant hemisphere. The statistical technique of cluster analysis indicated that hysterics were closer to schizophrenia than to normals. The hysterics were characterized by, along with the conversion parameter, imprecise verbal communications and a subtle form of affective incongruity (Flor-Henry et al., 1981).

The behavioral theories of conversion phenomena stress that the patient has learned methods to communicate feelings of helplessness and to elicit environmental changes through his/her symptoms. Thus there has been a learned helplessness by these patients who, as children, were reinforced for frailty, seductiveness, and passivity. They have used this learned behavior as adults to manipulate and control their interpersonal relationships, including physicians (Halleck, 1967; Celani, 1976). It is also possible that certain physiologic responses, both of the voluntary and autonomic nervous system, are learned through prior experiences and then evoked as conversion disorders in response to certain stimuli (Barr and Abernethy, 1977).

Psychoanalytic theories stress the importance of the symbolic communication of the conversion phenomenon, and assert that the symptoms provide a compromise between the instinctual drives and their prohibitions.

Hollender has proposed that conversion symptoms and some other forms of hysterical phenomena such as culture-bound syndromes, are nonverbal or pantomine responses that occur when more direct forms of expression are blocked (Hollender, 1972, 1976). "(Hysteria) . . . is the dramatization of a forbidden wish or impulse, its prohibition, or some compromise between the two. Usually the dramatization, being a form of pantomine, involves the body" (Hollender, 1972).

Engel (1970) suggests that the conversion symptom has four unconsciously determined aims. They are (1) to permit expression of the forbidden wish but disguised in such a manner as not to be recognized by the person nor by the person for which it was intended; (2) to impose punishment through suffering and disability for having such a wish; (3) to remove the person from a threatening or disturbing life situation; and (4) to provide a new method of relating to others, the sick role.

The Diagnosis of Conversion

The diagnosis of conversion disorders is fraught with difficulties. Periodically articles are published with the aim of helping to differentiate between organic neurologic disease and "hysteric" symptoms (Bowlus and Currier, 1963; Silverstein, 1976; Weintraub, 1977). Although the various techniques suggested to have value in ascertaining the baseline of objective findings, they still fall short of making definitive diagnoses. Not infrequently there is a complex interweaving of genuine organic disease and the patient's use of the illness for psychological purposes (Caplan and Nadelson, 1980). The patient may unconsciously exaggerate symptoms in an effort to convince the physician of their validity or as a way to obtain maximal gains. In either situation, the physician may diagnose the obvious simulation and fail to appreciate the more subtle evidence of organic disease.

The diagnostic criteria for "conversion disorder" as specified by the DSM III (American Psychiatric Association 1980) (see Table 2) stress the importance of secondary gains and are otherwise largely exclusionary in nature. To the contradiction of prior authorities (Engel, 1970; Ziegler et al., 1960), the DSM criteria exclude pain as a primary symptom ("psychogenic pain" is listed as a separate diagnosis in the DSM III).

Even the presence or absence of psychiatric symptoms, which are traditionally associated with conversion reactions, are difficult to interpret. "La belle indifference," a traditional classic sign in conversion reactions, is

TABLE 2. DSM III Diagnostic Criteria for Conversion Disorder

A. The predominant disturbance is a loss of or alteration in physical functioning suggesting a physical disorder.

B. Psychological factors are judged to be etiologically involved in the symptom, as evidenced by one of the following:
   1. there is a temporal relationship between an environmental stimulus that is apparently related to a psychological conflict or need and the initiation or exacerbation of the symptom
   2. the symptom enables the individual to avoid some activity that is noxious to him or her
   3. the symptom enables the individual to get support from the environment that otherwise might not be forthcoming

C. It has been determined that the symptom is not under voluntary control.

D. The symptom cannot, after appropriate investigation, be explained by a known physical disorder or pathophysiological mechanism.

E. The symptom is not limited to pain or to a disturbance in sexual functioning.

F. Not due to Somatization Disorder or Schizophrenia.

American Psychiatric Association, *Diagnostic and Statistical Manual of Mental Disorders*, Third Edition, p 247, Washington, D.C., APA 1980. Reprinted by permission.

actually of little use. This affective response of bland indifference to the symptom is found in a distinct minority of the patients (Chodoff, 1954; Stephens and Kamp, 1962; Weinstein et al., 1969). Some patients, particularly those who are older, may display some features of depression, and the "conversion" can be regarded as a defense against depression (Ziegler et al., 1960). Symbolism is frequently lacking or too obscure to be identified (Lewis and Berman, 1965), or at times there may be the imposition of secondary symbolism upon a genuine organic symptom (Fry, 1969). The correlation of conversion reactions with the hysterical personality is far from unity. Even when features of the hysterical personality are present, such personality characteristics do not convey an immunity from organic disease.

A further complication of the issues concerning diagnosis is that new advances in knowledge and more sophisticated laboratory examinations may demonstrate organic abnormalities for disorders previously believed to be hysterical (Roth, 1980). A well-publicized report by Slater (1965) indicated that in the majority of cases, neurologic disease emerges at a later date to explain symptoms originally called conversion reactions, even when the diagnoses were made by experienced neurologists and psychiatrists.

My experience suggests that hypnosis or an amytal interview may be useful adjuncts in the diagnosis of conversion. In a state of altered consciousness, the patient may verbally reveal the meaning of the symptom or, with suggestion, the symptom may remit. However, even with such apparently convincing evidence, the diagnosis of a conversion reaction should be interpreted with caution; the patient may still have a subtle underlying neurologic disability to which he was reacting with exaggerated symptoms.

Conversion is a phenomenon which *does* exist, and it is underdiagnosed. The paradox is that when it is diagnosed, the diagnosis is frequently inaccurate.

Illustrative Case History

A 34-year-old divorced cosmetic saleslady was being seen in supportive psychotherapy because of multiple somatic complaints of poorly defined etiology and her difficulty in establishing independence from her parents.

Prior to his annual vacation, the therapist anticipated that there might be problems due to his absence. The issue of separation was repetitively raised, but the patient denied any anxiety concerning the temporary interruption of therapy.

On the therapist's return to town there was an urgent call from the patient's primary physician who stated that the patient was hospitalized for paraplegia. All laboratory tests, including an electromyograph, had been normal, and it was assumed that the symptom represented a "hysterical paralysis."

The therapist interviewed the patient in the hospital and interpreted to her that she was angry at having been abandoned, envious that she had not accompanied him, and had felt that she "couldn't stand on her own two legs." The patient giggled at this interpretation and stated it was "ridiculous." However, the next day she walked from the hospital and was able to keep her next outpatient psychotherapy appointment, at which time she demonstrated no traces of the previous symptoms. A follow-up of eight years indicated no neurologic disease had subsequently developed.

The conversion symptom of paraplegia in the woman served to communicate feelings of anger and helplessness. In addition, the symptom provided the patient with the attention and gratification of dependency wishes which accompany hospitalization.

Treatment and Management of Conversion Disorders

The management of acute conversion disorders often appears deceptively simple; most remit spontaneously and/or with minimal suggestion. Other symptoms often yield to psychotherapy (either by the primary care physician or a psychiatrist), hypnosis, an amytal interview, or by environmental manipulation (e.g., discharge from military service). One study indicated that all patients with conversion reactions responded to a treatment program which incorporated an apparently ineffective but harmless somatic therapy (e.g., faradic stimulation) with suggestion. Contrary to popular wisdom, most of the patients in the study did not have symptom substitution over the follow-up period of one year (Hafeiz, 1980).

Conversion reactions that do not remit quickly may have been misdiagnosed and actually represent neurologic disease or may be associated with massive secondary gains which perpetuate the symptom. In the latter situation, a referral to a psychiatrist is indicated; frequently psychiatric inpatient care is required to break up the reinforcing cycle of symptom and secondary gain.

Despite the fact that the conversion symptom usually remits fairly quickly, there remain several important questions to ask. Are there chronic underlying emotional problems which may result in other symptoms if left unattended? Does the conversion represent a symptomatic expression of another psychiatric illness such as depression or incipient schizophrenia? Will symptomatic treatment of the symptom lead to a reinforcement of conversion as a behavioral pattern or, in other words, is one helping the patient learn to manipulate the environment through the use of bodily symptoms?

The answers to these questions will determine the management of the patient. Obviously if the symptom is reflecting an underlying psychiatric illness, that illness needs specific treatment, for example, the institution of antidepressant therapy for depression. If there are unresolved emotional or family problems, then these will also require attention; a referral for psychotherapy or family counseling may be indicated.

Management of the acute problem by the primary care physician will to some extent determine the patient's propensity for subsequent use of conversion to resolve emotional problems in the future. Management to be effective must take into account the psychological nature of the complaint. There must be as little reinforcement of the symptoms as is possible, and secondary gains must be minimized. Repetitive conversion symptoms are usually associated with Briquet's syndrome and require the techniques of management associated with that disorder.

BRIQUET'S SYNDROME

Modern efforts at developing more objective criteria for the diagnosis of hysteria began with the work of Purtell and his associates (1951). These investigators based their clinical descriptive study on earlier work by the French physician Briquet and the English physician Savill. The study of Purtell and colleages, which was conducted on the medical service of a New England hospital, compared patients with physical symptoms but no determinable disease, and diagnosed hysterics, to control groups of women from various sources (postpartum, healthy working women, women with chronic diseases). Women who had been assigned the diagnosis of hysteria differed from the controls in that the former had a significantly greater prevalence of a large number of symptoms such as headaches, blurred vision, and sexual indifference. The authors concluded that hysteria probably has a characteristic clinical picture, which includes an age of onset before 35 years; it occurs almost exclusively in women (if compensation cases are exluded); it is never monosymptomatic, exhibiting a multiplicity of symptoms, including a history of excessive surgical operations. These authors also noted that the hysterics were typically friendly and overly talkative during the examinations and had a dramatic way of describing past symptoms and illnesses. They quoted patients as characteristically saying such things as "I vomit every ten minutes. Sometimes it lasts for two to three weeks at a time. Can't even take liquids. I even vomit water. I can't stand the smell of food."

A research group of investigators at Washington University (St. Louis, Mo.) who are interested in hysteria have followed up on the original work of Purtell and collaborators and have done much to further knowledge about the phenomenology of the disorder. Perley and Guze (1962) demonstrated that when the diagnosis was based on defined clinical criteria (which included a dramatic or complicated medical history beginning before age 35 and a minimum of 15 medically unexplained symptoms in 9 of 10 groups), there was a 90% probability that the clinical picture would remain unchanged over a number of years and that no other disorder would develop that might explain the original symptoms.

As the St. Louis group further delineated the diagnostic criteria for research in hysteria, Guze (1967) proposed the eponym "Briquet's syndrome" for the specific group of patients they were diagnosing as hysterics. This was done in an attempt to develop a nonpejorative term and, at the same time, carefully define a specific clinical syndrome. There was a perceived need to have reliable diagnostic criteria in order that investigators from different research centers could compare findings. Although the creation of the new term has met with criticism (Briquet's syndrome or hysteria, editorial, Lancet, 1977), the concept of specific diagnostic criteria is essential for meaningful clinical research. Because the syndrome, as described, has clinical validity the eponym Briquet's syndrome has found increasing acceptance in the medical-psychiatric literature.

The Diagnosis of Briquet's Syndrome

The diagnostic criteria for Briquet's syndrome (hysteria) as specified by Woodruff and colleagues (1971) are listed in Table 3. A definitive diagnosis consists of at least 25 symptoms in 9 of the 10 groups. A probable diagnosis is indicated by at least 20 symptoms in 9 of the 10 groups. It is important to note that it is the manner in which a patient answers the questions in a medical history, rather than actual fact, that determines the criteria for the diagnosis of Briquet's syndrome. The patient with Briquet's syndrome has a characteristic manner of responding with positive answers to nearly all the questions concerning physical symptoms. This is probably closely related to the patients' suggestibility and their dramatic way of presenting their medical histories.

The recently published Diagnostic and Statistical manual, Third Edition (DSM III) of the American Psychiatric Association (1980) has based a new diagnosis on the research generated in reference to Briquet's syndrome. The new diagnosis has been labeled "somatization disorder"; diagnostic criteria are included in Table 4. Although there are similarities, the criteria for the two diagnoses are by no means identical. Unfortunately validity and reliability for the new diagnosis have yet to be established.

The 58-item checklist for Briquet's syndrome often proves to be a time-consuming interview depending upon the number of positive responses (experience at Vanderbilt Hospital has indicated a variation from about 15 minutes to two hours). In an attempt to shorten the interview time, Reveley et al. (1977) have reported upon use of a shortened 14-question screening interview. This brief test can be administered in a few minutes. Initial experience with the shortened screening interview indicates that about 14% of women patients will be false positives and require the more extensive original interview to either confirm or rule out the diagnosis. The authors found no false negatives.

A relationship between Briquet's syndrome and hysterical personality has

TABLE 3. Diagnostic Criteria for Hysteria (Briquet's Syndrome)

Diagnostic criteria are
1. complicated or dramatic medical history, with onset prior to the age of 35 years;
2. minimum of 25 symptoms in at least nine of the ten symptom groups;
3. at least 25 of the symptoms in a minimum of nine groups had no known medical explanation.

Symptom groups are

Group 1
Headaches
Sickly most of life

Group 2
Blindness
Paralysis
Anesthesia
Aphonia
Fits or convulsions
Unconsciousness
Amnesia
Deafness
Hallucinations
Urinary retention
Ataxia
Other conversion symptoms

Group 3
Fatigue
Lump in throat
Fainting spells
Visual blurring
Weakness
Dysuria

Group 4
Breathing difficulty
Palpitation
Anxiety attacks
Chest pain
Dizziness

Group 5
Anorexia
Weight loss
Marked fluctuations in weight
Nausea
Abdominal bloating
Food intolerance
Diarrhea
Constipation

Group 6
Abdominal pain
Vomiting

Group 7
Dysmenorrhea
Menstrual irregularity
Amenorrhea
Excessive bleeding

Group 8
Sexual indifference
Frigidity
Dyspareunia
Other sexual difficulties
Vomiting nine months pregnancy
   or hospitalized for hyperemesis
   gravidarum

Group 9
Back pain
Joint pain
Extremity pain
Burning pains of the sexual organs,
   mouth, or rectum
Other bodily pains

Group 10
Nervousness
Fears
Need to quit working or inability
   to carry on regular duties because
   of feeling sick
Crying easily
Feeling life was hopeless
Thinking a good deal about dying
Wanting to die
Thinking of suicide
Suicide attempts

Adapted from Woodruff, R.A., Clayton, P.J., and Guze, S.B., 1971, Studies of diagnosis, outcome and prevalence. JAMA 215:425–428. Copyright 1971, American Medical Association; reprinted by permission.

TABLE 4. DSM III Diagnostic Criteria for Somatization Disorder

A. A history of physical symptoms of several years' duration beginning before the age of 30.

B. Complaints of at least 14 symptoms for women and 12 for men, from the 37 symptoms listed below. To count a symptom as present the individual must report that the symptom caused him or her to take medication (other than aspirin), alter his or her life pattern, or see a physician. The symptoms, in the judgment of the clinician, are not adequately explained by physical disorder or physical injury, and are not side effects of medication, drugs, or alcohol. The clinician need not be convinced that the symptom was actually present, e.g., that the individual actually vomited throughout her entire pregnancy; report of the symptom by the individual is sufficient.

   Sickly: Believes that he or she has been sickly for a good part of his or her life.

   Conversion or pseudoneurological symptoms: Difficulty swallowing, loss of voice, deafness, double vision, blurred vision, blindness, fainting or loss of consciousness, memory loss, seizures or convulsions, trouble walking, paralysis or muscle weakness, urinary retention or difficulty urinating.

   Gastrointestinal symptoms: Abdominal pain, nausea, vomiting spells (other than during pregnancy), bloating (gassy), intolerance (e.g., gets sick) of a variety of foods, diarrhea.

   Female reproductive symptoms: Judged by the individual as occurring more frequently or severely than in most women: painful menstruation, menstrual irregularity, excessive bleeding, severe vomiting throughout pregnancy, or causing hospitalization during pregnancy.

   Psychosexual symptoms: For the major part of the individual's life after opportunities for sexual activity: sexual indifference, lack of pleasure during intercourse, pain during intercourse.

   Pain: Pain in back, joints, extremities, genital area (other than during intercourse); pain on urination; other pain (other than headaches).

   Cardiopulmonary symptoms: Shortness of breath, palpitations, chest pain, dizziness.

American Psychiatric Association, *Diagnostic and Statistical Manual of Mental Disorders*, Third Edition, pp 243–244, Washington, D.C., APA 1980. Reprinted by permission.

been described. Liskow and colleagues (1977) compared the MMPI scores of 29 patients diagnosed as having hysterical personality with the scores of 21 patients diagnosed as having Briquet's syndrome. The only differences in the profiles were that the Briquet's syndrome patients had a higher average L (lie) score and a higher average Hs (hypochondriasis) score. It should be remarked that the Briquet's syndrome patients were of a higher average age. Kimble and colleagues (1975) found that of 10 subjects diagnosed as hysterical personality, 9 met the criteria for Briquet's syndrome. However, teenage girls were deliberately excluded from the Kimball study because they had observed that teenagers with a clinical diagnosis of hysterical personality rarely met criteria for Briquet's syndrome. This observation is compatible with that of Liskow et al. (1977) in that Briquet's syndrome might reflect a natural progression of the hysterical personality; that is, somatic complaints increase with age.

In the following discussion the terms Briquet's syndrome or hysteria will be used consistent with the way in which the authors reporting their work used the terms. Often "hysteria" and Briquet's syndrome have been used interchangeably.

An Illustrative Case History

The following actual case history will serve to demonstrate many of the features of Briquet's syndrome. The patient met the diagnostic criteria of Briquet's syndrome and had 30 symptoms in 10 of 10 groups.

A 31-year-old twice-married Caucasian female when last seen in psychiatric consultation had already amassed the following medical history, the investigation and treatment of which had cost the responsible insurance company a sum in excess of $100,000.

As a result of complaints of double vision, dizziness, abdominal pains, headaches, menstrual complaints, fatigue, depression, and other vague symptoms, the patient had been hospitalized a minimum of eight times for extensive diagnostic studies. Her diagnoses included reactive hypoglycemia, migraine headaches, and spastic colitis, but none of these diagnoses had been made on objective criteria and no treatment regimen had been effective. She had been demanding of both narcotic-type medications and minor tranquilizers. Addiction to diazepam, which she obtained from multiple sources, was suspected on several occasions. She obtained a hysterectomy for questionable indications from the third gynecologist from whom she insistently sought consultation; she had previously seen two different gynecologists each of whom had stated that she had no evidence of gynecologic disease. A brief course of psychotherapy was not only ineffective, but she emphatically proclaimed that the failure of her physical symptoms to improve after seeing a psychiatrist only proved that the problems were not "in my head."

Her psychosocial history was remarkable. She was the tenth of 10 children born to the family of an alcoholic father who physically and sexually abused his children. The mother, a martyred woman, worked six days a week and refused to divorce her husband "for the good of the children." When the patient was about 12, her next older sister contracted tuberculosis and was sent to the state tuberculosis sanitarium for two years. The patient's recollection of this was that the sanitarium was a clean, pleasant place in comparison to home. Probably more important was that each Sunday, the only day she did not work, the mother would make the trip to spend the day at the sanitarium with the sister.

Largely to escape home, the patient married at age 17 to a man who drank to excess and abused her. She eventually left him and moved to another state where shortly thereafter she met her second husband, a kindly but passive, physically deformed man who made minimal sexual demands of her. The couple then had two children, and the responsibility for them overwhelmed the patient. Subsequent to the birth of the children, she spent most of her time on the livingroom couch, complaining that she felt ill, or hospitalized while the children were cared for by her mother-in-law and husband. The secondary gains of her illness relieved her of her responsibilities as wife and mother.

The Phenomenology of Briquet's Syndrome

Prevalence, Age, Sex, and Socioeconomic Status. The prevalence of Briquet's syndrome, based on studies of hospitalized postpartum women, is estimated to be between 1 and 2% of the female population (Farley et al, 1968; Woodruff et al., 1971). While there have been no comparable studies, the prevalence in men is believed to be much lower. In one investigation, 50 male psychiatric inpatients were surveyed, and when rigid criteria were utilized no men were found to have the disorder (Kroll et al., 1979). Males who fulfill the diagnostic criteria have been reported as single case studies (de Figueiredo at al., 1980; Kaminsky and Slavney, 1976; Rounsaville et al., 1979). Most reports of men believed to be "hysterics" have involved persons involved in litigation following injuries or some other form of compensation (Allodi, 1974), but, despite the use of the term, diagnostic criteria were not described.

It is commonly believed that patients with Briquet's syndrome are of lower socioeconomic status, lower education, or generally less psychologically sophisticated. The data on this are very scanty, but one study does support that view. Guze and associates (1971a) found that patients who reported conversion reactions as well as those diagnosed as "hysterics" were much less likely to have completed more than one year of college.

Although lower socioeconomic status among hysterics may be a statistical finding, it by no means excludes the more highly educated. The Consultation-Liaison Service of Vanderbilt University Hospital has seen in psychiatric consultation women who met the specific diagnostic criteria for Briquet's syndrome and who were college graduates and/or from the upper middle class.

That the onset of Briquet's syndrome occurs before age 35 is determined by the definition. However, the ages of women presenting with the syndrome may vary considerably. The syndrome may be well established by the late teens or still present and diagnosed in old age. The Psychiatric Consultation-Liaison Service, Vanderbilt University Hospital, Nashville, Tenn., uses rigid research criteria for the diagnosis, and the age range of patients who have met these criteria has varied from 17 to 71 years of age. This is an important point to note because the patient with Briquet's syndrome (hysteria) is often characterized as a young, seductive female. These patients do grow old, and there is no reason to believe that their behavior patterns change with age. In fact, the diagnosis appears to be quite stable as the next section will illustrate.

Stability of the Diagnosis. Guze and Perley (1962; Perley and Guze, 1963) in a retrospective review of patients who met the criteria for Briquet's syndrome found that 6–8 years later 90% continued to meet the criteria for the diagnosis. When the diagnosis had been originally rejected, because of failure to meet the criteria, then other clinical disorders had emerged to explain the original symptoms.

Of the group of 25 patients originally diagnosed as hysterics (Briquet's syndrome), 92% continued to consult physicians and 92% continued to complain of one or more of the symptoms of headaches, vomiting, or pain; 76% of the women continued to have sexual maladjustment problems, and 31% had problems leading to marital separation or divorce in the ensuing 6–8 years. It was also notable that during this time span, the group had a total of 53 hospitalizations (exclusive of childbirth) for an average of 2.1 hospitalizations per patient.

Family and Marital Histories. Arkonac and Guze (1963) obtained information concerning the primary relatives who were over 15 years of age of 21 index cases of hysteria. Hysteria was found in 15% of the female relatives interviewed, a figure considerably higher than the 1–2% expected by chance. Anxiety neurosis was diagnosed in 9% of the relatives, very close to the estimated 10% prevalence in the general population. Of the male relatives 24% presented a history of alcoholism, and an additional 9% of the males were given a diagnosis of sociopathy. Thus 33% of the male relatives interviewed had alcoholism or sociopathy. The results of this study were tentative because of the small numbers but suggested an increased prevalence of hysteria among the female relatives of hysterics and an increased prevalence of alcoholism and sociopathy among their male relatives.

In a larger study, Woerner and Guze (1968) extended the investigation to more cases and also included the husbands into the study. Their findings again, albeit with a small sample, indicated an increased prevalence of hysteria in the female relatives and a similar increased prevalence of alcoholism and sociopathy in the male relatives.

Of interest was the information concerning the husbands of the hysterics. Alcoholism and sociopathy were frequently found and most probably contributed to the characteristic marital and sexual discord experienced by their wives.

The Relationship to Sociopathy and Alcoholism

Guze and colleagues (1967) studied the families of convicted male criminals. Of the index subjects (the male criminals) the only psychiatric diagnoses found more frequently than in the general population were sociopathic personality, alcoholism, and drug addiction. Most relatives proved to be free of psychiatric illness, and the only diagnoses which were more frequent than that expected by chance in the general population were sociopathic personality, alcoholism, drug addiction, and hysteria. The first three were found chiefly among male relatives, and hysteria was found only among the female relatives. Whether it was the index subject, or the relative, the three disorders of sociopathy, alcoholism, and drug addiction were frequently found in the same individual.

A series of investigations by the St. Louis group continued to disclose a relationship between sociopathy and hysteria. Cloninger and Guze (1970a, 1970b) studied a group of 66 convicted women felons who were on parole. Of this group, 50% had served at least one prison term; the most frequent crime had been homicide. Many of these subjects fit the criteria for more than one diagnosis (i.e., alcoholism and sociopathy, sociopathy and hysteria, etc.). The most frequent diagnosis was sociopathy (65%); alcoholism was also notably frequent (47%); and the third most common diagnosis was hysteria (41%). Sociopathy was associated with hysteria 40% of the time, and antisocial symptoms had begun after the hysterical symptoms in 67% of the subjects who received both diagnoses.

Of the 27 cases of hysteria, 60% demonstrated histrionic personality features such as dramatic overstatement, seductive and manipulative behavior, and ostentatious grooming and dress.

The hysterics, when compared to subjects without the diagnosis, had a history of significantly more hospitalizations, 4.3 per woman for the hysterics compared to 1.6 for the other women.

An unexpected and very interesting difference between the hysterics and the other subjects was the hysterics' tendency to deny guilt (67 v 10%) or to offer extenuating circumstances to mitigate their guilt (30 v 15%). They were also more likely to claim illegal arrest, an unfair trial, or cruel treatment in prison or while on parole.

The investigators observed that hysteria and/or sociopathy was present in 80% of their subjects, and the two diagnoses frequently occurred together. They noted that sociopathy is generally a diagnosis made in men, and hysteria is a diagnosis made in women. They speculated that dependent upon the sex of the individual the same etiologic and pathogenic factors may lead to different, although sometimes overlapping, clinical pictures.

Aspects of the subjects' personal and family backgrounds were also investigated. Their socioeconomic origins tended to be of lower status; the head of the household during childhood was an unskilled laborer in 56% of the cases. The parental home had been frequently unstable, and only 35% of the subjects reported having both parents permanently in the home until age 18. Parental antisocial behavior was frequent, and the father, or his surrogate, was reported as a heavy drinker by over half the women; cruel or abusive behavior by him was reported 12% of the time. The mother, or her surrogate, was reported as a heavy drinker in 21% of the cases, and having demonstrated cruel or abusive behavior in 12% of the cases. On the basis of the family history, a suspected diagnosis of sociopathy or suspected alcoholism was made for 55% of the fathers and 27% of the mothers.

The patients frequently had school difficulties of a behavioral nature, and low academic achievement was common despite adequate intellectual resources. Work histories, as evidenced by menial positions with low pay and frequent changes, were similarly poor.

Sexual problems were frequently reported and marital histories were chaotic and unstable. Of those who married, 72% had married at least one sociopathic or alcoholic husband, and 64% reported fighting with their husbands or to have been beaten by them. Of the children these women had borne, 37% of those living did not live with their mothers.

What was remarkable in this study was that there was little difference between the women diagnosed as sociopathic and those diagnosed as hysteric. They came from similar backgrounds and had similar lifestyles except for those features that are part of the diagnostic criteria for the two disorders.

Another approach to studying relationships between sociopathy and hysteria involved comparing two diagnostic samples (hysteria and anxiety neurosis) derived from a large series of psychiatric clinic outpatients. The past histories of the hysterics had a significantly greater incidence of delinquent and antisocial behavior. They also had a larger percentage of first- or second-degree relatives who had a positive history of antisocial behavior or criminalty (Guze et al., 1971a, 1971b).

In summary, there appears to be a significant relationship between hysteria and sociopathy. Some caution, however, must be observed in interpreting the above data. The investigations of the St. Louis group have to a large extent focused upon lower socioeconomic status subjects. It is possible that poverty and limited resources may be the common denominator in determining these behavioral patterns rather than either psychodynamic factors or heredity.

The Relationship to Polysurgery and Polysurgical Addiction

Excessive surgery is a major complication and/or manifestation of hysteria. Cohen and colleagues (1953) found that hysterics, when compared to hospitalized sick women controls, had experienced twice as many major operations, were 7 times as likely to have had a gynecologic operative procedure, and were more than 6 times as likely to have had a minor surgical procedure or diagnostic manipulation. A Scandanavian study (Lindberg and Lindegård, 1963) indicated that women patients (but not men) with hysteroid personality features (manifested by characteristics such as strong suggestibility, impressionability, and histrionics) were much more likely to have had a surgical operation and almost twice as likely, when compared to nonhysteroid subjects, to have had multiple surgical procedures. Similarly, hospitalized psychiatric patients who meet the criteria for Briquet's syndrome had been shown to have experienced significantly more operations, particularly of a gynecologic nature, when compared to women psychiatric patients who do not meet the diagnostic criteria for Briquet's syndrome (Bibb and Guze, 1972).

Exploring the question of multiple operations from another vantage point Martin and coworkers (1977) found that of a series of randomly selected women undergoing hysterectomy for noncancerous indications, 27% met the diagnostic criteria for Briquet's syndrome. In another investigation DeVaul and Faillace (1980) investigated differences between patients who had experienced five or more surgical operations and a control group matched for age, sex, marital status, and type of medical insurance. The subjects, however, did not represent a random sample of hospitalized patients because they were obtained from a pool of women for whom psychiatric consultation had been requested. Of the multiple surgery group (who had experienced an average of 9.8 operations) 74% were determined to have Briquet's syndrome. In addition to noting the high prevalence in their patients the investigators also regarded many of their patients to comprise a subset of chronic pain patients. For example, 18 of the 23 patients had similarities to the pain-prone personality previously described by Engel (1959), and many patients had experienced multiple physican contacts which had resulted in disappointing therapeutic outcomes.

The term polysurgery and polysurgical addiction originated with Menninger (1934), who described several patients of both sexes who had experienced multiple operations for unclear indications. These surgical operations had apparently been sought out by the patient. Menninger hypothesized that the need to seek repetitive surgery was unconsciously determined by one or more of several factors, which included the need for punishment.

Wahl and Golden (1966) reported upon a series of 16 polysurgical patients and noted that there were recurrent common themes in their psychodynamics and background histories. Most patients were women who reported a lack of parental affection as children or a relationship with a parent which was sadistic and/or seductive. Usually the mother had a history of vague chronic illnesses and multiple surgical operations. The patients had not been successful in forming warm and gratifying relationships with others, and, while superficially compliant, they often demonstrated anger in more indirect ways. The medical histories were often vague, circumstantial, and contradictory, and the patients rejected any suggestions that the symptoms were psychogenic.

In summary, it is apparent that patients with Briquet's syndrome experience a significant number of surgical operations, particularly of the pelvic area and perhaps without clear medical indications. If patients with multiple surgical operations are psychiatrically investigated a significant number, more than would be expected by chance, meet the diagnostic criteria for Briquet's syndrome. Whether or not a diagnosis of Briquet's syndrome is appropriate, there are notable similarities in the personal histories of patients with Briquet's syndrome and/or polysurgery. Many patients with surgery proneness can also be described as pain-prone personalities with chronic pain syndromes. Phenomenologically both Briquet's syndrome and chronic pain syndrome have considerable overlap both in the symptom of polysurgery and in the psychological descriptions of these patients.

The Characteristic Clinical Presentation of Briquet's Syndrome

From the above phenomenologic descriptions, there emerges a fairly consistent clinical history of the typical patient with Briquet's syndrome. She most commonly comes from a childhood home which was inconsistent and not emotionally supportive; one or both parents may have been alcoholic or sociopathic. Schoolwork and social adjustments were poor and a history of adolescent delinquency is common. Menarche was often regarded as fearful and menstrual periods thereafter have been associated with discomfort. Sexual activity frequently began at a young age but is not usually regarded as enjoyable. Marriages are unstable, and often multiple, with husbands frequently described as alcoholic or sociopathic. Problems with drug addiction or alcoholism are frequently observed in the patient herself. A pattern of multiple physical complaints beginning in adolescence or young adulthood takes her repetitively into physicians' offices, and despite a lack of objective medical disease she is frequently hospitalized and subjected to multiple surgical operations, particularly in the pelvic region of the body (Cohen, 1953). Frequently, but by no means always, the patient with Briquet's syndrome dresses and grooms herself in an exhibitionistic manner and relates her symptoms in a talkative and dramatic style. She is frequently glib and her history is disorganized with a blend of fantasy and fact; as a result an accurate and well-organized medical history is difficult, if not impossible, to obtain.

The long-term natural outcome of Briquet's syndrome is not known. Patients of all ages have been diagnosed with the disorder. The symptoms appear stable and there is no reason to suspect that very many patients have spontaneous remissions. Medical management and psychiatric treatment are difficult.

Management and Treatment of Briquet's Syndrome

The essential part of the management of Briquet's syndrome is making the diagnosis. This, of course, requires a high index of suspicion because diagnosis is frequently not obvious. The patient with Briquet's syndrome often obtains her medical care from multiple sources, rather than from a single physician, and the patient's dramatic presentation of symptoms often creates a sense of urgency to take action. The interview that will establish the diagnosis takes time, approximately 45 minutes on the average, which is not easily obtained in a busy medical practice. However, when one considers the cost of not making the diagnosis, financially and in morbidity (and even mortality) in regard to unnecessary surgery and invasive diagnostic procedures, then it is obvious that the time spent in the interview is very cost effective.

Once the diagnosis has been established, there are a number of management techniques that can be employed. One must not be too optimistic about "curing" the disorder as it is often refractory to change. The major consideration is how to protect the patient from herself! As a rule the patient is usually best managed by the primary care physician; a referral to a psychiatrist may offer little besides confirmation of the diagnosis. The greater the number of physicians who become involved in the treatment, the greater the opportunity for the patient to engage in manipulation. As the primary physician becomes better acquainted with the patient's history, the physician will be better able to sort out relevant new information from old complaints.

Medications are a special problem in dealing with the patient with Briquet's syndrome. These patients often have medicine chests stuffed full of various drugs prescribed for questionable indications. This very number of drugs increases the likelihood of iatrogenic symptoms due to adverse drug reactions and/or drug interactions. Besides the problem about adverse reactions (and impulsive overdoses of unusual medications), a major problem in dealing with these patients is their propensity to abuse habituating drugs, narcotic analgesics, hypnotics, and minor tranquilizers. These medications should be used with great caution and prescribed in small amounts with nonrefillable prescriptions. However, despite the most conscientious precautions on the part of the primary care physician, the patient may still obtain these medications from other physicians. As a consequence, one must be always alert to the possibility that symptoms or findings are due to an excess dosage of medications (e.g., nystagmus secondary to hypnotics) or due to withdrawal from drugs to which the patient has become physiologically addicted (e.g., confusion and neurologic symptoms occurring 5–7 days after discontinuation of benzodiazepenes).

The cardinal rule in the management of patients with Briquet's syndrome is that *invasive diagnostic procedures and therapeutic interventions should be undertaken only on the basis of objective evidence rather than upon the subjective complaints of the patient.*

Useful suggestions in the management of the patient with Briquet's syndrome have been suggested by Morrison (1978) whose approach is basically one of behavioral modification. This management technique involves selective attention (or inattention) and verbal rewards. For example, dramatic presentations of symptoms such as hyperventilation should be ignored to the greatest extent possible and the family counseled as to take a similar approach. However, despite their potential usefulness such techniques should be used cautiously in view of two possibilities: (1) although the patient may "cry wolf" frequently, hysterics are by no means immune from genuine and serious disease; (2) if minor symptoms fail to achieve attention then the hysteric may escalate the seriousness of the symptoms and/or engage in acting-out behavior such as suicidal gestures.

Threats of suicide or similar behavior must be met with a firm stance. They must not be allowed to manipulate either the family or the physician. Brief admission to a psychiatric inpatient unit with a nongratifying restricted routine may serve to teach the patient that such complaints are taken seriously and will evoke the type of attention that she does not want.

Overall strategy involves the selective inattention to the patient's somatic complaints while redirecting the attention to her often genuine psychosocial complaints. A useful tactic to take with the patient with Briquet's syndrome is to communicate to her that the symptoms she experiences are due to stress. Because of the popular interest in "stress" this is often an acceptable explanation, and it avoids the fruitless and generally antitherapeutic confrontation that "it's all in your head." If the patient can accept that she is responding to the stresses in her life, then the groundwork for a therapeutic alliance has been established. Office visits can then center on how she is managing the stress at home (or the office), and rewards in the form of praise can be given for reports of efforts to move outside the somatization routine, into which she has been locked. Suggestions by the physician may include advice such as how to handle unruly children or how to become involved in social activities.

When the patient is frustrated with the physician or when angry because of a failure to receive an expected medication (narcotics, etc.), then there may be a threat that she will change physicians. Such a threat must be met with a kindly but firm statement that such action, while within the patient's rights and power, would be unfortunate because the physician has a long-standing relationship with the patient, knows her medical history well and this allows for providing the best medical care possible. Some patients will carry through on their threats and leave, but such an outcome is preferable and more therapeutic than reinforcing a pattern of manipulation.

Working simultaneously with the patient's family is an important, almost essential, component of the management of the hysteric. There are multiple reasons for this, including the fact that it may be necessary in order to obtain an accurate history. Direct communication with the family members will also reduce the opportunities for manipulation and misunderstandings. However, it must be kept in mind that the difficulties of the patient with Briquet's syndrome usually extend beyond her own particular behavioral patterns. She is often married to an alcoholic or sociopathic man, and the children also frequently have school and behavioral problems. Thus the entire family needs attention, and the problems of the patient cannot be treated in a vacuum. The primary care (or "family") physician is the health care professional best able to provide the type of care needed.

When psychiatric intervention is deemed necessary then consideration should be given to using a group therapy treatment technique. Valko (1976) reports that a group of patients, all with diagnosed Briquet's syndrome, had an overall favorable response to this treatment method. This was evidenced by their decreased use of medications, decreased use of psychiatric services, and increased function with their families. The therapists found that group therapy was associated with more enjoyment than was individual psycho-therapy in working with these patients. An important aspect of treatment was that patients learned to confront each other with the relationship of stress to symptoms, thereby reducing the demands on the therapist.

Psychotherapy techniques aimed at "getting the feelings out" are contraindicated in patients with Briquet's syndrome. These patients already rely too heavily on this behavioral pattern to the exclusion of thinking (Murphy, 1982).

SUMMARY

Hysteria, a form of illness behavior which has been described through several thousands years of medical history, proves to have a very elusive quality when there are attempts to specifically define it.

There are several paradoxes to note in the modern conceptual views of hysteria. The psychoanalytic theoretical formulations of hysteria were derived from a study of patients with conversion phenomenon but currently diagnostic descriptions of the "hysterical personality" (histrionic personality) do not include somatization but rather emphasize different forms of behavior. The diagnostic category of Briquet's syndrome was developed in a phenomenologic manner from patients who had conversion disorders. As a result of the fact that both of these concepts were ultimately derived from patients with conversion disorders there is considerable overlap and most patients with Briquet's syndrome can also be described as having a hysterical personality. But many, perhaps most, patients with conversion disorders do not meet the diagnostic criteria for either Briquet's syndrome or hysterical personality! Important theoretical and conceptual work based upon detailed phenomenologic research remains to be completed before the current confusion can be eliminated.

Awaiting the results of new investigations and theoretical constructs, clinicians will need to continue to treat "hysterical" symptoms on an empirical basis. The acute conversion symptom must be evaluated from the perspective that it may represent a solution to a psychological conflict, an underlying neurologic disorder, or both! Repetitive conversion phenomena (Briquet's syndrome) represent a characterologic method of coping with life stresses. Management techniques must take into account the pervasive disorganization in these patients' lives.

REFERENCES

Allodi, F.A. 1974. Accident neurosis: Whatever happened to male hysteria? Can Psychiatr Assoc J 19:291–296.

American Psychiatric Association. 1980. *Diagnostic and Statistical Manual of Mental Disorders,* 3rd ed. Washington, D.C.: APA.

Arkonac, O., and Guze, S.B. 1963. A family study of hysteria. N Engl J Med 268:239–242.

Barr, R., and Abernethy, V. 1977. Single case study: Conversion reaction: Differential diagnosis in the light of biofeedback research. J Nerv Ment Dis 164:287–292.

Bibb, R.C., and Guze, S.B. 1972. Hysteria in a psychiatric hospital. Am J Psychiatry 129:224–228.

Blinder, M.G. 1966. The hysterical personality. Psychiatry 29:227–235.

Bowlus, W.E., and Currier, R.D. 1963. A test for hysterical hemianalgesia. New Eng J Med 274:1253–1254.

Briquet's syndrome or hysteria (editorial).1977. Lancet 1:1138–1139.

Campbell, R.J. 1981. *Psychiatric Dictionary.* New York: Oxford University Press.

Caplan, L.R., and Nadelson T. 1980. Multiple sclerosis and hysteria: lessons learned from their association. JAMA 243:2418–2421.

Celani, D. 1976. An interpersonal approach to hysteria. Am J Psychiatry 133:1414–1418.

Chodoff, P. 1954. A re-examination of some aspects of conversion hysteria. Psychiatry 17:75–81.

Chodoff, P. 1982. Hysteria and women. Am J. Psychiatry 139:545–551.

Chodoff, P., and Lyons, H. 1958. Hysteria, the hysterical personality and "hysterical" conversion. Am J Psychiatry 114:734–740.

Cloninger, C.R., and Guze, S.B. 1970a. Female criminals: Their personal, familial and social backgrounds. Arch Gen Psychiat 23:554–558.

Cloninger, C.R., and Guze, S.B. 1970b. Psychiatric illness and female criminality: The role of sociopathy and hysteria in the antisocial women. Am J Psychiatry 127:303–310.

Cohen, M.E., Robins, E., Purtell, J.J., Altmann, M.W., and Reid, D.E. 1953. Excessive surgery in hysteria. JAMA 151:977–986.

de Figueiredo, J.M., Baiardi, J.J., and Long, D.M. 1980. Briquet's syndrome in a man with chronic intractable pain. Johns Hopkins Med J 147:102–106.

DeVaul, R.A., and Faillace, L.A. 1980. Surgery proneness: A review and clinical assessment. Psychosomatics 32:295–299.

Easser, B.R., and Lesser, S.R. 1965. Hysterical personality: A reevaluation. Psychoanal Q 34:390–405.

Engel, G.L. 1959. "Psychogenic" pain and the pain-prone patient. Am J Med 26:899–918.

Engel, G.L. 1970. Conversion symptoms. In Sign and Symptoms: Applied Pathologic Physiology and Clinical Interpretation (5th ed.), MacBryde, C.M., and Blacklow, R.S., eds. Philadelphia, Pa.: Lippincott, pp 650–668.

Farley, J., Woodruff, R.A., and Guze, S.B. 1968. The prevalence of hysteria and conversion symptoms. Br J Psychiatry 114:1121–1125.

Flor-Henry, P., Fromm-Auch, D., Tapper, M., and Schopflocher, D. 1981. A neuropsychological study of the stable syndrome of hysteria. Biol Psychiatry 16: 601–626.

Fry, W.F. 1969. Ulcerative colitis and the communication process. Am J Orthopsychiatr 39:484–492.

Guze, S.G. 1967. The diagnosis of hysteria: What are we trying to do? Am J Psychiatry 119:960–965.

Guze, S.B., and Perley, J.H. 1963. Observations on the natural history of hysteria. Am J Psychiatry 119:960–965.

Guze, S.B., Wolfgram, E.D., McKinney, J.K., and Cantwell, D.P. 1967. Psychiatric illness in the families of convicted criminals: A study of 519 first-degree relatives. Dis Nerv Sys 28:651–659.

Guze, S.B., Woodruff, R.H., and Clayton, P.J. 1971a A study of conversion symptoms in psychiatric outpatients. Am J Psychiatry 128:643–646.

Guze, S.B., Woodruff, R.A., and Clayton, P.J. 1971b. Hysteria and antisocial behavior: Further evidence of an association. Am J Psychiatry 127:957–960.

Hafeiz, H.B. 1980. Hysterical conversion: A prognostic study. Br J Psychiatry 136: 548–551.

Halleck, S.L. 1967. Hysterical personality traits. Arch Gen Psychiatry 16:750–757.

Havens, L. 1966. Charcot and hysteria. J Nerv Ment Dis 141:505–516.

Hollender, M.H. 1971. Hysterical personality. Comment Contemp Psychiatry 1:17–24.

Hollender, M.H. 1972. Conversion hysteria: A post-Freudian reinterpretation of 19th century psychosocial data. Arch Gen Psychiatry 26:311–314.

Hollender, M.H. 1976. Hysteria: The culture-bound syndromes. Papua New Guinea Med J 19:24–29.

Hyler, S.E., and Spitzer, R.L. 1978. Hysteria split asunder. Am J Psychiatry 135:1500–1504.

Jones, M.M. 1980. Conversion reaction: Anacronism or evolutionary form: A review of the neurologic, behavioral, and psychoanalytic literature. Psychol Bull 87:427–441.

Kaminsky, M.J., and Slavney, P.R. 1976. Methodology and personality in Briquet's syndrome: A reappraisal. Am J Psychiatry 133:85–88.

Kimble, R., Williams, J.G., and Agras, S. 1975. A comparison of two methods of diagnosing hysteria. Am J Psychiatry 132:1197–1199.

Kroll, P., Chamberlain, K.R., and Halpern, J. 1979. The diagnosis of Briquet's syndrome in a male population. J Nerv Ment Dis 167:171–174.

Lazare, A. 1971. The hysterical character in psychoanalytic theory. Arch Gen Psychiatry 25:131–137.

Lewis, W.C., and Berman, M. 1965. Studies of conversion hysteria. I: Operational study of diagnosis. Arch Gen Psychiatry 13:275–282.

Lindberg, B.J., and Lindegård, B. 1963. Studies of the hysteroid personality attitude. Acta Psychiatr Scand 39:170–180.

Liskow, B.I., Clayton, P., Woodruff, R., Guze, S.B., and Cloninger, R. 1977. Briquet's syndrome, hysterical personality and the MMPI. Am J Psychiatry 134: 1137–1139.

Ludwig, A.M. 1972. Hysteria: a neurobiological theory. Arch Gen Psychiatry 27: 771–777.

Mai, G.M., and Merskey, H. 1981. Briquet's concept of hysteria: An historical perspective. Can J Psychiatry 26:57–63.

Maloney, J.H. 1980. Diagnosing hysterical conversion reactions in children. J Pediatr 97:1016–1020.

Marmor, J. 1953. Orality in the hysterical personality. J Am Psychoanal Assoc 1:656–671.

Martin, R.L., Roberts, W.V., Clayton, P.J., and Wetzel, R. 1977. Psychiatric illness and non-cancer hysterectomy. Dis Nerv Syst 38:974–980.

Menninger, K.A. 1934. Polysurgery and polysurgical addiction. Psychoanal Q 3:173–199.

Morrison, J.R. 1978. Management of Briquet's syndrome (hysteria). West J Med 128: 482–487.

Murphy, G.E. 1982. The clinical management of hysteria. JAMA 247:2559–2564.

Perley, M.J., and Guze, S.B. 1962. Hysteria—The stability and usefulness of clinical criteria. N Engl J Med 266:421–426.

Proctor, J.T. 1958. Hysteria in childhood. Am J Orthopsychiatr 28:394–405.

Purtell, J.J., Robins, E., and Cohen, M.E. 1951. Observations on clinical aspects of hysteria: A quantitative study of 50 hysteria patients and 156 control subjects. JAMA 146:902–909.

Reveley, M.A., Woodruff, R.A., Robbins, L.N., et al. 1977. Evaluation of a screening interview for Briquet's syndrome (hysteria) by the study of medically ill women. Arch Gen Psychiatry 34:145–149.

Roth, N. 1980. Torsion dystonia, conversion hysteria, and occupational cramps. Compre Psychiatry 21:292–301.

Rounsaville, B.S., Hardin, P.S., and Weissman, M.M. 1979. Briquet's syndrome in a man. J Nerv Ment Dis 167:364–367.

Shapiro, D. 1965. Neurotic Styles. New York: Basic Books.

Silverstein, A. 1976. Hysterical neurological signs. Hosp Physician 12(8):16–19.

Slater, E. 1965. Diagnosis of hysteria. Br Med J 1:1395–1399.

Stephens, J.H., and Kamp. H. 1962. On some aspects of hysteria: A clinical study. J Nerv Ment Dis 134:305–315.

Valko, R.J. 1976. Group therapy for patients with hysteria (Briquet's disorder). Dis Nerv Syst 484–487.

Veith, I. 1965. *Hysteria, A History of a Disease.* Chicago, Ill.: University of Chicago Press.

Wahl, C.W.., and Golden, J.S. 1966. The psychodynamics of the polysurgical patient: Report of sixteen patients. Psychosomatics 7:65–72.

Weinstein, E.A., Eck, R.A., and Tyerly, O.G. 1969. Conversion hysteria in Appalachia. Psychiatry 32:334–341.

Weintraub, M.I. 1977. *Hysteria: A clinical guide to diagnosis.* Clinical Symposia Volume 29(6). New Summit, N.J.: CIBA.

Woener, P.I., and Guze, S.B. 1968. A family and marital study of hysteria. Br J Psychiatry 114:161–168.

Woodruff, R.A., Clayton, P.J., and Guze, S.B. 1971. Studies of diagnosis, outcome and prevalence. JAMA 215:425–428.

Ziegler, F.J., Imboden, J.B., and Meyer, E. 1960. Contemporary conversion reactions: A clinical study. Am J Psychiatry 116:901–909.

6

HYPOCHONDRIASIS

Although perhaps not as dramatic and colorful as that of hysteria, the history of hypochondriasis is nonetheless rich in its details. Traditionally the term originates with Galen and is related to the humoral theory of disease and temperament. Hypochondria literally means "beneath the cartilage" and refers to that anatomical area below the xiphoid cartilage and lower ribs. Abdominal organs were considered to be the source of black bile, thought to cause melancholia, and yellow bile, thought to cause mania (Adams, 1844).

Late during the 17th and 18th centuries, the diagnosis of hypochondriasis was very popular in England and the syndrome became known as the "English Malady." There was a presumed organic etiology of the disorder rather than the psychological etiology the term now connotes. A trip to the spa for treatment of "the vapours" was a fashionable therapeutic activity. The 18th century Englishman viewed hypochondriasis as a disease of civilization and claimed it with some chauvanistic pride (Fischer-Homberger, 1972).

In the early 18th century Bernard de Mandeville, a Dutch physician transplanted to England, authored *A Treatise of the Hypochondriack and Hysterick Passions*, a book consisting of a dialogue between a physician and his patient, a self-confessed hypochondriac (Shoenberg, 1976). Although not intended as an exposition of therapeutic technique the dialogue proves to be quite perceptive in terms of modern-day psychodynamic concepts of hypochondriasis. The patient related to the physician that he had family problems and demonstrated the qualities of being loquacious and clinging while simultaneously doubting the physician's skill. "But you think, perhaps, I'm a mad-man to send for a physician when I know before-hand that he can do me no good. Truly, Doctor, I am not far from it. But first of all, are you in haste, pray?" (Mandeville, 1730).

With the passage of time popular concepts of hypochondriasis changed from viewing it as a physical disease to seeing it as a psychogenic disorder. The term has frequently had a pejorative quality and at times has implied that the afflicted person was a malingerer. Recent formulations, as presented in this chapter, tend to reaffirm the ideas of the ancients in regard to the close relationship between hypochondriasis and depression (melancholia).

THE DIAGNOSIS OF HYPOCHONDRIASIS

Is hypochondriasis a diagnosis? Kenyon (1976), after an extensive review of numerous patients with hypochondriacal complaints, determined that it was not a diagnosis, but rather the term should be maintained only as an adjective to describe some forms of patient behavior. However, many, perhaps most, other authors have believed that there is a specific entity of hypochondriasis, although diagnostic criteria have not been very specific. Recent authors have generally used the definition of Gillespie (1928) or modifications of it such as that of Pilowsky (1970), "Hypochondriasis is defined as a concern with health or disease in oneself which is present for the major part of the time. The preoccupation must be unjustified by the amount of organic pathology and must not respond more than temporarily to clear reassurance given after a thorough examination of the patient."

The diagnostic criteria for hypochondriasis of the Diagnostic and Statistical Manual of Mental Disorders (DSM) (American Psychiatric Association 1980) are in essential agreement with the foregoing definition but exclude the diagnosis if there is any other mental disorder present (see Table 1).

The suggestion of Pilowsky that hypochondriasis be divided into two major categories, primary and secondary, has proven to be a therapeutically useful concept. The primary (or "true") form of the illness would meet the DSM III diagnostic criteria. Most importantly for a diagnosis of primary hypochondriasis there must not be any evidence of another underlying psychiatric disturbance to explain the hypochondriacal preoccupations of the patient. The secondary form of the illness exists when the hypochondriasis is a symptom (or a defense) of another underlying psychiatric disorder or when it is symptomatic of a transient adjustment reaction. The secondary form has been further subdivided into clinically useful categories by Idzorek (1975).

The various categories of primary (the "crock") and secondary hypochondriasis will be discussed in detail following descriptions of various different features of hypochondriasis in general.

TABLE I. DSM III Diagnostic Criteria for Hypochondriasis

A. The predominant disturbance is an unrealistic interpretation of physical signs or sensations as abnormal, leading to preoccupation with the fear or belief of having a serious disease.

B. Thorough physical evaluation does not support the diagnosis of any physical disorder that can account for the physical signs or sensations or for the individual's unrealistic interpretation of them.

C. The unrealistic fear or belief of having a disease persists despite medical reassurance and causes impairment in social or occupational functioning.

D. Not due to any other mental disorder such as Schizophrenia, Affective Disorder, or Somatization Disorder.

American Psychiatric Association, *Diagnostic and Statistical Manual of Mental Disorders,* Third Edition, p 251, Washington, D.C., APA 1980. Reprinted by permission.

THE PHENOMENOLOGY OF HYPOCHONDRIASIS

Prevalence, Sex, Age, and Social Status Distribution

The incidence of hypochondriasis has been reviewed by Kenyon (1965) and found in different investigations to vary from 3 to 14%. A study of the services provided by the outpatient department of a large health maintenance organization indicates that 11% of all patient visits were made by the "worried well," presumably hypochondriacal in nature (Garfield, 1976). However, the "worried well" constituted 29% of all patients who presented with symptoms (Garfield et al., 1976). If it is conservatively estimated that 3–10% of the visits to a physician are for hypochondriacal complaints then the condition is indeed common.

Distribution between the sexes has been reported as fairly equal by Kenyon (1964), while Pilowsky (1970) found a slight excess of men, and Altman (1975) describes the disorder as occurring primarily in postmenopausal women.

In one study the peak age group for males was found to be 30–39 years and for females to be 40–49 (Kenyon, 1964), while another report indicated a peak for both sexes in the 40s with females being slightly older (Pilowsky, 1970).

There does not appear to be a predominance of any one social class (Kenyon, 1964; Kreitman et al., 1965; Pilowsky, 1970). However, Busse (1976) believes hypochondriasis is more common in lower socioeconomic status elderly patients as a result of increased social stress.

The Nature of Presenting Complaints

Despite the anatomic description of the disorder, hypochondriacal patients complain most frequently of symptoms referrable to the musculoskeletal system (particularly the head and neck) (Kenyon, 1964; Pilowsky, 1970). Symptoms of the gastrointestinal system and the central nervous system are also frequently reported. Less frequently reported are symptoms referrable to otolaryngeal, genitourinary and cardiovascular systems. Pilowsky (1970) stated that complaints involving the skin, hair or appearance were relatively uncommon but when present showed a significant association with primary hypochondriasis.

Personality Types and Family Background

The most frequently found personality types of patients with hypochondriasis, according to Kenyon (1964) are "normal," anxious, and obsessional. Pilowsky (1970) has also reported that obessional and anxiety-prone personalities were common in the hypochondriacal patients whom he studied.

Different patterns of family histories have been reported. Pilowsky found a relationship between primary hypochondriasis in males and a family history of a hypochondriacal father, while Kreitman et al. (1965) found a greater similarity between the symptoms of the patient and that of the patient's mother.

PRIMARY HYPOCHONDRIASIS: THE "CROCK"

Clinical Features

The "crock" is a clinical phenomenon known to a physicians. There are a number of aliases, including "chronic complainers," "gourds," "turkeys," and "thick-chart patients," none particularly endearing. In fact it has been noted that it is particularly that very quality—dislike—which defines the crock. Cohen (1966) has noted that a crock is not a crock until a certain type of relationship has been established—namely, the patient fails to stimulate the physician's interest. "... The doctor should make up his mind to find at least one interesting thing about the patient, for the diagnosis is not made until the doctor has failed."

Treatment of the crock has been called "psychoceramic medicine," and an important diagnostic study has been the fanciful "serum porcelain." The patient's medical history has been called an "organ recital."

What makes the crock such a source of derision and why is so much anger engendered? The answers to these questions to a large extent explain the syndrome, for the patients have a capacity to tap into the physician's own conflicts about dependency and anger. Most simply stated, these patients are clinging, demanding at times, smothering, while at the same time ungrateful, angry, and complaining. They establish "hostile-dependent" relationships presenting their complaints with the resigned attitude of one who does not really expect much help (see quote from Mandeville above). They are frequently shuffled from doctor to doctor or clinic to clinic. Typically they are "unattractive middle-aged and old people. Young attractive individuals are not called crocks" (Cohen, 1966).

The complaints of the crock are offered to the physician in obsessive detail with little affect. It is not unusual for the patient to repetitively address the physician merely as "doctor" as if all doctors were interchangeable and the name of no consequence. However, despite the obsessive detail of the history and the frequent visits to the clinic or medical office which produce a thick chart, it is often remarkable how little history of a personal nature is communicated to the physician or ends up in the chart. This may result as much from the physician's efforts to stifle the patient's complaints as it is due to the patient's disinclination to talk about personal history (Lipsitt, 1970).

Typically the symptoms of these patients have extended over many years. Genuine organic disease may be admixed into the complex clinical presentation and complicate the diagnostic process. The patient's life may well have revolved around illness for a prolonged period of time. If the patient is socially isolated, then the relationship with physician, office nurses, and/or clinic personnel may be the most meaningful contacts with other people that the patient has. In a clinic setting it is common to see the patient arrive early and then stay around the clinic following their appointment time to talk with other patients or the receptionist.

Altman (1975) has described two types of patients with (primary) hypochondriasis. The first is consistent with the preceding discussion; and the second, regarded as less common, is characterized by a clinging, demanding patient who accepts authority and desires a passive childlike relationship with authority figures.

Primary Hypochondriasis: An Illustrative Case History

A 31-year-old thrice-married father of three children was admitted with complaints of weight loss, abdominal pain, complaints referrable to sinusitis, and atypical chest pain. The medical history indicated 10 prior hospitalizations over a 7-year period for diagnostic workups and treatment for sinusitis, peptic ulcer disease, and minor trauma. The medical records suggested complaints and concern by the patient in excess of the objective findings.

During his most recent hospitalization the patient received an extensive workup which revealed only minor abnormalities, insufficient to explain disabling symptoms. Despite reassurance, he remained convinced that he had serious ulcer disease and upon discharge conveyed the impression that he would continue to seek medical opinions until someone recommended gastric surgery.

The patient's past history was remarkable: He was the older of two sons born to a poor rural southern family. His younger brother had chronic respiratory problems, and the family's limited financial resources were diverted toward the care of this sickly sibling. The patient recalled that as a teenager he would be working in the tobacco fields of the family farm while his brother sat in an air-conditioned room watching television.

The patient worked his way through college and taught school for a while before starting his own small business. He was married twice prior to his present marriage, which he regarded as very satisfactory. His wife, a schoolteacher, has a regular income and is a steady, "logical" person whom he trusts completely. His dependency upon her was apparent to all of his health care team. Information obtained from the wife indicated that she was not nearly as satisfied with the marriage, and the patient's demands upon her drained her energy. The patient's illnesses and hospitalizations were, in retrospective analysis, always temporally related to stressful situations, particularly associated with problems in his business.

The patient related his history in a pleasant but obsessive manner, giving detailed medical explanations, using precise medical terminology. There was no evidence of clinical depression or psychosis, although there was an undercurrent of depressive themes.

A psychological test battery confirmed many of the clinical observations. The patient's full scale IQ was 109. Those MMPI scales elevated 2 standard deviations above normal were scale 9 (mania) and scale 1 (hypochondriasis). Projective testing suggested a tense person who had been frustrated in the attainment of high goals, and a great need to be productive was interpreted as a counterphobic denial of strong dependency needs. There were an excessive number of anatomic responses on the Rorschach test, which was completed in an obsessive, rather than hysterical, style.

During the period of hospitalization, both the patient and his wife paid lip service to the need for counseling to help in managing stressful situations. However, neither demonstrated any genuine motivation, and upon discharge they did not follow through with recommendations along this line. The patient expressed displeasure that no physical disorder was found and angrily insisted that he would seek further medical consultation.

The Management of Primary Hypochondriasis

There have been a number of suggestions offered by various authors in regard to management techniques to assist in the care of the hypochondriacal patient (Adler, 1981; Altman, 1975; Bender, 1964a, 1964b; Bittker, 1979; Brown and Vaillant, 1981; Idzorek, 1977; Ladee, 1966; Lipsitt, 1968; McCranie, 1979; Turnbull, 1974; Wahl, 1964; Walker, 1978; Webb, 1979). The following management techniques represent a synthesis of the recommendations of many of these clinicians.

First and foremost in establishing a relationship with the hypochrondriac is obtaining a complete history, personal as well as medical. The time and effort to obtain such a history may require multiple visits. Similarly an adequate physical examination and laboratory tests must be performed in order to rule out the possibility of underlying disease. This should be accomplished in a manner that will not reinforce the somatizing behavior. But, as noted by Ladee (1966), it is often a difficult task to avoid such reinforcement. "However, one acts, it is always a practically unavoidable danger that another use of words, or a different attitude, a somewhat altered method of examinations or prescription provides the hypochondriac with fresh food for his worry, doubt and mistrust . . . the hypochondriacal arsenal is richly filled by imaginary or real medical divergencies." Minor abnormalities must not be seized upon in order to explain away the patient's multiple complaints. As with the patient with Briquet's syndrome, invasive diagnostic–therapeutic procedures should be undertaken on the basis of objective evidence rather than on the basis of subjective complaints. All potentially dangerous diagnostic–therapeutic interventions must be judiciously evaluated. The patient who formerly had no disease can, by the physician's actions, develop genuine and incapacitating symptoms and disease.

The differentiation of primary from secondary hypochondriacal syndrome is very important because some of the technqiues utilized with the first group may actually reinforce somatizing behavior in the latter. In some types of secondary hypochondriasis (masked depression), the use of potent antidepressant medications is an important part of the treatment program. The use of any nonessential medications is contraindicated in primary hypochondriasis because the prescribing of medications reinforces somatic preoccupation.

The goal of treatment of the patient with primary hypochondriasis must be *care* rather than cure (Lipsitt, 1968). There must be no expectation by the physician nor promise to the patient that the symptoms will be completely removed. Instead, comments such as "It is remarkable how you are able to persevere with such pain" may well fit into the patient's masochistic view of himself/herself (Lipsitt, 1970). The offer of the physician to the patient should therefore be that the physician will attempt to help the patient, but symptoms are likely to continue, at least to some degree.

There must be attention to the physical complaints of the patient accompanied by warm acceptance of the patient as an individual. When the patient's complaints and symptoms are met with annoyance or the implication that the physician's time is too valuable to waste, then these attitudes reinforce and feed the pervasive anger that the patients experience toward physicians. On the other hand, it is necessary to convey to the patient that the relationship is not dependent upon the medical complaints, but rather the interest goes beyond the physical symptoms.

Any implication that the symptoms of which the patient complains are imaginary or "in the head" must be avoided. Such a confrontation will only create an adversary position and impede efforts to establish a therapeutic alliance. It is equally important that the physician does not use a fictitious (or irrelevant) diagnosis in order to humor the patient; the net result of such an action is to reinforce the somatizing behavior. Instead the physician can honestly make comments to both the patient and his/her family to the effect that the distress and discomfort is acknowledged. It can also be communicated that efforts are being directed toward eliciting the source of the distress and helping the patient feel more comfortable.

A major therapeutic technique with hypochondriacal patients is to allow patients to express their somatic complaints and to respond with increased interest and verbally or nonverbally reward the patients' willingness to talk about personal issues, particularly when such issues may involve the expression of feelings or longings. Over a period of time the patient may come to recognize that the relationship does not have to depend upon physical complaints. Along with this recognition there may be change in the patient's lexicon, words expressing emotion replacing those describing somatic sensations.

The physician, in accordance with the above principles, must accept that treatment of the hypochondriac is a lengthy undertaking. There is a necessity for regularly scheduled appointments irrespective of the presence of severity of complaints. The statement "Call me the next time you have a problem" is an open invitation for the patient to develop a new symptom in order to have a "ticket" to an office visit. Rather, each office consultation should end with the patient being given another appointment. The frequency of such appointments may vary. Early in the doctor–patient relationship, they may need to be quite frequent. Later, as the patient develops more trust and a sense that needs will be met, the frequency of visits can be reduced. Frequent telephone calls or an increasing urgency to the complaints are indications that the office visits are being scheduled too infrequently.

Group Therapy

Group psychotherapy is a treatment modality which has been recommended for hypochondriacal patients, and indeed from a theoretical viewpoint this form of treatment has many positive attributes. If one accepts as a basic tenet of hypochondriasis that the somatization represents an attempt by the patient to establish a relationship (albeit a neurotic one) with other persons (or the physician as a surrogate parent), then any treatment program must take that need into account. Group therapy does just that and in addition helps the patients, through relationships with fellow group members, expand their social networks. A group also provides the opportunity for the verbal expression of the angry feelings that the patient experiences and verbal expression of the desire for, and partial gratification of, dependency longings. Non-physicians such as nurse practitioners and psychiatric social workers have been proven to be effective therapists in this type of treatment for somatizing patients and have the potential of providing excellent and cost-effective care for these difficult patients (Ford and Long, 1977; Friedman et al., 1979; Roskin et al., 1980; Schoenberg and Senescu, 1966).

There are difficulties, of course, in developing group therapy programs for the somatizing patient. One of the most important is that of patient acceptability. Most patients will angrily reject any suggestion that their problems are psychiatric and that they should be referred for psychiatric treatment. There are two tactics which may to some extent cut through this resistance. The first is in the naming of the group. It can be called something to the effect of "Ways of Coping with Physical Distress" and educational and social support issues stressed as goals of the group rather than issues dealing with psychological insights. The second tactic is that the group should be scheduled to meet some place within the designated medical-surgical clinic area rather than in the psychiatric clinic. If at all possible, the primary care physician(s) should attend the meetings, at least on occasion, to demonstrate a continuing interest in and confidence of this form of treatment (Friedman et al., 1979). In regard to the basic technique of conducting the therapy sessions, the therapist must be willing to allow or even encourage considerable catharsis; complaints about the medical care system in general and physicians in particular are common. Other complaints concerning family, spouses, etc., will also be prevalent. At least initially the meetings often have the quality of "gripe sessions." Despite these complaints, the patients typically have difficulty in verbally expressing their feelings and can best be described as alexithymic (see below). The therapist, cautiously and gently, over a period of time, should help interpret to these alexithymic patients the emotional feelings they have difficulty in recognizing (Ford and Long, 1977). The therapist must be actively involved with group members, patient in terms of expectation of change, and cautious in what confrontations and interpretations are made. At least initially there is little place for complex psychodynamic interpretations for they may prove, in terms of the resistances they elicit, to be counterproductive.

Treatment results for groups of somatizing patients have been positive; not only do the patients achieve greater psychological comfort, but a reduction in the number of clinic visits for medical complaints has been reported (Friedman et al., 1979; Roskin et al., 1980; Schoenberg and Senescu, 1966).

From a pragmatic aspect, a group of somatizing patients is more easily established in the clinics of a teaching hospital or a health maintenance organization. However, the primary care physician who sees a number of these patients in his/her private practice is encouraged to make efforts to try this cost-efficient method of providing medical care. It offers an intellectually challenging break from the usual office routine. The physician can utilize a social worker or nurse practitioner as the primary therapist and need not attend the complete session.

SECONDARY HYPOCHONDRIASIS
Transient Hypochondriasis

Hypochondriasis may be the signal that one is experiencing external stress or an internal conflict (Idzorek, 1975; Turnbull, 1974). The symptoms may spontaneously remit if circumstances allow, or they may respond to brief psychotherapeutic intervention. Unfortunately "transient" syndromes can become long-standing or even lifelong problems if there is sufficient reinforcement. Such inadvertent reinforcement may come from persons in the patient's social system or from the patient's physician. Failure to recognize the underlying stress and misinterpretation of the patient's use of somatic, rather than verbal, communication can lead to multiple diagnostic–therapeutic procedures. The resultant implied message is that the patient is sick. Thus the patient's fears become confirmed, sick role behavior is reinforced and a new maladaptive method of coping is elaborated. Two brief clinical examples will illustrate this sequence of events.

An 18-year-old college freshman away from home for the first time and experiencing adjustment difficulties to both the social and scholastic demands of college presented himself to the university student health center with vague complaints of fatigue and headaches. The well-meaning student health physician failed to obtain a psychosocial history and immediately launched into an extensive diagnostic workup. In addition the physician wrote a series of notes to instructors requesting special consideration for the student because of illness. Despite the fact that all diagnostic tests proved to be within normal limits the student became a frequent visitor to the student health service at times of stress throughout his college career.

A 48-year-old businessman was admitted to the hospital with a well-documented myocardial infarction. Initially his convalescence was unremarkable but on return home he became concerned about both his sexual capabilities and his deteriorating relationship with his younger wife. Preoccupied with the fear that every bodily symptom was the omen of further cardiac disease he sought repetitive consultations from his physician. Failing to recognize the underlying conflicts the physician responded with symptomatic treatment to each new physical complaint, thereby markedly extending the period of rehabilitation.

Transient physical symptoms accompanying stressful life events are common, e.g., a student's nausea and vomiting before an important exam. It is necessary that physicians, while not ignoring the possibility of significant organic disease, be cognizant of underlying emotional events and the potent influence that the physician may have upon the future course of the patient's illness behavior.

Depression ("Masked Depression")

Patients with depression, often of a severe degree, frequently present themselves to physicians with physical complaints instead of complaining of a mood disturbance.

During the past two decades, there has been an increasing recognition of the strong relationship between hypochondriasis and depression (Dorfman, 1968; Jacobs et al., 1968; Katon et al., 1982a, 1982b; Kenyon, 1964; Kreitman et al., 1965). The comprehensive review by Katon and colleagues documented the association of depression and hypochondriasis and noted the high frequency of situations where physicians missed the diagnosis of depression in hypocondriacal patients.

According to Katon et al. the major factors that contribute to somatization, instead of complaints of a mood disorder, are sociocultural and childhood experiences. Children do not distinguish between emotional and physical distress. It is the reactions of the child's caretakers, which by evaluating, explaining, and labeling, teach the child to identify different mood states and to distinguish between psychological and somatic symptoms. Thus in some cultures (or families, which are in themselves subcultures) emotional experiences may be disvalued and persons learn to differentially attend to the somatic components of affective experience rather than the perception of psychological distress. A patient with a nonpsychological orientation is more likely to perceive and complain of symptoms such as sleep disturbance, appetite disturbance, and gastrointestinal distress than to complain of a depressed mood.

The somatizing person's family or social network may not be receptive to the use of emotional symptoms as an entry to the sick role, yet will accept somatic illness without question. Similarly, third-party payers frequently reimburse for somatic illness without any questions but may deny benefits for any disorder labeled as "psychiatric."

Patients who are more likely to somatize their depressions include those who are of rural backgrounds, who have less education, or who are from a non-Western culture (Katon et al., 1982a).

Alexithymia is another feature which is often correlated with persons who somatize (Ford and Long, 1977; Lesser et al., 1979). This term was initiated by Sifneos (1972) and means "without words for mood." The concept of alexithymia has been reviewed by Lesser (1981) and is similar to conditions described previously such as "emotional illiteracy" (Mally and Ogston, 1964). Patients with alexithymia do not use words to communicate their emotional feelings, are not psychologically introspective, do not have active fantasy lives, and, interestingly, do not tend to remember their dreams. Instead, these people use what has been called "operational thinking," a mechanical type of thought process preoccupied with details rather than with subjective experiences. It is easy to see that an alexithymic person who has vegetative symptoms of depression (e.g., constipation and anorexia) would focus upon details of the physiologic changes rather than verbally communicate emotional feelings. Consistent with the observations by Katon et al. (1982a), that persons who somatize their depression are often of lower socioeconomic status, is the finding that alexithymia is more prevalent in the lower socioeconomic classes (Lesser et al., 1979).

The following case history illustrates how someone with depression may enter the health care system under the guise of physical illness because of hypochondriacal behavior.

A 64-year-old Caucasian male presented to his physician with symptoms of a "sick feeling," gastrointestinal distress with nausea, an 18-pound weight loss, and a vague sense of nervousness. A complete gastrointestinal workup was within normal limits except for diverticulosis of the colon. The patient repetitively returned to his physician and received symptomatic therapy for a period of several months. There was no change in his complaints. After an episode of bright red rectal bleeding, the patient was referred to a university hospital for further evaluation.

On hospitalization, the only positive physical findings were EKG evidence of an old myocardial infarction and an anal fissure on proctoscopic examination, presumably secondary to the patient's severe constipation. Psychiatric consultation was obtained. Further symptoms elicited included sleep disturbance, decreased interest in the patient's usual activities of hunting and fishing, and a complaint of a decreased ability to concentrate. Intelligence was judged to be average. Depression was denied, and the patient seemed somewhat confused by repetitive requests to describe his feelings. He was pleasant and cooperative, answered questions in detail, but never used affective words except to complain of having some problems with his "nerves."

Personal history indicated that the patient was raised in the rural south, had worked for a while in a northern factory but retired to the area in which he has been raised. His retirement life had centered around his favorite activities of fishing and hunting. With the exception of the recent death of a close friend, the patient's life had seemed unremarkable in both distant past and recent past events.

A presumptive diagnosis of unipolar depression was made and the patient was started on antidepressant medications. Several weeks later, the patient's mood had obviously brightened and his vegetative symptoms had remitted. When questioned, he stated that "I must have been depressed if you say so, doctor," but he continued to have no psychological awareness of his experience with depression.

This man represents a patient whose limited psychological sophistication led him to interpret the symptoms of his endogenous depression wholly within a somatic framework. He clearly demonstrated the features of alexithymia. He cooperated with his physicians in an antidepressant treatment regimen and depressive symptoms remitted without the patient ever obtaining a psychological interpretation of what had occurred to him.

Lesse (1967, 1968, 1977, 1980) has been a leading advocate of the concept of "masked depression." He has described a large number of patients with various symptomatic presentations whose depression had been masked by the patients' preoccupation with physical symptoms. The hypochondriacal behavior had often been present for many years before the diagnosis of depression was established.

According to Lesse, patients with masked depressions are more frequently women than men, and the age distribution is clearly concentrated in middle age with a peak in the 40s. These patients are much more frequently encountered by the medical-surgical physician than by psychiatrists because the patients have little or no understanding of, nor apparently even words for, their emotional states. They relate their symptoms with great circumstantiality, emphasizing how disabled they are as a result of these physical complaints. Not uncommonly among their mutliple complaints are statements that memory is also poor. Of note is the fact that these patients with masked depression are often even more socially disabled than patients with well-defined severe organic illness. A complicating factor is that these depressed patients may in fact have a mild organic ailment which served as a focus of attention to the patient and the physician. This attention may have contributed to an iatrogenic reinforcement of the symptoms.

Once a masked depression is suspected, and a high index of suspicion is required with these difficult patients, the physician must not be too quick to confront the patient. Rather, it is necessary to gain the patient's confidence by allowing the recitation of the complex medical history. The diagnosis can be confirmed by the elicitation of symptoms such as insomnia, anorexia, persistent fatigue which is more marked in the morning, agitation with floor pacing, hand wringing, bruxism, sexual difficulties, and other symptoms consistent with anxiety and/or depression. As confidence in the physician is increased she (he) is then likely to talk of feelings of hopelessness, often to the extent of suicidal ideation, crying spells, and of suffering. The mood disturbance is usally described by euphemisms such as "feeling blue."

The patient with masked depression is typically an intelligent and capable person with personality traits that include perfectionism and a need to aggressively dominate the environment. The latter can be interpreted as an attempt to compensate for lifelong feelings of inadequacy and self-degradation. Family histories also indicate that, as a rule, one or both parents, most typically the mother, was a dominant person and not uncommonly had one or more medical problems. The patient frequently finds himself/herself in long-standing conflict with the dominant parent and feeling both anger and guilt about the relationship.

Multiple office visits may be required before the physician and, then secondarily, the patient are convinced that the basic problem is one of depression. At that time a treatment program needs to be instituted. These patients can rarely be induced to enter into intensive psychotherapy (Dorfman, 1968) and because of their nonintrospective and alexithymic characteristics (see above), such therapy may not be indicated. Patients with masked depression do tend to respond to a supportive relationship combined with antidepressant medications. The prognosis for a favorable response is related to the duration of the symptom complex prior to the initiation of therapy. The longer the symptoms have been present, the more refractory the depression is to treatment. Monoamine oxidase inhibitors have been reported to achieve excellent results with these patients (Lesse, 1977).

Another form of affective disorder which frequently presents with hypochondriacal symptoms is "psychotic depression," probably a more extreme symptomatic expression of either unipolar or bipolar depression. The patient with a depression of a psychotic magnitude typically has delusions dealing with the body and in addition may have delusions of guilt. Somatic delusions include statements such as "I'm rotting inside," "My brain is shriveling and dissolving." The patient with psychotic depression is very difficult to manage and represents a significant suicide risk. These are patients that the primary care physician will want to refer for psychiatric treatment. Aggressive treatment interventions such as pharmacotherapy or electroconvulsive therapy (ECT) can best be undertaken on an inpatient psychiatric unit where the patients can also be protected from their destructive impulses.

HYPOCHONDRIASIS IN OLD AGE

Hypochondriasis is frequently observed as part of the symptoms of illness in the elderly. Previous tendencies toward hypochondriacal preoccupation may intensify with age or hypochondriasis may appear for the first time in old age (Busse and Reckless, 1961).

That hypochondriacal concerns are common in old age is not unexpected. Essentially all diseases become more frequent with increasing age. As a consequence one might anticipate a person would become more concerned with bodily function as a way of scanning for the possibility of underlying desease and/or the changes of age. However, all elderly patients are not hypochondriacal and in one well-designed study elderly patients did not, on the average, complain of more physical symptoms than younger patients (Denney et al.1965). Hypochondriacal behavior should not, therefore, be considered a normal aspect of aging but rather a symptom of another underlying problem, usually depression or some other form of a poor psychological adjustment (Costa and McCrae,1980; Gianturco and Busse, 1978).

Hypochondriasis when it occurs in old age, as with younger patients, has many facets. It can be utilized as a way of obtaining the sick role, as a way of avoiding certain social responsibilities and as a way of explaining failures (Busse,1976). In addition to serving as a safeguard to self-esteem hypochondriasis can also be used as an interpersonal tactic to get attention and sympathy from others and as a means of manipulation (Brink et al. 1979,1981). Goldstein and Birnbom (1976) have noted that hypochondriasis may serve as a distress signal and as a way of asking for reassurance and support. Elderly patients often have difficulty in conveying their feelings directly and honestly to their "significant others," and somatic complaints of a hypochondriacal nature may be a way of expressing anger and provoking guilt in family members.

It has been noted that hypochondriasis in the elderly may represent a transient adjustment reaction in response to an external stress such as a change in residence or unfamiliar social situation (Busse, 1976; Goldstein and Birnbom, 1976). Patients who are hypochondriacal often perceive themselves as passive recipients of outside events beyond their control (Brink et al. 1981). Relatively brief psychotherapeutic intervention consisting of short but frequent supportive visits to a physician have been shown to be effective in helping elderly patients master the acute stressful event and allow them to discard the hypochondriacal symptoms (Goldstein and Birnbom, 1976). Family therapy has also been described as a very effective therapeutic intervention in altering hypochondriacal symptoms which accompany depression in old age (Goldstein and Birnbom, 1976).

In conclusion, hypochondriasis in old age may be a continuation of lifelong patterns, accompany depression, or represent an acute adjustment reaction. For the last two items the prognosis for a good response to well-timed treatment is excellent. The primary care physician is in a position to quickly identify, and respond to, the needs of elderly patients.

MONOSYMPTOMATIC HYPOCHONDRIASIS

In a recent review article Bishop (1980a), consistent with the European psychiatric literature, included three previously described syndromes into a general classification, monosymptomatic hypochondriasis. These three syndromes are dysmorphophobia, delusions of bromosis, and delusions of parasitosis. These disorders share the common feature that each may be the symptomatic expression of another underlying psychiatric illness and for that reason they may be also considered to represent forms of "secondary hypochondriasis." For ease of organization each of these syndromes will be discussed separately and followed by a discussion of treatment techniques.

Dysmorphophobia

Patients with dysmorphophobia believe that their bodies are deformed in some manner and repetitively seek medical attention in order to remedy the situation. Because the complaint is usually one of believing oneself to be ugly (e.g., an unattractive nose) it is the plastic surgeon to whom the complaints are most usually made and from whom remedial treatment is desired. One study indicates that approximately 2% of the patients who come to a plastic surgeon requesting plastic surgery have dysmorphophobia (Connolly and Gipson, 1978).

The term dysmorphophobia was originally coined by Morselli in 1886, but as has been correctly noted by Bishop the term is inappropriate in that there are no phobic symptoms but rather an obsession with the appearance of the body. Frequently the patient's complaints about appearance are not discernible to others, or if there is a defect if is usually of an inconsequential magnitude. The most common complaints are those directed toward the face (particularly the nose), hair, breasts, and genitalia (Hay, 1970). Patients cling tenaciously to their complaints and cannot be dissuaded that they are not deformed in some manner.

Data as to demographic information concerning patients with dysmorphophobia are limited, but these patients are typically in their late teens or 20s (Hay, 1970) and are frequently unmarried (Andreasen and Bardach, 1977). No consistent sexual distribution has been demonstrated.

Underlying psychiatric illness of a moderate to severe degree is frequently reported in patients with dysmorphophobia. Psychiatric study of a series of 17 patients yielded the following distribution of psychiatric diagnoses: 11 severe personality disorders, 5 schizophrenics, and 1 depressive illness (Hay, 1970). Andreasen and Bardach (1977) described patients with dysmorphophobia whom they had seen as usually being young and having personality traits of perfectionism and narcissism and a tendency toward being schizoid. Zaidens (1950) has regarded the diagnosis underlying the complaints of dysmorphophobia to be that of "pseudoneurotic schizophrenia."

One way of assessing the extent of the underlying pathology in dysmorphophobia is to follow and reevaluate those patients who have received cosmetic rhinoplasty (Connolly and Gipson, 1978). In one study a series of 86 patients who received cosmetic rhinoplasty were compared to a group of 101 patients who received rhinoplasty for disease or injury. This study, which was conducted an average of 15 years after surgery, indicated that of the 86 patients who had received cosmetic rhinoplasty, 32 were found to be severely neurotic and 6 were schizophrenic at the time of follow-up. Of the control group, only 9 were found to be severely neurotic and 1 schizophrenic at follow-up. These differences might have been even greater if those patients with obvious psychopathology who were seeking cosmetic surgery had not been denied, on initial contact, the operation they had desired and therefore were not included in the study.

Delusions of Bromosis

Some patients may seek repetitive medical consultation with the complaint that they emit an offensive odor. These patients may engage in rituals which include frequent bathing, change of clothes, and use of perfumed substances or deodorants (Bishop, 1980b). A case reported by Bishop (1980a) suggested that a patient can fix upon a mild variation of body odor and can become obsessed with it to a delusional degree.

Patients with delusions of bromosis are usually male, unmarried, and comparatively young (20s). Underlying psychiatric disorders may include depression, schizophrenia, and temporal lobe epilepsy (Pryse-Phillips, 1971).

Delusions of Parasitosis

The belief that one is infested with worms, skin vermin, and other forms of parasites has been reported numerous times in the literature (Hopkinson, 1973; Munro, 1978c; Schrut, 1963; Wilson and Miller, 1976). Physicians who specialize in parasitology indicate that they receive a number of consultations from these persons who will not accept reassurance that they are not infested. These patients almost invariably reject psychiatric referral and instead make repetitive visits to their physicians carrying with them bits of fiber, skin, and other particulate matter which they present as evidence of their infestation.

The typical patient with delusions of parasitosis is a middle-aged married woman. The underlying psychiatric disturbances which have been described include such varied entities as affective disorders, schizophrenia, tactile hallucinosis caused by toxins or drugs, folie a deux, and organic brain syndromes (Hopkinson, 1973; Wilson and Miller, 1946).

Treatment of the Monosymptomatic Hypochondriasis

Treatment of the monosymptomatic hypochondriacal syndromes is very difficult. The primary problem is the extreme resistance of these patients to accept any consideration that there may be a psychiatric component to their illnesses. They not only refuse any efforts to refer them to psychiatrists, but they are also reluctant to take any prescribed medications they consider to be psychotropic. However, even if patients were more accepting of a referral to a psychiatrist, problems with treatment would remain. A major consideration is that of diagnosis; even within the subgroups such as dysmorphophobia a wide range of underlying diagnostic impressions have been described. Some patients with monosymptomatic hypochondriasis may have a variant of true paranoia (Hopkinson, 1973; Wilson and Miller, 1946), a disorder which is almost totally refractory to treatment. Even when depression appears to be the underlying disorder there may be difficulty in effecting a good response.

Somewhat more promising than the above information are the reports that a new antipsychotic agent being used in Europe and Canada is very effective in the treatment of monosymptomatic hypochondriasis. Pimozide, not yet released in the United States, is a diphenylbutylpiperidine, a drug closely related to the butyrophenones. Pimozide is reported to achieve remarkable symptomatic relief, but the effect is suppressive rather than curative (Munro, 1978a, 1978b, 1978c). Although the early reports are promising, increased clinical experience is required to determine how effective (and with which subgroups of monosymptomatic hypochondriasis) pimozide proves to be.

HYPOCHONDRIASIS AND BRIQUET'S SYNDROME

There are many similarities between Briquet's syndrome (hysteria) and hypochondriasis. Because Briquet's syndrome is a diagnosis made solely on symptoms, not on interactional behavior with the physician or psychodynamic constellations, there is the possibility of diagnostic overlap. There are several possibilities to consider as to the relationship between "hysteria" and hypochondriasis. The first of these is that there essentially is no difference and that it is the physician's attitude which determines whether a patient will be called a hysteric or a crock. A young, attractive, interpersonally engaging woman may be labeled a hysteric while an old, unattractive, complaining woman may be called a crock. According to this hypothesis, age then becomes the important diagnostic issue: young hysterics become old crocks.

The sex of the patient may be regarded as the important differential between hysteria and hypochondriasis. Syndenham in the 17th century regarded hysteria as a disease of women and hypochondriasis a disease of men (Fisher-Homberger, 1972). Briquet took strong exception to this view and stated that nothing could be more the antithesis of hysteria than hypochondriasis, the latter being a condition where the sensations are imaginary and where there are constant fears of sickness, the future, and death (Mai and Merskey, 1981).

An important difference between hysterics and hypochondriases may be that of cognitive style. I have been impressed by the obsessive features and attention to detail that characterize the hypochondriac. In fact, it is not unusual to find a hypochondriac who maintains elaborate notebooks filled with the medical information and diagnoses that he/she has been given. This obsessive quality, tinged with depression, is compatible with Briquet's clinical description of hypochondriasis stated above. In contrast, the typical patient with Briquet's syndrome is a poor and inaccurate historian. The hysterical cognitive style relies on emotion and intuition; facts may be changed to suit the audience and dates are often forgotten. The medical history of the hysteric is dramatized. The abdominal pain which resulted in the removal of a normal appendix is retold as a "ruptured appendix" with surgery saving her from death "in the nick of time."

A third explanation of the difference between hypochondriasis and Briquet's syndrome is that the determination of the diagnosis rests upon the clustering of certain symptoms or characteristics that transcend all somatizing behavior. Thus somatizing behavior would be seen as a single entity with a wide range of symptomatic expression. The diagnosis of hypochondriasis would depend upon the clustering of several specific features. Similarly the diagnosis of Briquet's syndrome would be dependent upon the clustering of several factors.

SUMMARY

The term hypochondriasis is a description encompassing a wide variety of patient behavior. Hypochondriacal behavior may be the overt manifestation of depression, psychosis, transient stress situations (types of secondary hypochondriasis), or what essentially constitutes a personality disorder (primary hypochondriasis or the "crock").

Although it is very important to differentiate among the specific diagnoses underlying hypochondriacal behavior, it frequently requires several office visits before sufficient information has been collected in order to make an accurate diagnosis. When depression is the underlying diagnosis, the prognosis of response to antidepressant medication is fair to excellent, dependent upon the length of time the symptoms have been present. The prognosis of response to antipsychotic medication, when psychosis is the underlying diagnosis, is less favorable. However, there is promise that a new butyrophenone (Pimozide), not yet released in the United States, may be much more effective in the treatment of these refractory patients. The transient hypochondriacal states are best managed by quickly elucidating the underlying stress and redirecting the patient toward other techniques of solving life crises.

The patient with primary hypochondriasis represents a challenge; these patients reject help at the same time that they are demanding it. However, the physician needs to understand that the behavior is not personalized but instead represents the patient's reenactment of old conflicts. With this understanding a variety of management techniques, including the possibility of group therapy, can make the treatment of these patients very gratifying.

REFERENCES

Adams, F. 1844. *The Seven Books of Paulus Aegineta*, vol. 1. London: Sydenham Society.

Adler, G. 1981. The physician and the hypochondriacal patient. N Engl J Med 304:1394–1396.

Altman, N. 1975. Hypochondriasis. In *Psychological Care of the Medically Ill*. Strain, J.J., and Grossmann, S., eds. New York: Appleton-Century-Crofts.

American Psychiatric Association. 1980. *Diagnostic and Statistical Manual of Mental Disorders*. Washington, D.C.: APA, p. 251.

Andreasen, N. C., and Bardach, J. 1977. Dysmorphophobia: Symptom or disease? Psychiatry 134:673–676.

Bender, D. 1964a. A reexamination of the crock. In *New Dimensions in Psychosomatic Medicine*. Wahl, C. W., ed. Boston: Little Brown.

Bender, D. 1964b. Seven angry crocks. Psychosomatics 5:225–229.

Bishop, E. R. 1980a. Monosymptomatic hypochondriasis. Psychosomatics 21:731–741.

Bishop, E.R. 1980b. An olfactory reference syndrome—Monosymptomatic hypochondriasis. J Clin Psychiatry 41:57–59.

Bittker, T.E. 1979. The "worried-well": How to manage the somatizing patient. Behavioral Med 6(Nov):34–37.

Brink, T.L., Capri, D., DeNeeve, V., Janakes, C., and Olveira, C. 1979. Hypochondriasis and paranoia. J Nerv Ment Dis 167:224–228.

Brink, T.L., Janakes, C., and Martinez, N. 1981. Geriatric hypochondriasis: Situational factors. Am Geriatr Soc J 29:37–39.

Brown, H.N., and Vaillant, G.E. 1981. Hypochondriasis. Arch Intern Med 141:723–726.

Busse, E.W. 1976. Hypochondriasis in the elderly: A reaction to social stress. Am Geriatr Soc J 24:145–149.

Busse, E.W., and Reckless, J.B. 1961. Psychiatric management of the aged. JAMA 175:645–648.

Cohen, A. 1966. The physician and the "crock". In *Practical Lectures in Psychiatry for the Medical Practitioner*, Usdin, G.L., ed. Springfield, Ill.: Charles C Thomas.

Connolly, F.H., and Gipson, M. 1978. Dysmorphophobia—A long-term study. Br J Psychiatry 132:568–570.

Costa, P.T., and McCrae, R.R. 1980. Somatic complaints in males as a function of age and neuroticism: A longitudinal analysis. J Behav Med 3:245–257.

Denney, D., Kole, D.M., and Matarazzo, R.G. 1965. The relationship between age and the number of symptoms reported by patients. J Gerontol 20:50–53.

Dorfman, W. 1968. Hypochondriasis as a defense against depression. Psychosomatics 9:248–251.

Fischer-Homberger, E. 1972. Hypochondriasis of the eighteenth century—Neurosis of the present century. Bull Hist Med 46:391–401.

Ford, C.V., and Long, K.D. 1977. Group psychotherapy of somatizing patients. Psychother Psychosom 28:294–304.

Friedman, W.H., Jelly, E., and Jelly, P. 1979. Group therapy for psychosomatic patients at a family practice center. Psychosomatics 20:671–675.

Garfield, S.R., Collen, M.G., Feldman, R., et al. 1976. Evaluation of an ambulatory medical-care delivery system. N Engl J Med 294:426–431.

Gianturco, D.T., and Busse, E.W. 1978. Psychiatric problems encountered during a long-term study of normal aging volunteers. In *Studies in Geriatric Psychiatry.* Isaacs, A.D., and Post, F., eds. Chicester, England: Wiley.

Gillespie, R.D. 1928. Hypochondria: Its definition, nosology and psychopathology. Guy's Hosp Rept 78:408–460.

Goldstein, S.E., and Birnbom, F. 1976. Hypochondriasis and the elderly. Am Geriatr Soc J 24:150–154.

Hay, G.G. 1970. Dysmorphophobia. Bri J.Psychiatry 116:399–406.

Hopkinson, G. 1973. The psychiatric syndrome of infestation. Psychiatr Clin 6:330–345.

Idzorek, S. 1975. A functional classification of hypochondriasis with specific recommendations for treatment. South Med J 68:1326.

Idzorek, S. 1977. A practical approach to hypochondriasis. Resident Staff Physician 23(December):95–100 en passim.

Jacobs, T.J., Fogelson, S., Charles E. 1968. Depression ratings in hypochondria. N Y State J Med 68:3119–3122.

Katon, W., Kleinman, A., and Rosen, G. 1982a. Depression and somatization: A review, Part I. Am J Med 72:127–135.

Katon, W., Kleinman, A., and Rosen, G. 1982b. Depression and somatization: A review. Part II. Am J Med 72:241–247.

Kenyon, F.E. 1964. Hypochondriasis: A clinical study. Br J Psychiatry 110:478–488.

Kenyon, F.E. 1965. Hypochondriasis: A survey of some historical, clinical and social aspects. Br J Med Psychol 38:117–133.

Kenyon F.E. 1976. Hypochondriacal states. Br J Psychiatry 129:1–14.

Kreitman, N., Sainsbury, P., Pearce, K., and Costain, W.R. 1965. Hypochondriasis and depression in outpatients at a general hospital. Br J Psychiatry 111:607–615.

Ladee, G.A. 1966. *Hypochondriacal Syndromes.* London: Elsevier.

Lesse, S. 1967. Hypochondriasis and other psychosomatic disorders masking depression. Am J Psychother 21:607–620.

Lesse, S. 1968. Masked depression–a diagnostic and therapeutic problem. Dis Nerv Syst 29:169–173.

Lesse, S. 1977. Psychotherapy in combination with antidepressant drugs in patients with severe masked depressions. Am J Psychother 31:189–203.

Lesse, S. 1980. Masked depression – the ubiquitous but unappreciated syndrome. Psychiatr J Univ Ottawa 5:268–273.

Lesser, I.M., Ford C.V., and Friedmann, C.T.H. 1979. Alexithymia in somatizing patients. Gen Hosp Psychiatry 1:256–261.

Lipsitt, D.R. 1968. The "rotating" patient: A challenge to psychiatrists. J Geriat Psychiatry 2:51–61.

Lipsitt, D.R. 1970. Medical and psychological characteristics of "crocks." Psychiatry Med 1:15–25.

McCranie, E.J. 1979. Hypochondriacal neurosis. Psychosomatics 20:11–15.

Mai, F.M., and Merskey H. 1981. Briquet's concept of hysteria: An historical perspective. Am J Psychiatry 26:57–63.

Mally, M.A., and Ogston, W.D. 1964. Treatment of the 'untreatables.' Int J Grp Pschother 14:369–374.

Mandeville, B. 1976. A Treatise of the Hypochondriack and Hysterick Diseases (1730). Delmar, N.Y.: Scholars' Facsimiles and Reprints, p2.

Munro, A. 1978a. Monosymptomatic hypochondriacal psychoses: A diagnostic entity which may respond to Pimozide. Can Psychiatr Assoc J 23:497–500.

Munro, A. 1978b. Monosymptomatic hypochondriacal psychosis manifesting as delusions of parasitosis. Arch Dermatol 114:940–943.

Munro, A. 1978c. Two cases of delusions of worm infestation. Am J Psychiatry 135:234–235.

Pilowsky, I. 1970. Primary and secondary hypochondriasis. Acta Pschiatr Scand 46:273–285.

Pryse-Phillips, W. 1971. An olfactory reference syndrome. Acta Psychiatr Scand 47:484–509.

Roskin, G., Mehr, A., Rabiner, C.J., and Rosenberg, C. 1980. Psychiatric treatment of chronic somatizing patients: A pilot study. Int J Psychiatry Med 10:181–187.

Schoenberg, B., and Senescu, R. 1966. Group psychotherapy for patients with chronic multiple somatic complaints. J Chron Dis 19:649–657.

Schrut, A.H. 1963. Psychiatric and entomological aspects of delusory parasitosis. JAMA 186:429–430.

Shoenberg, P.J. 1976. A dialogue with Mandeville. Br J Psychiat 129:120–124.

Sifneos, P.E. 1972 Short-term Psychotherapy and Emotional Crisis. Cambridge, Mass.: Harvard Univ. Press.

Turnbull, J.M. 1974. The hypochondriacal patient. In Psychosocial Basis of Medical Practice, Bowden, C.L., and Burstein, A.G., eds. Baltimore, Md.: Williams & Wilkins Co.

Wahl, C.W. 1964. Psychodynamics of the hypochondriacal patient. In New Dimensions in Psychosomatic Medicine, Wahl, C.W., ed. Boston: Little Brown.

Walker, J.I. 1978. How to help your hypochondriac patients. Behaviorial Med 5 (February):30–32.

Webb, W.L. 1979. Hypochondriasis: Difficulties in diagnosis and management. South Med J 72:37–39.

Wilson, J.W., and Miller, H.E. 1946. Delusions of parasitosis. Arch Dermatol Syph 54:39–54.

Zaidens, S.H. 1950. Dermatologic hypochondriasis. Psychosom Med 12:250–253.

7

CHRONIC PAIN SYNDROMES

"Pain" is a word and experience so commonplace as to make definitions and explanations seem superfluous. Although a necessary component of human life, and the inability to experience pain is considered pathologic, for some persons chronic pain can make life seem worthless. A definition of pain offered by Merskey and Spear (1967) is that of an "unpleasant experience we primarily associate with tissue damage or describe in terms of tissue damage or both." Sternbach (1968) provides a tripartite definition to characterize pain. This concept includes a personal private sensation of hurt; a stimulus that signals current or pending tissue damage; and a pattern of responses that operate to protect the organism from harm. This comprehensive view of pain takes into account stimulus, perception, and response. Although these operational definitions are useful they still fall short of all the various meanings of pain and the need for a more global concept which incorporates the affectual components of pain. "Pain" is frequently used in everyday speech to communicate emotional experiences: "You have hurt me by your remarks." "The death of my mother has caused me great pain." It is apparent that in its broadest meanings pain is used to express any type of discomfort, whether or not there is actual tissue damage. In fact, until the advent of physiologic research delineating peripheral pathways for pain stimuli, pain was regarded to be an emotional experience rather than merely a disturbance located in the body (Merskey, 1980).

One point on which all agree is that pain is a *subjective* experience. There is no way to measure it: no dynes or serum mg%. No one ever really knows what someone else is experiencing in the way of pain. Pain can be inferred by verbal report, nonverbal behavior (wincing, etc.) or by reflex activity such as withdrawal responses, but no one ever knows exactly what another "feels" in the way of pain. There are, however, a number of adjectives commonly used to describe pain and a general consensual agreement to types of pain and their intensity (Melzack and Torgerson, 1971). Certain types of diseases have characteristic pain patterns (their "signatures"), and if a patient describes pain characteristic of this pattern or "signature" then a physician may be convinced that he understands the nature of the discomfort. For examples, the characteristic "sharp," "shooting" pains radiating down the leg which are characteristic of sciatica, or the steady "crushing" chest pain typical of a myocardial infarction. However, to jump to the conclusion that a certain disease is present presumes that the patient is accurately reporting the somatic sensations. In fact, patients may consciously or unconsciously perceive and describe symptoms compatible with previous illnesses or their ideas of what other persons close to them have experienced.

Can pain—experienced as a somatic disorder—exist in the absence of some peripheral stimulus? Can it be "all in the head?" The answer to these questions is apparently yes. But that does *not* mean that the pain is not real! It may be every bit as uncomfortable when generated from central mechanisms as when initiated from peripheral stimulation. Some brief examples will illustrate this point. First, a peripheral stimulus which is *not* inherently painful can be interpreted as such in certain emotional contextual situations. A two-year-old boy when in good nature is swatted across the bottom while playfully roughhousing with his father may squeal in delight and attempt to reciprocate similarly. However, if the father, when angry, and with the intent to punish, hits the child with the same degree of physical force (an identical peripheral stimulus), the boy now cries in pain and may run away. Another situation is that of phantom pain. It is well established that the loss of an external body part (limb or breast) frequently results in the persistence of the sensation that the body part is still there (Kolb, 1975). This may include the sensation of movement or pain. Phantom pain may be so severe as to be disabling. From these examples it is apparent that pain can indeed exist in the absence of peripheral stimulus or that the perception of pain may vary markedly with identical inputs of peripheral stimulation.

The reasons for the variation in the perception of pain most probably lies in the neuroanatomic nature of the brain and the numerous associative pathways linking sensory cerebral cortex and the limbic system (Snyder, 1977). The anatomic connections suggest a close relationship between pain and emotions. The sensation of pain can be stored as a memory and recalled as an isolated perception (similar to dreaming or hallucinations) or the experience (via memory) of pain may be evoked because of closely associated emotional experiences.

THEORIES OF PAIN PERCEPTION

The following theoretical constructs about pain represent different ways of looking at the same phenomenon. Each emphasizes a different aspect of the pain process. None by itself totally explains pain, and it is important to recognize they are not mutually exclusive. It is likely that each pain experience incorporates to some degree one or more of these concepts, although to different degrees with different events. Thus one or another of these proposed mechanisms may be the primary variable in different patients or with the same patient at different times.

Neuroanatomic and Physiologic Theories

It is beyond the scope of this book to review in any detail the physiologic and neuroanatomic information available in regards to the activation of receptor sites, transmission and the conscious awareness of stimuli which are perceived as painful. Recent research which has identified endorphins has led to more understanding of the central perception of pain (Snyder, 1977). The "gate theory" has also led to new concepts of pain control. Very briefly the gate theory holds that pain impulses are transmitted by different sized fibers at different speeds. The activation of some fibers may cause inhibition in the firing of other fibers thereby creating a "gate," which influences the intensity of stimuli, which are transmitted to higher CNS structures (Melzack and Wall, 1965).

Most neuroanatomic descriptions of the transmission of pain stimuli involve the specificity theory or some variation of it. The specificity theory has been compared to a telephone communication system, a concept of pain widely accepted by both physicians and patients. The specificity theory states that the intensity of the pain (signal transmitted) is roughly proportional to the amount of tissue damage that occurs peripherally. This view of pain infers the possibility of several therapeutic interventions for the control of pain; and indeed there are several clinical applications. The various therapeutic interventions are (1) to eliminate the cause of pain, e.g., treat the pathologic process; (2) to eliminate or diminish the sensitivity of the receiver or initial transmission system, e.g., the use of local anesthetics; (3) to intercept the transmission lines, e.g., "nerve blocks"; and (4) to reduce or eliminate the sensitivity of the receiver (cerebral cortex), e.g., use of anesthesia or centrally acting analgesics.

It is the specificity theory which offers apparent rationale to surgical procedures such as cordotomies, rhizotomies, and cingulectomies, with the view that pain can be eliminated if the capacity to transmit the peripheral signal is reduced or eliminated.

In clinical situations involving acute pain the specificity theory usually provides a satisfactory explanation on which to base therapeutic interventions. Local anesthesia for tooth removal is an effective symptomatic intervention. Anesthesia effectively blocks the conscious awareness of massive tissue damage in major surgery and analgesics such as morphine are effective in reducing the pain of acute trauma. However, there are important differences between acute and chornic pain, and it is in the experience of *chronic pain* that the specificity theory fails. Although a cordotomy should effectively end all painful sensations distal to it (and may do so temporarily) the pain frequently persists or returns after some transient relief (Melzack, 1974). In a situation such as this the specificity theory fails to explain the pain, and it is necessary to evoke other theoretical explanation.

Psychodynamic Theories

Psychodynamic theories of pain have been expounded by G.L. Engel (1959) and Pilowsky (1978b). These explanations are derived from the meanings of pain in the context of important infantile and childhood experiences, primarily with parents. For example, pain may be associated with hunger or with other discomfort such as a wet diaper. The resultant crying brings the mother who resolves the problem and simultaneously provides closeness and affection. Later when the child falls and scrapes an elbow or bumps his head, he runs crying to mother who "kisses the wound and makes it well." Thus in the situations such as those described pain may come to mean the expectation of care and affection. With parents who offer little in the way of loving affection but who perfunctorily tend to their children's basic needs, it is easy to see how children may learn to unconsciously view pain as a way of obtaining more parental involvement.

Another important meaning of pain is that of an association with punishment. Guilt and punishment (with resultant pain) are closely linked. Guilt brings with it the expectation of punishment, and conversely punishment often evokes a sense of guilt ("What have I done to deserve this?"). Parents may cause pain in their children through punishment. For some children the pain may be severe, such as that secondary to severe beatings and/or other forms of child abuse. Clinical experience indicates that children who have experienced such attacks from their parents often have rigid, punitive superegos. Unconsciously they have incorporated the feeling that to have deserved such punishment they must indeed be bad. (It is very difficult for the young child to perceive the parent as bad or sick because of the universal need of small, and therefore helpless, children to view the parents as omnipotent.) Children who have experienced physical abuse typically grow up to feel pervasively guilty and therefore in need of punishment (translated as pain). Another contributing factor to the need for pain that these children experience is that the parent who loses control and physically abuses a child often subsequently experiences feelings of guilt and then compensates by being particularly affectionate or generous with the child. As a consequence the experience of pain may have a reward in terms of a reunion with the parent and the punishment may be well tolerated in order to receive the desired "payoff".

From the above psychodynamic formulations one can postulate that some persons have unconscious determinants which make them "pain prone." These persons may use pain as an unconsciously determined punishment for

real or fantasied guilt or as a symptom which will reunite them to people
with whom they would like to be close.

Pain as a Learned Behavior

The use of learning theory to explain chronic pain has been expounded by
Fordyce (1974, 1978). The following concepts are largely derived from
reports of his work with pain patients at the University of Washington,
Seattle.

Utilizing learning theory, the diagnostician proceeds differently than with
the disease model (which may also incorporate psychodynamic etiologic
explanations). Rather than search for the etiologic factors the behaviorist
evaluates the relationships between the patient and his environment as
determined by the presence or absence of pain.

There are two major classes of responses or actions that an organism can
take: respondents and operants. Respondents are actions which are under
the control of antecedent stimuli. When there is an adequate stimulus then
the response occurs automatically, e.g., the Pavlovian dog. These responses
are largely reflexive in nature and reflect activity of the autonomic nervous
system. Operants, in contrast, involve actions of the organism which are
under voluntary control and as a consequence largely reflect activity of the
striated musculature. Operants, while capable of being elicited by antecedent
stimuli, are also influenced by the consequence of the action taken.
Therefore there is the possibility that the behavior will be affected by either
positive or negative feedback and therefore reinforced or diminished in
intensity. In the situation of pain, the experience of pain with movement may
cause the development of a behavior which is predicated on avoiding pain;
e.g., relative immobility. Such a behavior may be as either a respondent or an
operant dependent upon whether it is reflexive or voluntarily initiated.
Learned behavior may persist even when the underlying cause of the pain no
longer exists.

One's response to pain, such as grimacing and moaning may affect
persons in the environment who then behave differently in response to his/
her signals of pain. The pain with its signals, in order to maintain this
different behavior of others, may persist as a learned behavior. Fordyce notes
that most pain behaviors are operants which elicit many responses such as
attention or solicitous behavior from others, or which may result in the
obtaining of medications such as narcotics or in receiving financial
compensation. Pain behaviors may be negatively reinforced such as the
termination or avoidance of aversive situations (e.g., work) or they may be
positively reinforced (e.g., increased attention from spouse). The same pain
behavior may be under the influence of both types of reinforcement.

Pain behaviors do not require the presence of pain (the organic or concrete concept of pain) to persist. Fordyce (1974) states that " . . . with regard to the positive reinforcement of pain behavior, or the successful avoidance of pain, it is not at all necessary to postulate some kind of emotional or personality pathology. . . . "

Treatment strategies employing learning theory (behavioral modification) involve reducing or eliminating reinforcers which have been maintaining the behavior or to increase the rate of a behavior which is incompatible with the one which is to be decreased. An important clinical point to note is that pain behavior, particularly when under the influence of intermittent reinforcement, may not decrease (and may even transiently increase) for a long period of time. Therefore a failure to achieve immediate results should not be misinterpreted to mean that treatment is ineffective (Ferster and Skinner, 1957).

"Painsmanship"

The meaning and use of pain in interpersonal relationships has been pointed out by Szasz (1957). Sternbach (1974), utilizing the transactional analysis concepts of Berne, has expanded the idea that pain may be used as a form of interpersonal manipulation and control: "Painsmanship." There are several common games which can be readily recognized by physicians who work with these patients. These games may occur whether the pain is primarily psychogenic or somatogenic. The pain becomes the "currency" of interpersonal transactions and may be used to obtain narcotics, disability, or some type of advantage in a relationship with another person.

Sternbach notes that there are many possible games and recommends alternative responses that the physician can make in order to alter the outcome.

A Systems Theory Concept of Pain

General systems theory, which is being increasingly utilized in psychiatry as a way to conceptualize multiple simultaneous phenomena and incorporate different theoretical perspectives (Meir, 1969), provides an excellent framework by which to investigate pain. Systems theory presumes that the universe is comprised of a hierarchial series of subsystems interacting among themselves and that the interaction of these systems is governed by certain general principles, such as the tendency to maintain stability (e.g., homeostasis). For example, a person is a subsystem of his interpersonal contacts (society) but is comprised of psychological and physiologic subsystems. A symptom (e.g., pain) can be viewed as evidence of strain upon the system and/or an effector which attempts to maintain stability of the systems or subsystem.

Concepts developed by Miller (1973a, 1973b) by which systems theory can be used in psychiatric consultation are referable to the evaluation and treatment of pain. Acute pain can serve to warn of danger to the stability of the system and thereby effect changes which will ultimately preserve it. This situation is best demonstrated by the reaction of withdrawal, thereby preserving part of the body, in response to touching something hot. Another situation is that of a chronic pain syndrome where pain itself may serve to preserve stability in the system, for example, to maintain the continuous flow of disability payments. Using a systems theory approach to evaluate pain, one must look simultaneously at all of the identified component subsystems and determine the meaning that the pain has to each individual subsystem and to the larger system as a whole. Pain may simultaneously effect the physiologic subsystem, the intrapsychic subsystem, the inter-personal subsystems, and a more general societal subsystem such as the place of employment. A different term, tertiary gain, has been also used to describe the effects of the social system in maintaining a symptom or illness (Bokan et al., 1981, Dansak, 1973). Pain may serve the purposes of a variety of persons in the patient's environment, and they may be reluctant to allow the patient to discard the symptom.

FACTORS INFLUENCING ACUTE PAIN

Because the experience of pain is to a large extent subjective it is influenced by a number of personal "host" factors.

Age, Sex, and Race

In a study in which over 40,000 persons were subjected to a test of measured pain tolerance (pressure on the Achilles tendon) statistical differences were found among several groups (Woodrow et al., 1972). The largest differences were between men and women; men were able to tolerate a considerably greater amount of pain stimulus than women. Less striking but still statistically significant were racial differences. Whites were able to tolerate the greatest degree of pain stimuli, orientals the least, and blacks an intermediary position between the two former groups. Pain tolerance was found to decrease with age for both women and men and for all racial groups. The research team noted that the pain which they were ex-perimentally investigating was not the same as clinical pain, and their findings could not be necessarily translated into the medical situation. They also noted that their pain stimulus was that of "deep pain" and that it had been previously demonstrated that tolerance to superficial (or cutaneous) pain tends to increase with age.

Ethnic Factors

Differences between ethnic groups in regard to their behavior toward pain have been reported by Zborowski (1958). His descriptions, which have been frequently referenced, indicated that Italians and Jews are very sensitive to pain and very emotional in their responses to it. In contrast the Irish are described as denying pain or being very stoical about it, and "Old Americans" (white Protestants established in the United States for several generations) are described as being emotionally detached while offering objective descriptions of their pain sensations. An "Old American" may become more emotionally expressive concerning his pain when by himself and for that reason may tend to become more socially isolated when experiencing severe pain.

Zborowski attributed the ethnic differences which he observed to cultural differences in child raising. He suggested that "Old American" mothers support the efforts of their children to resist pain, thus emphasizing masculinity. In the Italian family the mother inspires the child's emotionality, while in Jewish families both parents express attitudes of worry and concern which are transmitted to the children.

A recent investigation (Flannery et al. 1981), which compared pain responses to an episiotomy, found no differences among the five ethnic groups of the postpartum women studies. The five ethnic groups included Anglo-Saxon Protestant, Afro American, Jewish, Irish, and Italian patients. All women were at least third-generation American, and the authors opined that if there were ethnic differences in the expression of pain such differences disappear through acculturation.

What is important to recognize is not that there may be differences in ethnic groups, but that different families may inculcate varying attitudes and encourage varying pain behaviors in their offspring. As a consequence the physician must be aware of the fact that the expression of pain may differ considerably from patient to patient irrespective of the patient's ethnic background.

Psychological Factors

Several different psychological factors which affect the perception of pain have been identified in experimental and clinical situations. Patients who are described as "extraverted" have more tolerance to pain while patients who demonstrate neuroticism are less tolerant of pain (Lynn and Eysenck, 1961; Bond, 1976).

Anxiety is an important factor influencing the perception of pain. The physiologic responses to pain are essentially identical to those found in anxiety and include increases in heart rate, blood pressure, respiration, peripheral blood flow, palms sweating, pupillary diameter, and muscular tension (B.T. Engel, 1959). Anxiety is such an important variable that in the experimental situation there may be no consistent relationship between the intensity of pain stimulus and the magnitude of the pain response (Sternbach, 1968). Increasing anxiety will enhance pain responses and decreasing anxiety will reduce such responses.

In the clinical situation anxiety and other emotional factors often influence the perception of pain. Dentists frequently go to great lengths to design their offices and procedures in such a manner to make patients as comfortable (and ultimately as pain-free) as possible. In a more dramatic illustration Beecher (1956) reported that soldiers at the Anzio beachhead frequently expressed no sensation of pain despite having suffered massive tissue damage. Beecher interpreted this response to the immense psychologic relief that the soldiers experienced in finding that they were still alive and would as a consequence of their injuries have an acceptable exit from the war.

CHRONIC PAIN SYNDROMES

Chronic pain differs from acute pain in many respects. If the pain continues, the physiologic responses which accompany acute pain attenuate over a period of weeks to months. In their place there is an emergence of the vegetative symptoms which often accompany depression. Patients then report symptoms such as insomnia, loss of appetite, decreased sexual interests, irritability, and an increased preoccupation with their bodies (Sternbach, 1978b). There is a high degree of congruence between depression and pain syndromes. Lindsay and Wyckoff (1981) found that of a series of 300 pain center patients 87% were depressed and of a series of 196 depressed private practice patients 57% had recurring benign pain.

The changes in mood (and personality) which accompany chronic pain are so frequently observed that it has been opined that the neurotic features of chronic pain are the consequence rather than the cause of chronic pain (Reuler et al., 1980). However, despite acknowledgment that chronic pain does indeed have the capability of eliciting psychological reactions, many clinicians who have studied patients with intractable chronic benign pain (as opposed to pain associated with malignancies or other disorders with ongoing tissue changes) are impressed that these patients do fit certain psychological profiles, and these psychological characteristics predated the onset of the pain syndrome.

In 1959 G. L. Engel published a paper on psychogenic pain and the pain-prone patient. This paper, now regarded as a "classic," is oft-quoted, and his descriptions have served as the basis for subsequent clinical investigations. Because of the clinical importance of Engel's work the features of the pain-prone patients as described by him will be reviewed in detail before proceeding to discuss findings of other investigators in regard to proneness to pain.

The Pain-Prone Patient

Engel observed that the chronic pain patients he studied did not represent a homogeneous group but, as a rule, shared many features in common. Frequently they were depressive, pessimistic individuals who unconsciously did not believe that they deserved success or happiness and felt that they must pay a price for it. Their life histories were replete with instances where they had been hurt, defeated, or humiliated. Many of these situations could have been avoided, yet the patient did not seem to learn by experience. Pain-prone individuals often developed pain at times when things appeared to be going well in their lives as if they felt they did not deserve happiness.

The developmental backgrounds of pain-prone patients often disclosed descriptions of aggression, pain, and suffering in the childhood home. One or both parents, perhaps alcoholics, were frequently verbally or physically abusive to the child. Attention to the child may have occurred only when the child was sick or suffering. A parent or other close relative may have had an illness or pain for which the child, often because of aggressive fantasies, may have felt responsibility.

According to Engel the first episode of pain in the pain-prone patient often occurs in adolescence and is associated with guilt about sexual impulses. Women in particular may offer a history of dysmenorrhea or other gynecologic symptoms; a history of an appendectomy for questionable indications is common. The pain may subsequently occur when external circumstances fail to satisfy the unconscious need to suffer or as a response to real threatened or fantasied loss (see Case 1 below). Pain symptoms may also occur when guilt is evoked by intense aggressive or forbidden sexual feelings.

The location of pain in the pain-prone patient is determined by a variety of factors. The pain may be similar to that of pain experienced by the person in the past, or it may be similar to a pain experienced by someone else (or which the patient fantasied the other person to have experienced) with whom the patient had a close relationship. At times the location of the pain may be determined by symbolism associated with guilt concerning a conscious or unconscious wish that another person suffer pain.

In Engel's opinion the psychiatric diagnoses to which pain-prone patients may be assigned are variable, including such diverse conditions as conversion reactions, depression, schizophrenia, hypochondriasis, or admixtures of the foregoing disorders.

From their careful study of a series of 234 pain patients (compensation cases excluded), Blumer and Heilbronn (1981) found many psychological characteristics in their patients similar to those characteristics of the pain-prone patients described by Engel. These authors were impressed that the patients fit into a fairly homogeneous group, and they differed from Engel in that they thought the patients should be assigned to a specific diagnostic category: the "pain-prone disorder." The most characteristic feature of their pain-prone patients was that related to the patients' expression of emotions. They were characterized as alexithymic (see Chapter 6) with little ability to verbalize feelings, stoic, overly controlled, and action oriented. [Pinsky (1978) has similarly emphasized the alexithymic characteristics of chronic pain patients.] These patients, in addition to their alexithymic features, had a tendency to idealize their families (often in the presence of fairly obvious conflict) and also demonstrated a tendency to be good-natured and conscientious rather than angry and resentful. Although depression, as such, was usually denied, many patients had depressive symptoms. Features of guilt, dependency, and masochism were common and combined with a preoccupation with somatic suffering. Similar to the descriptions offered by Engel, these chronic pain patients frequently had been exposed to models of pain and disability in their early life experiences.

The experiences of other writers in regard to the heterogeneity–homogeneity of pain patients would support the view that these patients are a very diverse group. Prokop and colleagues (1980) studied a large number of pain patients with the Minnesota Multiphasic Personality Inventory (MMPI). Utilizing the statistical technique of multivariate cluster analysis, they found a number of distinct and separate subgroups of pain patients. Consistent findings by investigators who have studied chronic pain patients by use of the MMPI include usual elevations of the clinical scales Hs (hypochondriasis), Hy (hysteria), and D (depression) (Blumetti and Modesti, 1976; Jamison et al. 1976; Prokop et al., 1980; Strassberg et al., 1981). Using multiple personality tests to evaluate a series of unselected chronic pain patients, Timmermans and Sternbach (1974) found that a major factor in these patients was interpersonal alienation and manipulativeness.

One subgroup of pain clinic patients which has been reported are those with narcissistic features (Blazer, 1980). This subgroup represented slightly more than 20% of a consecutive series of pain patients. The narcissistic patients were typified by the manner in which they distrusted and disregarded others, while at the same time they craved prestige and admiration. The quality of their interpersonal relationships was superficial. Other features of these narcissistic patients included a frequent history of excellent health prior to a sudden and unexpected event causing injury (such as an automobile accident) which left the patient with an unaccustomed feeling of helplessness and anxiety. As a result of the narcissistic injury suffered these patients typically developed anger toward family members and health care personnel who were viewed as unconcerned and incompetent.

In their study of a group of patients who complained of severe pain, Swanson and Maruta (1980b) found these patients, when compared to pain patients who complained of less severe pain, to be more frequently female, to have longer histories of pain, to have been disabled longer, to have had more surgical procedures and hospitalizations, to be more dependent on drugs and to be less responsive to therapy. Interestingly, this group of severe pain patients did not demonstrate a greater degree of objective organic disease. Swanson and Maruta interpreted the complaints of the severe pain patient as an effort to say that life was very difficult and not to make demands. They also noted that the declaration of extreme pain is rarely relinquished.

Timmermans and Sternbach (1976) found (using a tourniquet pain test to evaluate the severity of pain) that the higher a patient overevaluated his subjective pain the more life was centered around it and the more it affected daily functioning. However, as the actual intensity of pain increased, there was increased depression which was regarded as a reaction to the pain.

My personal clinical experience favors a multidimensional view of the phenomenon of chronic pain. The complaint of chronic intractable pain has been observed in patients who met diagnostic criteria for widely varied disorders and personality types. In some patients it appeared that the etiology of the pain was determined by intrapsychic conflicts; Case 1 below is such an example. Other patients have been significantly depressed and the pain represented a depressive equivalent. The complaints of pain from still other patients have been maintained because of expectations from the environment; learning theory or systems theory may best explain the persistence of their symptoms (see Case 2 below). The etiology of the pain of other patients has been interpreted to such varied causes as a defense against murderous impulses (Ford et al., 1974).

Illustrative Case Histories

CASE 1. A 28-year-old mother of two small children was referred for psychiatric consultation and treatment following two years of disabling back pain. Numerous consultations with her internist and orthopedist had failed to find a cause for her distress. Symptomatic therapy had brought only transient relief.

The patient's history and the etiology for her pain emerged during once-a-week psychotherapy extending over several months. She was the elder of two children born into a middle-class but very socially ambitious family. She recounted numerous childhood battles with her mother over her weight; there was a demand that she remain attractive in order to "make a good marriage." The mother was often cruel in her comments to the patient and would engage in sadistic behaviors such as feeding dessert to her younger brother while denying it to the patient. Adolescence was stormy; the patient engaged in acting-out behavior including an out-of-wedlock pregnancy which precluded the "social wedding" desired by the mother. The patient subsequently married, was abused by her husband, divorced, and remarried. The second marriage was more stable.

When the patient's mother became ill with metastatic breast carcinoma the patient, feeling guilty, returned to the mother's home to care for her during her terminal illness. During this time the mother was critical, domineering, and demanding. Because of the mother's behavior the patient began to secretly hope that "she would die and get it over with." During the mother's final hospitalization the patient, while in the hospital coffee shop, received word via telephone that her mother had just died. The patient recounted that her severe back pain began at that moment.

It was interpreted to the patient that she had taken on the back pain as punishment for her secret wishes that the mother would die. The patient accepted this interpretation and then stated (previously unmentioned) that her mother's principal symptoms has been due to metastases to the vertebrae. The patient's pain remitted over the next week and several psychotherapy sessions were then spent working through her ambivalent feelings toward her mother. The patient's pain did not recur during a five-year follow-up period.

The diagnostic impression of this woman's symptoms was that of a *conversion disorder*. The symptom was reflective of an intrapsychic conflict and had only minimal reinforcement from the environment. With resolution of the conflict the symptom could be quickly discarded.

CASE 2. A 55-year-old married male accountant was referred for psychiatric evaluation because of severe disabling neck pain extending over 18 months. Findings on physical examination included spastic posterior neck muscles which had palpable fibrotic nodules. The patient appeared mildly depressed, although he denied it, and the only positive mental status finding was his lack of verbalized emotion (alexithymia). Despite these findings his disability seemed excessive; he spent most of each day (and night) propped up in bed watching television. His salary was paid by a disability insurance plan at his place of employment.

The patient's past history was fairly unremarkable. Although his father had died during his childhood, his mother had remarried and a stable, although fairly unemotional homelife, had been provided for him. His work history was good, and his marriage of many years was reported as solid and uneventful. His wife was described as strong and the dominant force in the marriage.

Psychotherapy and an attempt at treatment with tricyclic antidepressants were not successful in altering the symptoms. The patient continued to be bedridden except when he made the hour trip, each way, to see his physician. Because therapy appeared stalemated he was asked to bring his wife for conjoint sessions. These sessions clearly indicated that the wife was actively promoting the disability because she made repetitive statements to the effect that the patient should stay in bed because of his pain. No amount of encouragement for him to assume more activity could budge her reinforcement of his immobility.

The reasons for the wife's reinforcing behavior were not clear until one day when she commented about his "alcoholism" (a topic never mentioned previously by the patient). The story emerged that he had been arrested 18 months previously for drunk driving after an office party. The wife had had to bail him out of jail and was humiliated by the experience; she was a teetotaler and came from a family which regarded drinking as a sin. Although this episode was the only instance of known alcohol abuse on the part of the patient, she had determined that it would never again recur. Her reinforcement of the pain syndrome was motivated by her desire to keep him away from alcohol. Another problem which then emerged was that the wife was covertly depressed. Her focused preoccupation on the patient's pain syndrome and "alcoholism" appeared to be a defense against the awareness of her own depression. With the above information out in the open, and the wife receiving treatment for her depression, therapy progressed. The patient, although he continued to have some pain, once again became active.

This case is best viewed from a systems theory perspective. The patient did have organically based pain, but the disability resulted from his wife's reinforcement of the pain, his inherent passivity, and the secondary gain of continued salary through disability insurance. The pain served some of the wife's intrapsychic needs, and until these had been dealt with, therapy was stalemated. Thus we can see how a symptom (pain) serves to maintain stability in a system which is itself comprised of subsystems.

THE TREATMENT OF CHRONIC PAIN

There is a multiplicity of treatments for chronic pain, presumptive evidence that none of them are highly effective with all patients. That one specific treatment does not always alleviate chronic pain is not surprising when we consider the complexity of the various organic etiologies, the intrapsychic and interpersonal uses of pain, and behavior patterns which intitially result from pain and later reinforce its persistence. A wide variety of therapeutic techniques are necessary to treat the different types of patients who present with chronic pain. Because the etiology of pain is usually multideterminal any one patient will generally require several different types of therapeutic interventions (Pilowsky, 1978a). A complete review of the therapeutic techniques proposed to treat chronic pain would fill several volumes, therefore those techniques more readily available to the practicing physician will be highlighted here.

Therapeutic Strategy

The typical pain patient has seen multiple physicians without any lasting relief from his/her pain. The patient's perspective is that the pain is caused by a somatic process and that a competent physician should be able to find the cause and then institute a specific effective treatment which will relieve the pain and immediately restore the patient to his/her imagined normal state of health. If the physician also takes this stance—and assumes that the previous physicians were incompetent in their inability to help the patient—then the "game" has once again been engaged. The physician will be the eventual loser and the pain will be the victor. Instead of engaging the symptom in a contest, a new therapeutic strategy is necessary in order that the previous "games" are outflanked.

The initial contact with the chronic pain patient is a vital part of the overall management. The patient must not be promised complete relief from his pain. To the contrary, he must be told that complete relief is unlikely and that a major task for the patient is to learn to live with some pain (in National Football League parlance, "to play hurt"). This news comes as a surprise to some patients who expect total relief from pain and have continued to search for the doctor with the correct diagnosis and the "right treatment. Upon learning that chronic pain may not have a magical cure, some patients return to work without requiring any further medical intervention (DeVaul and Zisook, 1978).

It is necessary to establish a therapeutic contract with the patient starting with the first visit. One of the issues to be negotiated is whether or not the patient really wants to get better. Although the physician may believe that this wish is implied by the seeking of consultation, Sternbach (1978a) notes that pain patients frequently use their symptoms as a way to blame and manipulate others. He recommends that an open committed statement from the patient that he/she wishes to get better is necessary before instituting treatment.

Patients must also be told, during the initial consultation, that psychological problems are essentially always present with pain syndromes and that management must take them into account. This information must be transmitted from the first contact so that when psychological treatments are brought into the picture the patient does not react with feelings of rejection or with anger for having been deceived. Experience in the past (and almost all chronic pain patients have seen multiple physicians) has most likely been a series of somatic treatments which have failed, and then the patient was told that he should see a psychiatrist. The latter has almost always been rejected by the patient. The pain patient can be told, and quite honestly, that pain itself may be the cause for some of the psychic problems which have been experienced, and that to be effective, treatment must be comprehensive including both the body and emotions.

Patients must also be warned that the treatment of pain is often a lengthy undertaking which will demand efforts from them, not just something done to them by the physician, and that they should not expect immediate results.

In summary, the strategic approach is to change the patient's orientation from that of an acute disease, with all which implies in terms of the sick role, to that of a chronic problem. The goal of treatment must be the rehabilitation of the patient rather than the cure of pain (DeVaul and Zisook, 1978).

Somatic Therapeutic Interventions

The traditional treatment for pain is a prescription for an analgesic. Often these have been prescribed despite the fact they have been ineffective (or the patient would not be complaining of pain). The patient has continued to take them and may even be addicted. A secondary problem may be present in that the patient's depressive symptoms may be due to the iatrogenic effects of narcotics or other CNS depressants. Narcotics are rarely indicated in the treatment of chronic benign pain. [Narcotics do have a major role in the treatment of pain associated with malignancy and paradoxically they are often underutilized for cancer patients (Hammond, 1979; Marks and Sachar, 1973).]

A group of medications that are useful adjuvants in the management of chronic pain patients are the tricyclic antidepressants. These drugs often afford pain relief at a dosage below that generally believed to be effective for depression. From this observation it would appear that they may have some specific analgesic action independent of the antidepressant effect. However, because depression very commonly accompanies chronic pain the use of antidepressant medication may be "killing two birds with one stone." A suggested treatment regimen is to start with 30–100 mg daily of either amitriptyline or imipramine, and if that amount is not effective then slowly raise the dose to the usual antidepressant dosage range. If there is still no response after several weeks then a switch to another tricyclic antidepressant is indicated before abandoning the treatment (Moore, 1980).

Neuroleptics have also been recommended for the treatment of chronic pain and may be effective (Maltbie et al., 1979). However, caution is indicated because treatment for chronic pain is a lengthy undertaking and the neuroleptics can cause tardive dyskinesia.

Other psychotropic medications have been periodically recommended as effective with selective patients. Again caution is indicated because many of these drugs such as the benzodiazepenes and stimulants have addictive potential when used over a long period of time.

Transcutaneous nerve stimulation (TNS) has been demonstrated to help some patients, particularly those with pain in their lower extremities or back. The effect of TNS is hypothetically explained by the gate theory. The transcutaneous stimulation causes firing of the cells of large diameter nerve fibers, which then effect an inhibition of the activation of the small diameter nerve fibers which transmit sensations interpreted as pain. In one investigation, TNS was shown to be initially effective in 78% of pain patients but only 12.5% received long-term benefit (Loeser et al., 1975).

Dorsal column stimulation is another pain relief method which has proposed to function with a similar principle to that of TNS. Dorsal column stimulation requires surgical placement of the electrodes in dorsal column of the spinal cord and therefore requires the expertise of a neurosurgeon. This technique is replete with complications, and one surgeon who has extensively used the procedure views it as having value only for selected patients (Shealy, 1974).

Acupuncture appears to have about the same effectiveness as TNS, and it appears that the mechanism of action is due either to the release of endorphins or by inhibition of pain fibers in a manner similar to that proposed for TNS (Reuler et al., 1980). Expertise with acupuncture is not readily available in the United States.

Nerve blocks are a technique primarily for anesthesiologists or other physicians who are skilled in the technique and knowledgeable about anatomy. They may be of therapeutic or diagnostic use (Bonica, 1974b), but as a long-term treatment they, along with the surgical ablative procedures, are usually ineffective because the pain almost inevitably returns after 6–18 months (Sternbach, 1978b).

Biofeedback techniques have become popular in recent years, and these do appear to be helpful, particularly in muscle tension states such as tension headaches (Peck and Kraft, 1977). It is not clear if the benefit is from the overall behavioral modification implied in the use of biofeedback or the specifically learning of how to identify and modify a somatic physiologic state (Sternbach, 1978b).

Nonsomatic Therapeutic Interventions

The failure to achieve lasting beneficial effect from any of the somatic therapies currently available has led most physicians working in the treatment of pain, at the very least, to supplement their treatment programs with a variety of nonsomatic therapies such as behavioral modification and/or psychotherapy.

Behavioral modification plays an important role in the treatment of chronic pain. The goals are to extinguish pain behaviors and to shape new behaviors which are pain-incompatible. In order to determine the nature of the patient's various pain behaviors (and presence or absence of "well" behaviors), the maintenance of a detailed diary over a two-week period is very useful. From the diary the behavior therapist can identify certain patterns and then, with the patient and family, establish goals and techniques for modification. Examples of common behaviors which are desirable to modify include decreased activity, pain behaviors evocative of protective action by others, excessive reliance on pain medications, and decreased social activities (Fordyce, 1978).

Exercise is a central issue in modifying behavior and a therapeutic program may be established to progressively increase the patients level of exercise. Health care staff can respond with increased attention and praise (positive reinforcement) to the patient's activity and "well" behaviors while providing minimum social attention for pain behaviors (Fordyce, 1978).

Behavioral modification was the primary treatment modality utilized for a series of 200 chronic pain patients treatment in an inpatient psychiatric setting by Swanson and colleagues (1979). The mean length of hospitalization was 20.3 days. At time of discharge, 50% of the patients had achieved moderate improvement or better, and after one year 65% of those who were successfully treated continued to do well.

Psychotherapy is another treatment technique used for chronic pain patients. Traditional individual insight-oriented psychotherapy does not appear to be a useful or cost-effective means of treatment for most of these patients, although there are dramatic exceptions. These exceptions are usually patients who have well-defined intrapsychic conflicts or minimal behavior changes (see Case 1).

Group therapy has been described for chronic pain patients, and for most patients may be more useful than individual therapy. Pinsky (1978) reported that chronic pain patiens respond unexpectedly well to intense short-term group psychotherapy offered in a pain center inpatient service. The patients volunteered the information that the group helped them to become more confident in social activities and to begin to enjoy a more active life whether or not the pain experience itself was changed. Other clinicians have also indicated that group therapy, in groups comprised exclusively of pain patients, is an effective adjuvant to other treatment techniques for chronic patients (Hendler et al., 1981). Long-term outpatient group psychotherapy seems to facilitate the emergence of self-reliance.

Irrespective of the type of treatment intervention utilized there must be attention to the patients's marital and family situation. The spouse frequently suffers from significant psychiatric distress and this finding has implications for the treatment program (Standfield et al., 1979). Interestingly when there is a high congruity between the patients report of pain and the family's perception of the patient's pain there are more management problems and poorer treatment results (Swanson and Maruta, 1980a). What is suggested is that these families have a high degree of an undesirable mutuality, or enmeshment, and that the patient's symptom of pain serves a psychological purpose within the family. These observations, concerning spouses and families, are consistent with general systems theory in relationship to the symptom of pain as described earlier. Conjoint marital therapy or family therapy may be necessary in order to favorably modify a chronic pain syndrome.

Pain Clinics

The complex diagnostic and therapeutic needs of the chronic pain patient frequently require a multidisciplinary approach. Such comprehensive care can be afforded by a pain clinic comprised of a number of different medical specialists, physical therapists, psychologists, and other health care givers. Needed services, including a behavioral modification program and other psychological—psychiatric therapies, can be provided at one location. This increases communication among the caregivers and reduces the possibility of manipulation or noncompliance by the patient. Pain patients are very accepting of the pain clinic concept, perhaps because the very name addresses their problem. Within the context of comprehensive treatment they are more willing to accept psychological interventions than when such recommendations are made by their personal physicians. The number of pain clinics extant is rapidly increasing and many are based on the pioneering work of Bonica and his colleagues (1974a). In fact, the demand for pain clinics has been so great that many have been founded by health care providers without sufficient expertise in the area of pain. To be effective (and ethical) a pain clinic should provide comprehensive service and be comprised of persons who are recognized as competent within their own disciplines.

The goals of a pain clinic (which may be administered primarily by either an anesthesia or psychiatry service) are to decrease the pain experience by the patient, to decrease the amount of medications taken by the patient, to restore functioning, to decrease the use of medical facilities and to help the patient develop insight into his situation (Hudson and Pratt, 1979).

SPECIFIC PAIN SYNDROMES

The preceding discussion has focused upon chronic pain syndrome in general. Several specific pain syndromes are well recognized and each will be discussed separately.

Chronic Pelvic Pain

The symptom of chronic pelvic pain has been the subject of a number of studies involving fruitful collaboration between psychiatrists and gynecologists. These investigations have consistently indicated a significant degree of psychopathology in women who complain of chronic pelvic pain (Benson et al., 1959; Gross et al., 1980; Gidro-Frank et al., 1960). There have been two major interpretations of these findings. The first is that the chronic pelvic pain is a "psychosomatic" condition where psychological issues may cause pelvic congestion and lead to pain (Taylor, 1954; Neubardt, 1973). The alternate interpretation, which is more widely accepted, does not emphasize the presence of any organic pathology, but rather centers upon the pain as an expression of the woman's conflicts over sexuality (Beard et al., 1977; Gidro-Frank et al., 1960; Gross et al., 1980). In addition to the patients' complaints of chronic pelvic pain, often described as a dull continuous sensation, there are also frequent complaints of dysmenorrhea and dysparunia.

A question to consider is why do women have chronic pelvic pain and men do not? A possible explanation is that a man's genitalia ordinarily bring only pleasure—pain syndromes are rare except when associated with organic disease. On the other hand, a woman's genitalia bring both pleasure and pain within the extent of normal physiologic function. Menstruation, childbirth, and increased susceptibility to painful infection are examples of potential pain. There is little wonder then that a woman's pelvic organs may be ambivalently regarded and subject to psychic conflicts (Gidro-Frank et al., 1960).

Problems with ambivalence and conflicts over femininity and sexuality are frequently reported by authors who have investigated pelvic pain. The women's past histories are marked by a variety of chaotic experiences, and any type of stability would be the exception rather than the rule. The childhood family life was not secure, and the traditional two-parent home is found in a minority of the histories. Typically there was not a satisfactory relationship with the mother who is often described as strict, critical, and controlling and imparting attitudes that sex is nasty, unpleasant, and to be avoided. A striking finding by Gross et al. (1980) was that 36% of their chronic pelvic pain patients revealed a history of childhood incest!

Sexual histories of these pelvic pain patients indicate that the women were frequently rebellious in nature with many short but unsatisfactory sexual contacts. Premature and impulsive ventures in sexual activity often proved disappointing, traumatic, and destructive. The women report feelings of guilt about their sexual behavior and a high frequency of orgasmic dysfunction. Marriages, on the whole, have not been gratifying. The women are not likely to be satisifed in the role of homemaker, and their adult lives have been a continuation of their unstable childhoods (Gidro-Frank et al., 1960; Gross et al., 1980; Castelnuovo-Tedesco and Krout, 1970).

The psychiatric diagnoses of these women are varied, but severe character pathology is frequently present. Hysterical borderline, passive-aggressive, and antisocial personalities are frequently described (Castelnuovo-Tedesco and Krout, 1970; Gidro-Frank et al., 1960; Gross et al., 1980; Benson et al., 1959).

Women with chronic pelvic pain often eagerly seek out a physician who will operate upon them, and in one series (Castelnuovo-Tedesco and Krout, 1970) 40% had received a hysterectomy at the time of follow-up. However, following the hysterectomy other symptoms had been substituted for the chronic pain, often of a psychological nature such as pain.

Despite acknowledgment of severe psychopathology in their series of patients with chronic pelvic pain, Gross and colleagues (1980) were optimistic about the efficacy of "crisis intervention." They reported that 74% of their patients were improved or asymptomatic 6–12 months after evaluation, and they attributed this good result to the large amount of time spent with the women during the evaluation part of their study. Benson and colleagues (1959) found that about half of their patients with chronic pelvic pain were amenable to short-term psychotherapy, and of these half were significantly benefited by the treatment. Beard et al (1977) also reported that most women who accepted psychiatric treatment or sexual counseling were cured of their symptoms or markedly improved. Henker (1979) found that few women with pelvic pain remained in psychotherapy but those who did had a good symptomatic response.

Phantom Pain

Phantom phenomena occur very frequently following amputation, in almost 100% of patients who have lost a limb (Kolb, 1975) and in greater than 50% of women following mastectomy (Jamison et al., 1979). This sensation, that the body part is still present, is a normal process by which the lost part is mourned and the body image is reorganized (Kolb, 1975). One must also keep in mind that the stored memories for the lost body part remain intact in the brain, and therefore there is neuroanatomic explanation for persistence of sensation.

There are certain characteristics of limb phantoms, and their course over time, that are so common that they must be regarded as normal (Kolb, 1975). The phantom sensations are increased in the distal portion as opposed to the proximal portion of the missing limb. Typically there is a sensation of pins and needles when the neuromata on the stump is stimulated, but this pain is perceived as different than phantom phenomena or phantom pain. The person with an amputation may forget the absence of his/her limb and start to walk or move as if it were present. There may also be the sensation that the phantom is penetrating solid objects if the stump is moved in such a manner so as the missing distal portion would have to move through an object. As the phantom begins to disappear the more proximal parts go first. The great toe, thumb, little and index fingers are retained the longest. In general, this is in relationship to the amount of representation in the "homunculus"; those parts with the largest representation in the cerebral cortex remain the longest. There is, consequently, a telescoping effect, but this effect is never complete, and the phantom may be restored to its former extent when the stump is stimulated. When an acute illness affects the level of consciousness, there may also be a reemergence of the phantom. Most patients have the normal phanton phenomenon described; however, some patients develop a chronic pain syndrome which involves the phantom.

A study of phantom pain, following an amputation of a limb, disclosed that after one year 61% of the amputees continued to have some pain, although the pain was rated moderate or severe in only 30% of the patients (Parkes, 1973). The persistence of pain was correlated to the personality characteristics of the patient. Rigid and/or compulsively self-reliant persons continued to have phantom pain and their outward appearance of adjustment was more apparent than real, the pain being the tip of an iceberg of discontent! Other factors were also associated with a persistence of phantom pain. The pain was more likely to continue if the patient had stump pain during the first month after the operation or persisting illness with threat of life or remaining limbs after the operation. If the patient had been ill for greater than one year before the operation, persistent phantom pain was more likely to occur.

That phantom pain is not exclusive to limbs is demonstrated by a report of phantom ulcer pain following gastric surgery (Szasz, 1949) and phantom breast sensations following mastectomy (Jamieson et al., 1979). In regard to phantom breast syndrome, Jamieson and colleagues reviewed previous reports and described their clinical experiences with a sample of 41 postmastectomy women. Over half of their subjects experienced phantom breast syndrome, and yet the majority did not report their symptoms to their physicians! Those women who had phantom breast pain were those who did not receive much emotional support from their surgeons, who were younger, and those with a poorer relationship with their husbands. These women also tended to use more tranquilizers after surgery, to view their overall emotional adjustment as poorer, and to perceive their emotional problems as being due to the mastectomy.

Kolb (1975) has stated that the failure to adequately mourn the lost body part will result in psychological maladjustment. It appears from the foregoing discussion that phanton pain represents a failure to have mourned the lost part and to have accepted a new body configuration. The pain represents both the hurt of the loss and very concretely a denial of the loss. If it still hurts, how can it be gone? In addition, the pain represents an angry statement of the injustice of the injury. This is demonstrated by the fact that pain occurs more frequently in those women who feel less support from their husbands and surgeons. Thus the pain represents both the pain of loss (depression) and an angry indictment of others.

A suggestion that magical thinking about the lost part remains prominent is implied by the case report of an amputee whose "burning" phantom pain was related to learning that his disposed limb had been cremated against his wishes (Solomon and Schmidt, 1978).

The treatment of phantom pain begins with prophylactic measures. It is important that the surgeon communicates to the patient information concerning phantom phenomena and facilitates the patient's expression of emotions concerning the loss (Parkes, 1973; Jamison et al., 1979). The patient's wishes for disposal of the body part must also be respected (Kolb, 1975; Solomon and Schmidt, 1978). Although the surgeon's provision of a supportive relationship may be helpful, some patients will nevertheless experience phantom pain. These patients must be helped to express their grief (including anger) and work through the necessary changes in body image and lifestyle. The use of phenothiazines, tricyclic antidepressants, and other somatic treatments for pain may be useful adjuvants.

Low Back Pain

Back pain is one of the most common symptoms experienced; one study indicates that 18% of the population between ages 18 and 64 have persistent back pain (Nagi et al., 1973). The majority of these complaints relate specifically to the lower back.

With a symptom as common as back pain one would not anticipate that there would be a specific psychiatric illness or psychological constellation associated with it. Studies of large unselected populations, such as industrial workers, indicate no increase in psychopathology in those complaining of back pain when they are compared to matched controls (Crown, 1978). Yet when study samples are drawn from clinics or general hospitals, it is found that a sizeable proportion of these patients have psychic disorders (Gentry et al., 1974). Descriptions such as tension, anxiety, and neuroticism and diagnoses such as malingering, hysteria, and depression are common. This discrepancy between surveys of nonpatients and the descriptions of chronic back patients can be interpreted in the light of a recent investigation (Lloyd et al., 1979). It was demonstrated that psychological tests used at a patient's first clinic visit for the complaint of back pain demonstrated no predictive value in terms of persistent clinic visits. However, when those patients who were still attending the clinic after 90 days, continuing to complain of pain (approximately one sixth of the original group), were psychiatrically evaluated it was found that 35% of this group (approximately 4% of the original number) had a definitive diagnosis of depression. It was concluded that back pain is a common symptom that occurs in a very heterogeneous population. One episode (or clinic visit) cannot be equated with psychiatric problems, but for the small proportion of patients who have persistent symptoms a significant number do have evidence of psychiatric illness.

A demographic study indicated there were significant differences between those persons who complained of persistent back pain and those who did not. Persons complaining of back pain were more likely to be female, older, more poorly educated, more likely to also complain of anxiety, more likely to view their health as poor, and likely to have a greater propensity to utilize health services (Nagi, 1973).

A combined psychiatric–psychophysiologic study demonstrated that back-ache patients had generalized increased muscular tension. The patients were described as anxious, restless people who tolerated idleness and inactivity poorly. These patients were also described as basically immature, insecure, sensitive, dependent, and quick to react to life situations with intense feelings of resentment, frustration, hostility, humiliation, and guilt. Hostile feelings were withheld rather than being expressed (Holmes and Wolff, 1952).

Patients who have chronic back pain and objective findings of physical abnormality tend to have abnormal psychological test scores as do those patients who do not have objective evidence of organic pathology. However, those patients who have the more abnormal psychological test scores (on test instruments such as the MMPI) do not respond to treatment as well as those who demonstrate less psychopathology. McCreary and Jamison (1975) reviewed a number of different studies relating psychological test scores to outcome of surgery in back pain patients and conclude that there is "... a general and fairly consistent tendency for indices of psychological well being or 'adjustment' to be positively correlated with a good response to medical and/or surgical intervention in chronic pain patients." Responding to this indication to look for better predictors as to candidates for surgical intervention, a preoperative screening test for chronic back pain is being developed; initial results suggest that it is a useful technique (Hendler et al., 1979).

In summary, low back pain is one of the most common symptoms presented to physicians. As an isolated episode, there is only a small probability that the symptom reflects a psychological problem. With persistent complaints, the possibility of an underlying psychiatric illness, usually depression, becomes more likely. Psychological tests, particularly the MMPI, have proved to be of value in predicting which patients are likely to be benefited by back surgery.

Atypical Facial Pain

Patients with a variety of different complaints concerning the facial area are seen frequently by dentists, physicians, and oral surgeons (Harris, 1974). The type and location of the pain may vary. Patients may complain of painful eyes, pain over the mandible or maxilla, or within the oral cavity. Symptoms may include complaints of a painful tongue (glossodynia) or sensitive teeth. The pain may be unilateral or bilateral, dull or sharp, nagging or burning. Not uncommonly the pain had its origin in a minor dental procedure but then persisted and changed in character over time. Symptoms may persist for many years and be of a disabling extent. Multiple somatic treatments may have resulted in having had all the teeth extracted, nerve blocks or resections and a variety of other operative procedures with resultant iatrogenic morbidity (Lesse, 1956).

Facial pain is not always of psychogenic etiology, and the physician must be suspicious of an etiology such as latent malignancy. However, in one series, 42% of patients presenting with atypical facial pain proved to have a psychogenic cause for their symptom (Gayford, 1969).

Most patients with atypical facial pain are women and the age when the symptoms begin is most frequently in the decade between 40 and 50 (Gayford, 1969; Lesse, 1956; Lascelles, 1966). The patients are most frequently described as obsessional or rigid and perfectionistic. Typically they had been hardworking prior to the onset of their disabling symptoms. Depression is almost always associated with the symptom complex (Lesse, 1956; Lascelles, 1966), and it is not uncommon for the pain syndrome to begin after an important life event, such as bereavement, marital disharmony, or the premature retirement of a successful husband (Harris, 1974). That the depression is severe and that this is not a benign condition is demonstrated by reports of suicide which have occurred among these patients (Bebbington, 1976; Lesse, 1956).

Treatment for patients with atypical facial pain is essentially the treatment indicated for depression. However, because of the focus upon the somatic complaint, the patient may be reluctant to accept psychiatric treatment or referral. When treatment is accepted the results appear to be very favorable.

Lascelles (1966) indicates that 39 of 53 patients had a complete or significant relief of symptoms with treatment for depression. Most were treated with a monoamine oxidase inhibitor, phenolzine (Nardil) in combination with chlordiazepoxide (Librium).

SUMMARY

The complaint of pain is most likely the most common presenting symptom in a physician's office. On close examination the concept of pain becomes very complex. At different times pain may signal somatic injury or psychologic distress or reflect learned behavior. At other times it becomes a means of communication or a way to manipulate interpersonal relationships. Because of these multiple simultaneous functions, pain can best be conceptualized from a systems theory perspective rather than from any one limited interpretation.

The experience and meaning of acute pain is very different from that of chronic pain. Physiologic and psychological mechanisms reflecting anxiety are reflected more in acute pain, while depression and associated vegetative changes are more prominent in chronic pain.

Chronic pain appears to occur more frequently in some persons who have been called "pain prone." Factors implicated in this proneness to pain include difficulty in directly expressing emotion, prior personal experience with pain or someone who had pain, and personality features reflecting elements of masochism.

Some pain syndromes such as atypical facial pain and persistent phantom pain appear to be closely linked to depression and the pain may respond favorably to active treatment of the underlying depression.

In general the treatment of the chronic pain patient emphasizes changing the patient's perspective from relief of pain to, instead, rehabilitation to restore former activities. Multiple therapeutic modalities are usually indicated and may include psychological therapies (both behavioral modification and psychotherapy) and somatic therapies, including entities such as pharmacologic agents and transcutaneous nerve stimulation.

Chronic pain syndrome is not a specific disorder but, rather, a generic term encompassing a wide variety of abnormal illness behaviors.

REFERENCES

Beard, R.W., Belsey, E.M., Lieberman, B.A., and Wilkinson, J.C.M. 1977. Pelvic pain in women. Am J Obstet Gynecol 128:566–570.

Bebbington, P.E. 1976. Monsymptomatic hypochondriasis, abnormal illness behavior and suicide. Br J Psychiatr 128:475–478.

Beecher, H.K. 1956. Relationship of significance of wound to pain experienced. JAMA 161:1609–1613.

Benson, R.C., Hanson, K.H., and Matarazzo, J.D. 1959. Atypical pelvic pain in women: Gynecologic-psychiatric considerations. Am J Obstet Gynecol 77:806–823.

Blazer, D.G. 1980. Narcissism and the development of chronic pain. Int J Psychiatr Med 10:69–79.

Blumer, D., and Heilbronn, M. 1981. The pain-prone disorder: A clinical and psychological profile. Psychological profile. Psychosomatics 22:395–402.

Blumetti, A.E., and Modesti, L.M. 1976. Psychological predictors of success or failure of surgical intervention for intractable back pain. In *Advances in Pain Research and Therapy*, vol. 2. Bonica, J.J., and Albe-Fessard, D., eds. New York: Raven Press.

Bokan, J.A., Ries, R.K., and Katon, W.J. 1981. Tertiary gain and chronic pain. Pain 10:331–335.

Bond, M.R. 1976. Pain and personality in cancer patients. In *Advances in Pain Research and Therapy*, vol. 2. Bonica, J.J., and Albe-Fessard, D., eds. New York: Raven Press.

Bonica, J.J. 1974a. Organization and function of a pain clinic. Adv Neurol 4:433–443.

Bonica, J.J. 1974b. Current role of nerve blocks in diagnosis and therapy of pain. Adv Neurol 4:445–453.

Castelnuovo-Tedesco, P., and Krout, B.M. 1970. Psychosomatic aspects of chronic pelvic pain. Psychiatry Med 1:109–126.

Crown, S. 1978. Psychological aspects of low back pain. Rheumatol Rehabil 17:114–124.

Dansak, D.A. 1973. On the tertiary gain of illness. Compre Psychiatr 14:523–534.

DeVaul, R.A., and Zisook, S. 1978. Chronic pain: The psychiatrists's role. Psychosomatics 19:417–421.

Engel, B.T. 1959. Some physiological correlates of hunger and pain. J Exp Psychol 57:389–396.

Engel, G.L. 1959. "Psychogenic" pain and the pain-prone patient. Am J Med 36:899–918.

Ferster, C.B., and Skinner, B.I. 1957. *Schedules of Reinforcement*. New York: Appleton-Century-Crofts.

Flannery, R.B., Sos, J., and McGovern P. 1981. Ehtnicity as a factor in the expression of pain. Psychosomatics 22:39–50.

Ford, C.V., Castelnuovo-Tedesco, P., Goodman, S.J., Bustamante, J.P., and Long, K. 1974. Chronic pain in a victim of attempted homicide. Int J Psychiatr Med 5:283–293.

Fordyce, W.E. 1974. Pain viewed as a learned behavior. Adv Neurol 4:415–422.

Fordyce, W.E. 1978. Learning processes in pain. In *The Psychology of Pain*. Sternbach, R.A., ed. New York: Raven Press, pp 49–72.

Gayford, J.J. 1969. Atypical facial pain. Practitioner 202:657–660.

Gentry, W.D., Shows, W.D., and Thomas M. 1974. Chronic low back pain: A psychological profile. Psychosomatics 15:174–177.

Gross, R.J., Doern, H., Caldirola, D., Fuzinski, G.M., and Ripley, H.S. 1980. Borderline syndrome and incest in chronic pelvic pain patients. Int J Psychiatr Med 19:79–96.

Gidro-Frank., L, Gordon, T., and Taylor, H.C. 1960. Pelvic pain and female identity. Am J Obstet Gynecol 79:1184–1202.

Hammond, D. 1979. Unnecessary suffering: Pain and the doctor–patient relationship. Perspect Biol Med 23:152–160.

Harris, M. 1974. Psychogenic aspects of facial pain. Br Dent J 136:199–202.

Hendler, H., Viernstein, M., Gucer, P., and Long D. 1979. A preoperative screening test for chronic back pain patients. Pychosomatics 20:801–805.

Hendler, N., Viernstein, M., Shallenberger, C., and Long, D. 1981. Group therapy with chronic pain patients. Psychosomatics 22:333–340.

Henker, F.O. 1979. Diagnosis and treatment of nonorganic pelvic pain. South Med J 72:1132–1134.

Holmes, T.H., and Wolff, H.G. 1952. Life situations, emotions and backache. Psychosom Med 14:18–33.

Hudson, J.S., and Pratt, T.H. 1979. Pain clinics: Their value to the general practitioner. South Med J 72:845–847.

Jamison, K., Ferrer-Brechner, M.T., Brechner, V.L., and McCreary, C.P. 1976. Correlation of personality profile with pain syndrome. In *Advances in Pain Research and Therapy*, vol. 1. Bonica, J.J., Albe-Fessard, D., eds. New York: Raven Press, pp 317–321.

Jamison, K., Wellisch, D.K., Katz, R.L., and Pasnau, R.O. 1979. Phantom breast syndrome. Arch Surg 114:93–95.

Kolb, L.C. 1975. Disturbances of the body image. In *American Handbook of Psychiatry*, 2nd Ed., vol IV. Arieti, S., ed. New York: Basic Books, pp 810–837.

Lascelles, R.G. 1966. Atypical facial pain and depression. Br J Psychiatry 112:651–659.

Lesse, S. 1956. Atypical facial pain syndromes of psychogenic origin: complications of their misdiagnosis. J Nerv Ment Dis 124:346–351.

Lindsay, P.G., and Wyckoff, M. 1981. The depression-pain syndrome and its response to antidepressants. Psychosomatics 22:571–577.

Lloyd, G.G., Wolkind, S.N., Greenwood, R., and Harris, D.J. 1979. A psychiatric study of patients with persistent low back pain. Rheumatol Rehabil 18:30–34.

Loeser, J.D., Black, R.G., and Christman, A. 1975. Relief of pain by transcutaneous stimulation. J Neurosurg 42:308–314.

Lynn, R., and Eysenck, H.J. 1961. Tolerance for pain, extraversion and neuroticism. Percept Motor Skills 12:161–162.

McCreary, C., and Jamison, K. 1975. The chronic-pain patient. In *Consultation-Liaison Psychiatry*. Pasnau, R.O., ed. New York: Grune and Stratton.

Maltbie, A.A., Cavenar, J.O., Sullivan, J.L., Hammett, E.B., and Zung, W.W.K. 1979. Analgesia and haloperidol: A hypothesis. J Clin Psychiatry 40:323–326.

Marks, R.M., and Sachar, E.J. 1973. Undertreatment of medical inpatients with narcotic analgesis. Ann Int Med 78:173–181.

Meir, A.Z. 1969. General system theory: Developments and perspectives for medicine and psychiatry. Arch Gen Psychiatry 21:302–310.

Melzack, R. 1974. Psychological concepts and methods for the control of pain. Adv Neurol 4:274–280.

Melzack, R., and Torgerson, W.S. 1971. On the language of pain. Anesthesiology 34:50–59.

Melzack, R., and Wall, P.D. 1965. Pain mechanisms: A new theory. Science 150:971–979.

Merskey, H. 1980. Some features of the history of the idea of pain. Pain 9:3–8.

Merskey, H., and Spear, F.G. 1967. The concept of pain. J Psychosom Res 11:59–67.

Miller, W.B. 1973a. Psychiatric consultation: Part I. A general systems approach. Psychiatry Med 4:135–145.

Miller, W.B. 1973b. Psychiatric consultation: Part II. Conceptual and pragmatic issues of formulation. Psychiatry Med 4:251–271.

Moore, D.P. 1980. Treatment of chronic pain with tricyclic antidepressants. South Med J 73:1585–1586.

Nagi, S.Z., Riley, L.E., and Newby, L.B. 1973. A social epidemiology of back pain in a general population. J Chronic Dis 26:769–779.

Neubardt, S.B. 1973. Pelvic congestion. Med Aspects Hum Sexuality 7:12–20.

Parkes, C.M. 1973. Factors determining the persistence of phantom pain in the amputee. J Psychosom Res 17:97–108.

Peck, C.K., and Kraft, G.H. 1977. Electromyographic feedback for pain related to muscle tension. Arch Surg 112:889–895.

Pilowsky, I. 1978a. Pain as abnormal illness behavior. J Hum Stress 4:22–27.

Pilowsky, I. 1978b. Psychodynamic aspects of the pain experience. In The Psychology of Pain. Sternbach, R.A., ed. New York: Raven Press.

Pinsky, J.J. 1978. Chronic, intractable, benign pain: A syndrome and its treatment with intensive short-term group psychotherapy. J. Hum Stress 4:1721.

Prokop, C.K., Bradley, L.A., Margolis, R., and Gentry, W.D. 1980. Multivariate analysis of the MMPI profiles of patients with multiple pain complaints. J Personality Assessment 44:246–252.

Reuler, J.B., Girard, D.E., and Nardone, D.A. 1980. The chronic pain syndrome: Misconceptions and management. Ann Int Med 93:588–596.

Shanfield, S.B., Heiman, E.M., Cope D.N., and Jones, J.R. 1979. Pain and the marital relationship: psychiatric distress. Pain 7:343–351.

Shealy, C.N. 1974. Six years' experience with electrical stimulation for control of pain. Adv Neurol 4:775–782.

Snyder, S.H. 1977. Opiate receptors and internal opiates. Sci Am 236 (#3):44–56.

Solomon, G.F., and Schmidt, K.M. 1978. A burning issue: Phantom limb pain and psychological preparation of the patient for amputation. Arch Surg 113:185–196.

Sternbach, R.A. 1968. Pain: A Psychophysiological Analysis. New York: Academic Press.

Sternbach, R.A. 1974. Varieties of pain games. Adv Neurol 4:423–430.

Sternbach, R.A. 1978a. Treatment of the chronic pain patient. J Hum Stress 4:11–15.

Sternbach, R.A. 1978b. Clinical aspects of pain. In The Psychology of Pain. Sternbach, R.A., ed. New York: Raven Press.

Strassberg, D.S., Reimherr, F., Ward, M., Russell, S., and Cole, A. 1981. The MMPI and chronic pain. J Consult Clin Psychol 49:220–226.

Swanson, D.W., and Maruta, T. 1980a. The family's viewpoint of chronic pain. Pain 8:163–166.

Swanson, D.W., and Maruta, T. 1980b. Patients complaining of extreme pain. Mayo Clin Proc 55:563–566.

Swanson, D.W., Maruta, T., and Swenson, W.M. 1979. Results of behavioral modification in the treatment of chronic pain. Psychosom Med 41:55–61.

Szasz, T.S. 1949. Psychiatric aspects of vagotomy IV. Phantom ulcer pain. Arch Neurol Psychiatry 62:728–733.

Szasz, T.S. 1957. *Pain and Pleasure*. New York: Basic Books.

Taylor, H.C., Jr. 1954. Pelvic pain based on vascular and autonomic nervous system disorder. Am J Obste Gynec 67:1177–96.

Timmermans, G., and Sternbach, R.A. 1974. Factors of human chronic pain: An analysis of personality and pain reaction variables. Science 184:806–808.

Timmermans, G., and Sternbach, R.A. 1976. Human chronic pain and personality: A canonical correlation analysis. In *Advances in Pain Research and Therapy*, vol. 1 Bonica, J.J., and Albe-Fessard, D., eds. New York: Raven Press.

Woodrow, K.M., Friedman, G.D., Siegelaub, A.B., and Collen, M.F. 1972. Pain tolerance: Differences according to age, sex and race. Psychosom Med 34:548–556.

Zborowski, M. 1958. Cultural components in responses to pain. In *Patients, Physicians and Illness*. Jaco, E.G., ed. Glencoe, Ill.: Free Press, pp 256–268.

8

MALINGERING

"... it cannot be denied that medical malingerings and intentional fraud is on the increase; indeed at the present time it is being practiced to an alarming extent...." These words appear appropriate for the 1980s when physicians are troubled by malicious and mercenary malpractice suits and insurance companies are frequently defrauded as a consequence of claims for exaggerated disabilities. However, this statement was actually written in 1903 (Punton), and the author detailed many instances of medical fraud which had been perpetrated against railroad companies. Thus malingering and its attendant problems for third-party payers is a long-standing problem and by no means merely a product of modern times.

The terms "malingering" and "factitial illness" are frequently used loosely and/or interchangeably. There are, however, subtle differences in their definitions which need to be addressed when considering this group of illnesses. According to *Webster's Third International Dictionary* (1961), malingering is defined as follows: (1) to pretend to be ill or otherwise physically or mentally incapacitated so as to avoid work or duty; (2) to deliberately induce, protract or exaggerate actual illness or other incapacity so as to avoid duty or work. Factitial (illness) is defined as follows: induced by deliberate human action with or without the intention to produce a lesion or disease.

From the definition of malinering, it can be seen that a crucial part of the definition rests upon the motivation of the individual involved. But, because one person's motivation cannot be determined for certain by another, it has been correctly pointed out by Szasz (1956) that malingering is an accusation rather than a diagnosis. Malingering is found in those situations which offer probable benefits for the presence of disease. These situations in western culture are the military, prison or court trial situations, and industrial and motor vehicle accidents which have the potential of litigation.

Malingering is probably as old as history. Galen, in the second century, wrote a short treatise on simulated disease and means used to detect them. Included among the simulated symptoms were hemoptysis, hematemesis, and bloody discharge from the bowels (Adams, 1846). All military organizations have had to cope with the problem of malingering. It is of historical interest that during World War II the Germans bombarded American servicemen fighting in Italy with "friendly" instructions as to how illnesses of various severity might be produced by the soldier (Liddle, 1970).

THE DIAGNOSIS OF MALINGERING

Malingering can be divided into three major categories: (1) pure malingering in which there is a deliberate deception by the description and/or production of nonexistent symptoms and signs; (2) partial malingering, which involves the conscious and voluntary exaggeration of symptoms of a real disease; and (3) the deliberate attribution of an actual disability to an injury or accident that did not cause it (Garner, 1965). Pure malingering is more rare, while the second two categories are seen frequently.

A wide variety of symptoms have been simulated by malingerers, including blindness, mutism, deafness, seizures, confusion, paralysis, pain, and loss of taste. Sophisticated diagnostic tests for various disorders have been developed, and these can frequently determine that in fact the patient is either consciously or unconsciously simulating a disability. For example, tests are available to determine that a "blind" patient can actually see (Kramer et al., 1979), that a "deaf" patient can actually hear (Robinson and Kasden, 1973), and that a dyspneic patient is voluntarily restricting expiration (Morgan, 1979).

The determination of whether the patient is consciously simulating the disorder or is presenting with a conversion reaction is far more difficult. In many cases the differential diagnosis between neurosis and malingering can be made with certainty only by the confession of the patients (Spaeth, 1930). Yet, as can be seen by the case history offered below, even that criterion may be of questionable benefit.

Garner (1965) states that one may suspect malingering if the patient demonstrates a lack of real sincerity or if there is incongruity or a lack of completeness to the symptoms. Exaggerated symptoms, in an effort to prove their validity, may also be a suspicious sign. Malingerers are reportedly less cooperative and more defensive or angry with examinations than are patients with conversion reaction and less likely to demonstrate "la belle indifference." They are also careless about their symptoms and may readily give them up when no one is watching. For example, the mute patient reported by Miller and Cartlidge (1972) who supposedly had not spoken for two years was noted to engage in an animated conversation during the train ride home from his physician's appointment. Because of this inconsistency, which would not be typical of the patient with conversion reaction who is attempting to deceive himself as well as others, insurance detectives are sometimes used to document that the disability disappears at times convenient to the patient.

Psychological tests may be useful in providing additional information as to the possibility of malingering. Unfamiliar with the meanings of these tests, the malingerer may respond with exaggerated and/or unusual patterns which are not characteristic of either mental health or any known psychiatric disorder. Patients may respond to the Minnesota Multiphasic Personality Inventory (MMPI) in a manner which reflects an exaggeration of the corresponding psychiatric disorder (Hunt, 1973). Similarly, reponses to the Rorschach may be excessive in number and unusually colorful or dramatic (Exner, 1978). In a study of patients who had been previously diagnosed as malingering a psychosis, psychological tests were able to identify the malingerers over 90% of the time. Tests used included the Wechsler Adult Intelligence Scale, the Rorschach, Bender-Gestalt, and others (Bash and Alpert, 1980).

My personal clinical experience indicates that the MMPI is an easily administered and useful test in the detection of malingering. Patients strongly suspected of malingering, irrespective of the type of symptom, almost invariably have MMPI profile scores that are inconsistent with the clinical presentation (e.g., MMPI findings consistent with psychotic disorganization in the presence of a normal mental status examination).

It should be kept in mind, as has been noted by Flicker (1956), that malingering is a symptom *not* a disease. "Malingering should no more be placed on the part of the chart as the final diagnosis than is the temperature in a case of pneumonia or the gastric analysis findings in a case of pernicious anemia." Consistent with opinions of Szasz (1956), Flicker states that a physician has no special qualifications to decide whether his patient is guilty of fraud.

CHARACTERISTICS OF MALINGERERS

Flicker (1956), from his experience of evaluating military draft inductees during World War II, estimated that about 5% of the inductees malingered. Despite this estimate the rate of official diagnosis was very small. Of those men who were detected to be malingering, 10% had no psychopathology which could be uncovered. When psychopathology was encountered, it was found in the presence of psychosis, sociopathic personalities, mental deficiency, neurosis, fear states, and morale deficiencies. In regard to the last-mentioned item, it was notable that during the first weeks following the attack at Pearl Harbor, when anger was high, malingering was almost unknown, and then as enthusiasm for war began to wane, malingering once again occurred with great frequency.

A close correlation between malingering and personality has been described by Garner (1965), who states that those who malinger often have a "rather weak sense of social and group responsibility." They may be inadequate, asocial, or immature persons who had a tendency toward delinquency or other acting-out in earlier life histories. Other features may be previous lawsuits, difficulties with law enforcement agencies, or a history of excessive lying.

Kramer and colleagues (1979) reported that patients who malingered eye symptoms tended to be young (usually in second or third decade), under some pressure, particularly associated with employment, and to frequently have suffered some trivial ocular insult in the recent past. Ocular "hysterics" tended to have a wider age range and also frequently displayed "la belle indifference."

Malingering is often thought to be closely related to hysteria, and Cameron (1947) has stated that "...the difference between hysteria and malingering must finally rest upon the criterion of self-deception.... There are (many cases) in which pretense and self-deception are so intermingled as to make clear distinction impossible." Cameron goes on to say that whether a patient is considered hysterical or a malingerer, he is in need of therapeutic help.

Other physicians have taken a view of malingerers which is less psychologically oriented and interprets the behavior more as a crime than as a symptom.

The "patient" described by Punton (1903) illustrates a "con artist" who used malingered symptoms as a livelihood. This man had a "cane and screw racket" in which he used a specially prepared cane to lossen the floorboards of trains and street cars. He would then pretend to fall over these loosened boards and institute a claim for the injuries (malingered) which were sustained. He stated that he made it a rule to employ only the very best doctors because he found that they were the most easily fooled while at the same time the companies he fleeced were better satisfied with their opinions. He also paid his doctors' bills promptly (even when he thought them to be exorbitant) in order to impress his physicians with his honesty.

Miller and Cartlidge (1972) have also been impressed with pecuniary motivations of the malingerer. They documented how frequently and rapidly a patient's symptoms may resolve following financial settlement. They note that, although simulation of an injury to the nervous system is common in young men, it is more prevalent in middle-aged men who have decided that it is no longer worthwhile to work, especially in jobs where the outlook for advancement is bleak.

Bash and Alpert (1980) failed to establish any distinctive characteristics among their subjects who had malingered psychosis. They opined that the difference between those who malinger and those who do not is determined by the behavior of malingering rather than by any other characteristic. They also suggested that the simplest explanation of why some individuals malinger and others do not is that the latter are deferred by their fear of being caught and a lack of confidence in their ability to be successful in their simulation.

AN ILLUSTRATIVE CASE HISTORY

That malingering is a complex and potentially multidetermined behavior is illustrated by the following case history.

A 53-year-old married man was seen in psychiatric consultation during a hospitalization initiated by the patient's numerous neurological and abdominal symptoms. All symptoms were subjective, and there were no objective abnormal findings on carefully performed physical and neurologic examinations. Extensive laboratory and radiologic tests, including computerized tomography of the head, were also within normal limits.

The patient, as was disclosed in psychiatric evaluation, was in the process of suing a firm which he claimed had negligently allowed an overhead door to fall on his head causing injury. This, however, was only one of multiple litigations in which the patient was currently engaged. He was a self-made man who had overcome his deprived background through very hard work. His small business, which in the past had been very financially successful, was recently doing poorly. Personality characteristics included paranoid traits, and the patient always carried a handgun because of fear of others.

Psychological testing was obtained, the results of which demonstrated inconsistent and nonreproducible findings. During the course of the psychological testing, the patient's wife told the psychologist that the patient had confessed to her that he was malingering his symptoms as well as the psychological testing. This was motivated by a desire to obtain a large settlement in his lawsuit. She also stated that he threatened to kill her if she told anyone what he had said.

Subsequently, during hospitalization, the patient became very demanding of narcotic medications, which were refused by his physician. He left the hospital against medical advice and signed into another hospital. His new physician then proceeded with an exploratory laparotomy in order to investigate the abdominal complaints. The patient died of postoperative complications. The autopsy did not disclose any abdominal pathology, but an unexpected finding was that of glioma in the frontal lobe of the brain.

The retrospective psychodynamic formulation was that this man had utilized a minor injury on which to focus his vague and subjective neurologic symptoms. In an effort to protect himself from the knowledge and fear of real disease, he malingered unconsciously motivated symptoms in order to restore his feelings of mastery over the situation. His use of projection and his initiation of litigations were consistent with lifelong personality patterns. Thus his malingered symptoms under his control, and consciously designed to obtain financial rewards, were in fact unconsciously determined and served as a screen to protect against fears of a disease he could not control. Similar explanations for other persons with malingered symptoms have been offered in previous reports (Bustamante and Ford, 1977; Schneck, 1962, 1970).

THE MANAGEMENT OF MALINGERING

Recommendations for "treatment" or the management of malingering vary according to attitudes as to whether malingering represents an illness or merely "bad behavior." Cameron (1947), who viewed malingering as closely related to conversion reaction, recommended therapeutic help for both. A rather opposite viewpoint is taken by Miller and Cartlidge (1972) who state that it makes little difference whether the patients's symptoms are due to conversion or malingering " . . . since experience shows that, whichever label is attached to the condition under discussion, it is almost certain to clear up after (financial) settlement."

Garner (1965) suggested that psychotherapeutic care may be offered to the malingering patient and that such psychotherapy should be a modification of behavior therapy. With this technique the therapist does not respond to, or ignores, the pseudoillness. There is a positive response to those aspects of the relationship which suggest that the patient is contacting the therapist at a more mature level.

Techniques suggested by Kramer et al., (1979) in reference to the ophthalmic malingerer include the gradual and subtle inference by the physician to the patient that there is knowledge of the simulation. The patient frequently responds with spontaneous improvement. In military situations, a hint of a suspicion of malingering may be combined with information that malingering is subject to a courtmartial. In this type of situation, the patients often demonstrate spontaneous improvement. Yet another treatment technique for acute episodes of malingering, which is also based on behaviorial modification principles, involves isolating the patient and providing minimal gratification, e.g., no radio, television, or reading material, and minimal interpersonal contact. The patient deprived of the usual benefits of the sick role almost always demonstrates dramatic improvement.

The management of the patient suspected of medical fraud raises ethical questions. To what degree is it appropriate to "treat" a patient who is known or suspected to be a malinger, and how much of this information should be shared with other parties such as courts of law. Some physicians believe that when malingering is suspected, this information should be given to the patient (Naish, 1979) and that no efforts should be made to actively or passively collaborate in the efforts to deceive insurance companies or governmental agencies (Alexander, 1980). It has been suggested that in situations where medical evidence is conflicting and malingering suspected, a judge should use an independent physician (or panel) to determine disability, and that the physicians should be bold enough to state a suspicion of malingering when indicated (Robertson, 1978).

Making the diagnosis of malingering can be dangerous. Serious psychiatric illness can masquerade as malingering, and there is more to emotional disturbance after injury than merely a quest for compensation. In Australia, an accident litigant, angered by the reports of four different orthopedic surgeons that he was fit for work, shot and killed two of them and wounded a third before killing himself (Parker, 1979).

SUMMARY

Physicians may come in contact with patients who are malingering symptoms in their attempts to avoid military conscription, obtain financial rewards in personal injury suits, or to obtain justification for continued disability benefits. Determination that the symptom is indeed malingered is only the first piece of detective work, for malingering is a symptom, or as Szasz (1956) would say, an "accusation," not a diagnosis. One must search beyond the symptom in order to determine its purpose. Is it indicative of psychosis, a defense against awareness of an even more serious illness, the equivalent of a conversion reaction complete with symbolic meaning, or is it criminal behavior with the purpose of defrauding an insurance company? It is wise to not be too hasty in coming to the diagnostic conclusion.

REFERENCES

Adams, F. 1846. *The Seven Books of Paulus Aegineta*, Vol. II. London: Syndenham Society.

Alexander, E., Jr. 1980. A 'truth in mending' act. JAMA 243:1239–1240.

Bash, I.Y., and Alpert, M. 1980. The determination of malingering. In *Forensic Psychology and Psychiatry*. Wright, F., Bashn, C., and Richer, R.W., eds. Ann NY Acad Sci 347:86–99.

Bustamante, J.P., and Ford, C.V. 1977. The Ganser syndrome: A case report. Psychiatric Opinion 14(5):39–41.

Cameron, N.A. 1947. *The Psychology of Behavior Disorders*. Boston: Houghton Mifflin.

Exner, J.E. 1978. *The Rorschach: A Comprehensive System*. New York: Wiley, pp 303–313.

Flicker, D.J. 1956. Malingering—A symptom. J Nerv Ment Dis 123:23–31.

Garner, H.H. 1965. Malingering. Ill Med J 128:318–319.

Hunt, H.G. 1973. The differentiation of malingering, dissimulation and pathology. In *Psychopathology: Contributions from the Social, Behavioral and Biological Sciences*. Hammer, M., Salzinger, K., and Sutton, S., eds. New York: Wiley, pp 441–455.

Kramer, K.K., LaPiana, F.G., and Appleton, B. 1979. Ocular malingering and hysteria: Diagnosis and management. Surv Opthalmol 24:89–96.

Liddle, G.G. 1970. An artifice of war. JAMA 212:785.

Miller, H., and Cartlidge, N. 1972. Simulation and malingering after injuries to the brain and spinal cord. Lancet 1:580–585.

Morgan, W.C. 1979. Clinical significance of pulmonary function tests: Disability or disinclination? Impairment of importuning? Chest 75:712–715.

Naish, J.M. 1979. Problems of deception in medical practice. Lancet 2:139–149.

Parker, N. 1979. Malingering: A dangerous diagnosis. Med J Aust 1:568–569.

Punton, J. 1903. Medical malingering and intentional fraud. Kansas City Medical Index-Lancet 24:273–280.

Robertson, A.J. 1978. Malingering, occupational medicine, and the law. Lancet 2:828–831.

Robinson, M., and Kasden, S.D. 1973. Clinical application of pure tone delayed auditory feedback in pseudohypocusis. Eye Ear Nose Throat Mont 52:31–33.

Schneck, J.M. 1962. Pseudo-malingering. Dis Nerve Syst 23:396–398.

Schneck, J.A. 1970. Pseudo-malingering and Leonid Andreyeus' "The Dilemma." Psychiatr Q 44:49–54.

Spaeth, E.B. 1930. The differentiation of the ocular manifestations of hysteria and of ocular malingering. Arch Opthalmol 4:911–938.

Szasz, T.S. 1956. Malingering: "Diagnosis" or social condemnation? Arch Neurol Psychiatry 76:432–443.

Webster's Third International Dictionary. 1961. Springfield, Mass.: G & C Merriam.

9

FACTITIOUS ILLNESS

There appears to be an increasing frequency of factitious disease, and this increase may be related to the fact that much of the cost of medical care is now being borne by third-party payers (Shafer and Shafer, 1980).

Factitious disease is defined by *Webster's International Dictionary* (1961) as that disease which is caused by deliberate human action, with or without the intention to produce a lesion or disease. In general usage the term refers only to patient-produced illness, as opposed to iatrogenic disease. Factitious illness differs, in definition, from malingering in that the latter is determined by the specific motivation of the individual for some personal gain such as relief from military duty or the obtaining of financial compensation (see Chapters 8 and 12). However, self-induced illness often occurs in situations where the gain to the patient is not immediately obvious and the motivation is not understood by the patient. Factitious diseases may be consciously, willfully, and with deliberate deceit produced in such a manner as to confuse all, including the physician, as to their origins. They can also be produced in a state of altered consciousness (such as a fugue state), and the patient may not be fully aware of their origins. Those factitious diseases in which there is no effort to deceive the physicians (e.g., neurotic excoriations) are often not viewed as factitious diseases per se but rather as a symptom of another disease such as a compulsive neurosis. It must also be kept in mind that a symptom produced by a patient may not be acknowledged, not because of a willful attempt to deceive, but rather, because of the embarrassment of admitting to socially unacceptable behavior.

Because of these various circumstances in the presentation of factitious disease, there can be no assumption (unlike malingering where motivation is a part of the definition) that the symptom is motivated by overt secondary gain. As can be seen by the following descriptions of the more common forms of factitious disease, the secondary gains are often impossible to determine and the diseases are often secondary to severe psychiatric disorders.

Factitious diseases have been described for widely varying and sometimes rare disorders. The correct diagnosis may be missed for long periods of time because these disorders are not a part of the usual differential diagnosis. For example, it took 7 months before it was discovered that the parotid "tumor" of a young female laboratory technician was actually caused by injection, via a syringe, of saliva into various areas of the face, including eyelids (Keane et al., 1981). Factitious disease can also occur in children as evidenced by the report of a 10-year-old boy who simulated passage of renal stones (Sneed and Bell, 1976).

Numerous naturally occurring diseases have been simulated (Shafer and Shafer, 1980), but some syndromes appear to be more common or dramatic than others. Instead of exhaustively reviewing all of the various reports the following discussion will focus upon five groups of the more frequently occurring (and reported) factitious illnesses. These are dermatitis artefacta, factitious endocrine disorders, factitious gastrointestinal diseases, factitial blood dyscrasias, and factitious fever. Each will be discussed separately followed by a discussion of the common characteristics among the five groups.

FACTITIOUS FEVER

One of the most easily simulated (or artificially produced) symptoms in medicine is that of a fever. Because it is ostensibly an objective finding, one is not inclined to question its validity as an indication of underlying disease, and the person with a fever is usually immediately afforded the sick role.

Patients with factitious fever have varied in age from infancy (with parents manipulating the temperature) to 59 years of age (Rumans and Vosti, 1978; Petersdorf and Bennett, 1957). In one unusual situation an unethical private duty nurse falsely elevated the temperatures recorded on the patient's chart in order to extend her period of employment (Petersdorf and Bennett, 1957).

In 1957 Petersdorf and Bennett (1957) reviewed a number of case histories of factitial fever previously reported and described an additional 14 new cases who had "pyrexia by fraud." Twelve of these patients were women; of those, five were nurses. Also noted was that several of these patients had a history of other factitious diseases at some prior time in their lives.

Following the classic paper of Petersdorf and Bennett, there have been several subsequent reports of series' of patients having factitious fever. Herzberg and Wolff (1972) described five children and adolescents with fevers of unknown origin (FUO) referred for evaluation at the National Institute of Health (NIH). These children varied in age from 11 to 17 years.

The authors stressed the importance of disordered family relationships as etiologically relevant to the diagnosis and the importance of the need for the family physician to consider the possibility of the diagnosis of factitious fever early in the workup for chronic unexplained fever in an adolescent. They advised early psychiatric consultation in suspected cases and indicated that therapeutic results have been favorable.

Reporting on the adult sample from the same NIH study of patients with FUO, Aduan et al. (1979) indicated that 9% of the total study sample referred to NIH for an FUO evaluation proved to have factitious fever. Twenty-five of the 32 patients were female, and nurses and other paramedical personnel were disproportionately represented (16 had an association, present or past, with the medical profession). The authors stressed the frequent finding that the adult patients with factitious fever could best be described psychiatrically as having borderline personalities. This severe personality disorder (specific diagnostic criteria are listed in Table 1) is characterized by hostility, dependency, intense but unstable personal relationships, a poor sense of personal identity, and, not uncommonly, poor impulse control particularly in the area of self-destructive behavior. The authors also noted that their

---

TABLE 1. DSM III Diagnostic Criteria for Borderline Personality Disorder

---

The following are characteristic of the individual's current and long-term functioning, are not limited to episodes of illness, and cause either significant impairment in social or occupational functioning or subjective, distress.

A. At least five of the following are required:
1. impulsivity or unpredictability in at least two areas that are potentially self-damaging, e.g., spending, sex, gambling, substance use, shoplifting, overeating, physically self-damaging acts;
2. a pattern of unstable and intense interpersonal relationships, e.g., marked shifts of attitude, idealization, devaluation, manipulation (consistently using others for one's own ends);
3. inappropriate, intense anger or lack of control of anger, e.g., frequent displays of temper, constant anger;
4. identity disturbance manifested by uncertainty about several issues relating to identity, such as self-image, gender identity, long-term goals or career choice, friendship patterns, values, and loyalties, e.g., "Who am I?", "I feel like I am my sister when I am good";
5. affective instability: marked shifts from normal mood to depression, irritability, or anxiety, usually lasting a few hours and only rarely more than a few days, with a return to normal mood;
6. intolerance of being alone, e.g., frantic efforts to avoid being alone, depressed when alone;
7. physically self-damaging acts, e.g., suicidal gestures, self-mutilation, recurrent accidents or physical fights;
8. chronic feelings of emptiness or boredom.

American Psychiatric Association, *Diagnostic and Statistical Manual of Mental Disorders*, Third Edition, pp 322–323, Washington, D.C., APA 1980. Reprinted by permission.

patients tended to fall into two distinct subgroups. The first group consisted of somewhat younger patients who manipulated their thermometers after a genuine acute febrile illness, apparently for secondary gain. The second group was somewhat older and had serious underlying psychiatric illness (usually of the borderline syndrome) and created disease by self-infection.

Another series of patients with factitious fever has been reported by Rumans and Vosti (1978). This series of nine patients ranged in age from 10 months to 34 years. The fevers of the two children in the series were presumably produced or fraudulently reported by their mother who herself had presented with an FUO which proved to be factitious. Similar to the other series reported above, nurses and other persons with paramedical experience were disproportionately represented. Relatively little psychiatric information concerning patients in this series was available, but one patient had been psychiatrically hospitalized on multiple occasions, one had recently broken up with her boyfriend, and another was diagnosed by the psychiatric consultant as a borderline personality.

The means by which patients produce their factitious fevers vary (Petersdorf and Bennett, 1957; Rumans and Vosti, 1978; Murray, 1979). Common methods utilized have included fraudulently recording the temperature on the hospital chart, switching the thermometer and heating or rubbing the thermometer on the bedsheets. It is claimed that some patients can produce sufficient friction by oral or rectal manipulation to cause an elevated reading (Hale and Evseichick 1943)! Other methods include rinsing the mouth with a hot liquid before placing the thermometer in the mouth and shaking the mercury column upward. Other patients create a genuine fever by producing factitial disease by injecting themselves with pyrogenic materials such as contaminated urine, feces, vaccines, thyroid hormone, and tetanus toxoid.

One of the important reasons to detect the presence of a factitious fever as quickly as possible is to spare the patient the risks of potentially dangerous and disfiguring procedures. The factitious fever literature is replete with unfortunate and bizarre examples of repeated and extended hospitalizations, unnecessary surgical operations, biopsies, etc., all undertaken in the search for a genuine disease (Murray, 1979). It is remarkable what these patients will accept in the way of diagnostic procedures for an illness of which they themselves know the etiology.

In the effort to detect factitious fever there are a number of factors which should alert the clinician to this possibility (Murray, 1979). These include (1) unexpected physical findings such as a slow pulse and cool skin despite high temperature; (2) a healthy appearance and no abnormal physical signs; (3) essentially normal laboratory findings such as CBC and ESR; (4) lack of the usual diurnal fever patterns; (5) unusually high temperatures; and (6) patient characteristics, such as an inconsistent history, previous factitious disease, paramedical or nursing education, psychiatric history, or an apparent personality disorder.

Several means to confirm the factitious nature of the fever have been described (Murray, 1979). These include (1) obtaining simultaneous oral and rectal temperatures; (2) use of an electronic thermometer which gives instantaneous readings; (3) recording and checking thermometer serial numbers, and (4) measuring the temperature of freshly voided urine to compare with the usual method of obtaining the temperature (Ellenbogen and Nord, 1972). Another means of establishing the diagnosis, but one that raises significant ethical issues (see below), is that of searching the patient's room and belongings for material and paraphernalia which might be used to produce a fraudulent fever (Murray, 1979).

DERMATITIS ARTEFACTA

Skin lesions self-induced by the patients are not uncommon. The patients may admit that he or she has caused them or may withhold this information thereby creating a diagnostic challenge.

Factitial skin lesions typically occur in readily accessible parts of the body and in right-handed persons the left side is usually involved. If the physician "suggests" that they may spread to certain areas the lesions often appear within a short time in the suggested area. Details of the types of lesions which can be produced have been described by Lyell (1972) and Waisman (1965). The appearance of the lesions may vary; some of the types described include simple erythema, vesicles, bullous lesions, gangrenous or ulcerating lesions, and their sequelae. The lesions often have the characteristic finding of a clearly demarcated edge adjacent to normal tissue. If the lesion were produced by an initiating chemical there may be telltale streaks extending downward from where the caustic substance was applied. The extent of lesions may be considerable, resulting in scarring and disfigurement, often to the apparent disinterest of the patient. The diagnosis may come from discovering the patients in the act of producing the lesions, finding paraphernalia used to produce the lesions, evidence of drips or stains on the nails or fingers, or from a favorable therapeutic response to occlusive bandages over the lesions.

In their extensive review of the medical literature in regard to factitial skin disease Hollender and Abram (1973) found descriptions of 130 patients with factitial skin lesions. Almost 90% of these patients were women and two thirds of the women were under 30 years of age. Of the 97 women for whom the marital status was known, 70 were single, 18 married, 2 widowed, 1 separated, and 1 divorced. Thus the most typical patient was an unmarried woman under 30. In regard to etiology, the authors found descriptions of two major categories of persons with factitial skin disease. The first was a group composed primarily of men who were attempting to escape arduous or dangerous duty or seeking to obtain financial gain. The second group consisted mainly of women who seemingly used their disability in an effort to elicit attention or to elicit sympathy or pity. These women were frequently described as having hysterical traits or an hysterical type of personality. Hollender and Abram suggested that the motivation of the women who engaged in behavior to create factitious skin disease was determined by their efforts to (1) seek the sick role to avoid everyday stresses; (2) obtain gratification of dependency wishes; (3) seek sympathy or pity; and (4) satisfy their needs for self-punishment secondary to masochistic personality characteristics.

In a report of four young women with factitial dermatitis who were evaluated at the National Institute of Allergy and Infectious Diseases, Herzberg (1977) noted that the onset of the illness in each had occurred in middle to late adolescence. Each patient acknowledged having experienced considerable stress at that time of her life in the form of a major conflict over issues such as sexuality, career choice, or leaving home. Three of the four women remembered having been beaten by their fathers around the time of their menarche. In addition, all of the patients had a special responsibility in relationship to a dependent or handicapped mother or spouse which they resented, and as a result of their dermatologic infirmity no longer had to fulfill.

Young female patients with factitial dermatological disease have also been described in detail by other authors (Curran, 1973; Ackerman et al., 1966). The case history reported by Ackerman and colleageues is particularly dramatic and illustrative and is summarized here.

A 15-year old girl presented to medical attention with fever and skin lesions. The lesions were raised, erythematous, firm, movable, slightly tender nodules 3–6 cm in diameter. By apearance and biopsy findings they were compatible with a diagnosis of Weber-Christian syndrome. The patients's hospital course was stormy and lengthy. At times she appeared moribund. During the 11th week of the hospitalization a nurse discovered a syringe and hypodermic needle in the patient's bed. It was learned that the patient had been injecting 5 cc of milk subcutaneously in order to produce the lesions and ensuing fever.

Psychiatric consultation was obtained and disclosed the information that the patient was second of six children born to a family of a rigid authoritarian retired Air Force sergeant. The mother was a diligent but nonempathetic nurse who also took care of foster children in order to supplement the family income. The patient was expected to help care for these foster children. The patient made few friends but seemed to entertain herself with her vivid imagination. She also told untruthful tales about her family which resulted in family embarrassment and subsequent subtle rejection by the parents who regarded her as the "bad child." The father had become worried about the patient's interest in boys when she was in the eighth grade and had her transferred from the public school to a church school.

The patient's behavior during psychiatric evaluation was described as that of demure coquetry. Her thought content was dominated by themes of having embarrassed her parents and an intense desire to avoid returning home. Her predominant emotional tone was that of depression tinged with desperation. She was somewhat indifferent, however, to her disfiguring skin lesions. Because of her characteristic behavior, her extreme use of repression and denial and her maladaptive reliance on fantasy she was diagnosed as an hysterical personality. Her response to psychiatric treatment was not provided in the published case history.

A subgroup of factitious skin disorders is that of neurotic excoriation. The patients with this disorder have the compulsive habit of digging or picking at their skin. Although they may conceal the habit because of embarrassment, it is not usually with the intent to deceive the physician. The obsessive compulsive nature of these patients was observed by Zaidens (1951), who also noted that there was often repressed anger and an underlying depression.

A psychological study utilizing the Minnesota Multiphasic Personality Inventory (MMPI) to evaluate patients who had neurotic excoriations was completed by Fisher and Pearce (1974). Their findings indicated that the most frequent diagnostic interpretation was that of involutional depression associated with obsessive-compulsive and introverted personality features. The patients in this investigation were for the most part middle-aged and fairly well educated. The investigators interpreted the skin mutilation as the symbolic equivalent of suicide and also noted the high hypochondriacal preoccupations suggested by the MMPI profile. There was some suggestion that the patients might benefit from antidepressant medication.

FACTITIOUS BLOOD DISEASE

Diseases of the blood are often dramatic and also provide for the possibility of symbolism. Evidence of this interest in blood is the popular interest in vampires and Dracula and the use of popular terms such as "bleeding heart." It is therefore not surprising that disorders of the blood have been frequently chosen to be simulated. The two major types of factitious blood diseases are anemia and bleeding dyscrasia. Each will be discussed separately.

Factitious Anemia

A number of patients with factitious anemia secondary to surreptitious self-induced bleeding have been reported (Barosi et al., 1978; Daily et al., 1963; Ratnoff, 1980; Tattersall, et al., 1972; Victor, 1972). Of these only the reports by Daily and Victor offered detailed psychological information. The self-induced bleeding was produced by a variety of means but usually by a syringe. One woman used a knitting needle to lacerate her colon and thereby simulate ulcerative colitis. The degree of anemia produced was often severe and required blood transfusions.

Most patients with factitious anemia have been younger women, usually single and there is a frequent history of an association with the medical profession. Psychiatric information, when obtained, has indicated severe emotional problems; one patient had suffered a psychotic depression; one was struggling with strong feelings of guilt and hostility; one had "strong suicidal tendencies," and one patient was described as having conflicts in the sexual area and hysteroid defenses. Follow-up information as to effectiveness of treatment or the ultimate fate of these patients with factitious anemia is unknown.

Factitious Bleeding Disorders

A number of patients who have either simulated bleeding disorders or who have surreptitiously ingested bishydroxycoumarin (Dicumarol) to create a bleeding disorder have been described. In their review of the literature Abram and Hollender (1974) found 36 cases in which anticoagulents had been used to produce factitious bleeding disorders. Most of these patients were nurses or in some other way associated with the medical profession or had been previously prescribed an anticoagulent. Most were comparatively young women in their 20s or 30s. Agle et al. (1970) reported in detail on three patients whom they had evaluated for the surrepetitious use of Dicumarol and contrasted these patients with one who had taken the drug in error. The latter patient, who had developed a bleeding disorder secondary to a pharmacist's error, had no evidence of psychopathology. The three patients who surreptitiously took Dicumarol were all unmarried nurses, between age 27 and age 30. They were all described as having evidence of hysterical and masochistic personality traits and all displayed pseudologia phantastica. The degree of the patients' masochism was seen not only in the self-punishing qualities of their presenting symptoms but also in other areas of their lives. They seemed to seek pain and a variety of painful or denigrating experiences. It is remarkable that all described experiences of punishing, overtly aggressive parents, and each described associations of beatings with bruising and blood. Each patient described a bleeding problem in the sadistic parent and a remembered association of bleeding with sexual trauma.

One of the three refused psychiatric treatment, but some improvement in her bleeding disorder followed a confrontation and continued medical management. The other two patients were followed in long-term supportive psychotherapy; medications were used as indicated by the patients' affective states. The authors found that the provision of psychological insight was often followed by a weakening of the patient's control of her self-destructive impulses. With the suportive treatment program these patients have had no further bleeding, and they have continued to work within their profession. However, they have continued to be socially constricted.

FACTITIOUS ENDOCRINE DISEASE

The availability of endocrine medications has made it possible for patients to simulate naturally occurring endocrinologic disease by the surreptitous ingestion of these compounds. At least three endocrinologic syndromes of factitious etiology have been described to date: factitious hypoglycemia (simulating an islet cell tumor), factitious hyperthyroidism, and factitious pheochromocytoma. With the multitude of endocrinologic agents available it is likely that in time a variety of other factitial endocrinopathies will be reported.

Factitious Hyperthyroidism

A review of the English language medical literature disclosed seven cases of factitial hyperthyroidism. Diagnosis was established by either finding the thyroid medication that the patient was surreptitiously ingesting (Hawkings et al., 1956) or establishing, by measurement of thyroxine kinetics, that the source of the hyperthyroid state was external (Gorman et al., 1970; Rose et al., 1969). The diagnosis of factitial hyperthyroidism can be made by laboratory examination. The 24-hour ^{131}I uptake is suppressed with factitial disease and increased in Graves disease. Concurrently the TSH (thyroid stimulating hormone) level is decreased in factitious disease and increased with Graves disease. It is interesting that those patients in whom an external source of thyroid was proven within all reasonable certainty continued to deny their ingestion of exogenous thyroid. Despite their denial the symptoms of some patients abated shortly after they were confronted with the knowledge of the factitious nature of their disease.

Of the three patients reported by Gorman et al. (1970) two refused psychiatric consultation, a 33-year old woman, who had actually allowed a subtotal thyroidectomy to be performed upon herself, and a 49-year-old man. The third patient, a 63-year-old housewife, was described by the consulting psychiatrist as hysterical and extremely hostile toward her husband. It is of interest to note that the patient had made a small doll representing one of her physicians, and she repetitively punctured it with a pin.

Rose et al. (1969) also reported a series of three patients with factitial thyrotoxicosis. Again, none of the patients ever admitted their use of thyroid but the diagnosis of surreptitious use was supported by the demonstration of an accelerated thyroxine turnover. These laboratory findings were comparable to those found in a patient with iatrogenic disease who was receiving large doses of thyroxine. One of the patients with factitious hyperthyroidism was a 46-year-old married woman who had been the ninth of 17 children in her childhood home. Psychological testing revealed depression in an immature and constricted woman who " . . . would go to any length to avoid facing the emptiness of her life." The second patient was a 49-year-old spinster who had become depressed after the death of her father. Psychological testing revealed the intolerance of weakness in herself and the repression of hostile feelings which threatened to break through her control. This patient was ultimately an apparent suicide. The third patient was a 36-year-old married woman who was noted to be depressed and hostile. Rose and colleagues stressed the importance of depression in their series of patients and recommended that factitious thyroid disease be treated as if it were a suicide attempt.

Factitial Pheochromocytoma

A 27-year-old nurse was referred to the Mayo Clinic with a presumptive diagnosis of pheochromocytoma. She had complained of recurrent attacks of tachycardia, anxiety, diapheresis, and dizziness. Laboratory examination revealed elevated levels of catecholamines in the urine. It was of note that the urinary catecholamines consisted of epinephrine only, an extremely rare finding. The patient's room was searched and an empty epinephrine vial found. The patient then admitted that she had added epinephrine to her urine samples. She refused psychiatric treatment but openly stated she enjoyed all the attention that she had received from friends and physicians (Brandenburg et al., 1979).

Factitious Hypoglycemia

Possibly reflecting the ready availability of insulin, and the dramatic nature of the symptoms, there have been a number of reports of patients with factitious hypoglycemia. Symptoms caused by factitious hypoglycemia can be manifested by acute and severe neurologic deficits and proceed, if the blood glucose is sufficiently reduced, to coma. Factitious hypoglycemia is usually induced by the self-injection of insulin but can also occur with the surreptitious use of tolbutamine or chlorpropanide. The latter situation appears to be increasing in frequency and the hypoglycemia induced by chlorpropanide can mimic an insulinoma both clinically and biochemically (Jordan et al., 1977). Recurrent severe hypoglycemia attacks may be indications of an islet cell tumor and many of these patients have allowed themselves to be operated upon; one patient went so far as to allow a pancreatectomy (Service and Palumbo, 1974).

Moore et al. (1973) reviewed the medical literature in regards to factitious hypoglycemia and found a total of 16 patients to which they added three cases of their own. Of the 19 patients, 16 were women. Age ranged from 16 to 48 years. Most patients had an association with the medical profession (all three patients reported by Moore et al. were nurses) or had experience with diabetes, either personal or through their families. Features of the hysterical personality were commonly noted as were histories compatible with childhood emotional deprivation. The patients demonstrated denial, inappropriate nonconcern, blandness, ever-cooperativeness in search for an organic etiology, an uncooperativeness when the quest turned toward looking for a psychiatric etiology.

In the well-documented history of a young woman with factitious hypoglycemia, reported by Burman et al. (1973), the authors offered the following formulation. "Consciously or unconsciously, her highly dangerous game is directed against her father and her mother who she felt never cared for her when she was healthy, and against the doctors who failed to detect her emotional needs. The resentment against the medical world is seen in her efforts to fool the doctors and to place them in a state of utter perplexity and confusion."

The diagnosis of factitial hypoglycemia can be confirmed by several means. Often it has involved searching the patient's belongings and finding a hidden bottle of insulin. The placing of ^{131}I-hippuran into the hidden vial and then monitoring the patient's urine for radioactivity has been described as a way of confirming the diagnosis (Berkowitz et al., 1971). If the person is not a diabetic and denies use of insulin, the presence of insulin antibodies (after approximately two weeks of use) will disprove that history (Palumbo et al., 1969). Because C-peptide is secreted in equimolar concentrations with insulin it can be used as a marker of beta cell secretory function. Therefore if plasma levels of insulin are significantly higher than those of C-peptide an exogenous source for the insulin can be presumed (Service et al., 1975). Burman et al. (1973) state that the occurrence of apparently spontaneous hypoglycemia in a patient who had previously required insulin for diabetes mellitus should raise the possibility that the hypoglycemia is factitious.

A method of differentiating between an insulinoma and the surreptitious use of sulfonylurea is to administer tolbutamide. This should result in a prompt rise of plasma insulin concentrations if the patient has an insulinoma (Walfish et al., 1975). The determination of sulfonylurea in the plasma of a patient who denies taking the drug is also a simple method to determine the factitious nature of the hypoglycemia (Duncan et al., 1961; Alberti et al., 1972).

Risk factors for the possibility of factitial hypoglycemia include female sex, single marital status, medical knowledge obtained from experience with diabetes or occupation (e.g., nursing), and features of the hysterical personality (Moore et al., 1973). When these characteristics coincide with clinical manifestations of hypoglycemia, a factitious etiology should be suspected. The diagnosis can be confirmed by the use of a number of different laboratory examinations. A high index of suspicion will help to prevent unnecessary and potentially disabling surgery.

FACTITIOUS GASTROINTESTINAL DISEASE

There are two major forms of self-induced gastrointestinal disorders: laxative abuse and psychogenic vomiting. Self-induced vomiting appears to be increasing in frequency, and it is often related to anorexia nervosa (Beumont et al., 1976). These two disorders will be discussed separately because of some important differentiating features, but many of the symptoms of both syndromes are similar because the end result of either chronic diarrhea or vomiting is an electrolyte inbalance.

Laxative Abuse

Chronic self-medication with one of the multitide of ubiquitously available laxatives may lead to a number of potentially serious complications. In addition to diarrhea, the symptoms of chronic laxative abuse may include multiple other complaints, including abdominal pain, vomiting, weight loss, skin pigmentation, and steatorrhea. The bowel may develop melanosis coli and may superficially resemble some of the radiologic findings associated with ulcerative colitis. A metabolic disorder occurs in 25–50% of patients who abuse laxatives. Features of this metabolic disturbance are hypokalemia, sodium and potassium depletion, increased renin and aldosterone secretion, impaired renal function, thirst, muscular weakness, and edema (Cummings, 1974). Because of the combined gastrointestinal and renal symptoms a diagnostic puzzle may result and elaborate diagnostic procedures, including surgical operations, may be undertaken in an effort to identify, and treat, the patient's illness. It is remarkable to what extent these patients, who know the etiology of their symptoms, will allow physicians to proceed in regard to potentially dangerous procedures.

Diagnosis is difficult because of the wide number and different types of laxatives available. The easiest laxative to detect is phenolphthalein. This may be demonstrated by alkalinization of either urine or stool; a purplish red color then develops. Chemical techniques to diagnose other laxatives are either too tedious or unavailable for routine clinical use. It has been suggested (Cummings, 1974; Cummings et al., 1974) that a search of the patient's locker and belongings should be made in order to confirm a suspected diagnosis. This procedure raises serious ethical questions, which are discussed below.

Patients with surreptitious laxative abuse are usually women, and not infrequently have an association with the medical profession such as nursing

(Cummings et al., 1974; Kramer and Pope, 1964). Age varies widely, from the 20 to the 60s. The psychiatric disorders associated with chronic laxative abuse include hysterical personality, anorexia nervosa, and depression.

When confronted with the fact that the physician is aware of the factitious nature of the illness some patients may seek medical care elsewhere, apparently preferring to live a life of ill health. For those patients who are willing to continue with the same physician medical management includes making efforts to wean the patient off those laxatives, which may damage the bowel, and substitute a high fiber diet and bulk preparations for those patients who may fear constipation. Patients who have developed the pathologic features of the cathartic colon may require a colectomy with a ileorectal anostomosis. Electrolyte problems must also be watched carefully and if the patient persists in the laxative abuse it may be more useful for the physician to continue the relationship and treat the metabolic problems with potassium supplements and spironolactone rather than have the patient start the cycle anew with another physician (Cummings, 1974).

Psychiatric treatment of these patients, as with all patients who have factitious illness, is very difficult. If depression appears to underlie the disorder then steps should be taken to institute antidepressant treatment. The prognosis may be better with depression which is a treatable disorder than with the severe personality disorders.

Self-induced Vomiting

Vomiting self-induced by the patient appears to be a disorder increasing in prevalence (Fairburn, 1980). It is frequently associated with anorexia nervosa, but all aspects of the anorexia nervosa syndrome are not always present (Beumont et al., 1976; Palmer, 1979). Some patients, particularly women, may have learned this method of controlling weight, and it progressively became a habit disturbance. Techniques to induce vomiting may include ingestion of an irritating substance (Rich, 1979), using fingers or something such as a rolled paper (Fairburn, 1980). I have seen patients who have learned to induce vomiting voluntarily as a "learned behavior." Therefore any difference between "psychogenic" and self-induced is moot.

The symptoms which accompany self-induced vomiting are those associated with recurrent emesis, irrespective of cause. They include electrolyte disturbance, particularly hypokalemia, esophageal tears, weight loss, pulmonary aspiration, thirst, and constipation (Fairburn, 1980). Problems specifically associated with hypokalemia include anergy and lassitude, peripheral paresthesias, and cardiac arrhythmias. Patients with surreptitious vomiting may present themselves with complex metabolic abnormalities which mimic organic renal diseases such as Bartter's syndrome (Ramos et al., 1980; Veldhuis et al., 1979; Wolff et al., 1968). The diagnostic studies to which patients may submit may include procedures such as renal biopsy.

The diagnosis can ultimately be established by measuring the chloride clearance and establishing that the electrolyte imbalance is not of renal origin (Ramos et al., 1980; Veldhuis et al., 1979).

Patients with self-induced vomiting are usually female. Ages of the patients vary but most range from the teens to the 40s. To use the symptom to seek the sick role does not appear to be a universal finding because some patients come to medical attention only as a result of the metabolic side effects of the vomiting. Most patients have hidden their habit [to the extreme that one hospitalized patient kept her vomitus in a suitcase (Fairburn, 1980)], but at least some have sought help for the habit (Rich, 1978).

A series of 18 patients with "psychogenic vomiting" who sought medical care and who allowed a psychological evaluation (6 patients refused psychological evaluation) was reported by Rosenthal et al. (1980). These authors were not impressed with the severity of the psychopathology in their series of patients but noted that 3 (17%) of the patients who allowed an evaluation were diagnosed as having a unipolar depression. One of .two patients reported by Rich (1978) was also diagnosed as being depressed and was successfully treated with phenelzine.

The symptoms of psychogenic vomiting have been reported to occur at times of psychological stress and it was noted that the patients expressed an intense dislike for confrontation and disagreement. "Vomiting seemed to resolve the conflict by symbolicaly purging the anger." (Rosenthal et al., 1980) Sexual problems have also been described in patients with self-induced vomiting (Fairburn, 1980).

Reports of response to treatment have varied. A favorable prognosis is suggested when the patient is open about the symptom and seeks help. Efforts at treatment are much more difficulty when the patient remains secretive about the symptom (Rich, 1978; Fairburn, 1980; Rosenthal, 1980).

The following case history is illustrative of many of the features frequently seen in patients with self-induced vomiting.

A 35-year-old single career woman was seen in psychiatric consultation after being referred from an internist who had seen her following a syncopal episode. Medical evaluation had initially disclosed a serum potassium of 1.8 mEq/liter, and a detailed metabolic workup indicated that the hypokalemia was extrarenal. When confronted with this information the patient confessed that she engaged in repetitive self-induced vomiting. The patient reported that she had started to self-induce vomiting over 15 years previously as a means to control her weight: This was in response to her disgust of an obese sister. The vomiting increasingly became a compulsive habit. At times she would find herself under intense inner tension which could be relieved only by vomiting. To the psychiatric consultant the patient appeared to be 10–20 pounds under ideal weight, but she did not perceive herself as underweight. She indicated to him that she often received what she interpreted as favorable comments to the effect, "How do you maintain your figure?"

Personal information of importance included the fact that the patient was a devout fundamentalist Protestant. She had never married and had experienced sexual intercourse only once, while intoxicated. She expressed profound guilt over both her intoxication and sexual behavior. In addition she made repetitive out-of-town trips, at considerable inconvenience and expense to herself, to care for a demanding and critical mother who had been allegedly dying of cancer over an extended period of time. She was unable to express any anger over her mother's obviously manipulative behavior.

The patient indicated that she often felt tearful but could not cry and that she had a sleep disturbance. She appeared mildly to moderately depressed. Appointments for follow-up treatment were made but then cancelled.

In summary, self-induced vomiting, with secondarily induced factitious disease, may be far more prevalent than is generally recognized. Most of these patients are women who became involved with the behavior as a method of weight control. However, with the passage of time the symptoms appear to obtain greater psychological significance. Difficulties with sexuality and the expression of anger are commonly noted and the symptom of vomiting may be used as a symbolic expression of hostility. A minority, but significant percentage of these patients, have a depression which can be treated. The degree of psychopathology in patients with self-induced vomiting appears to be correlated with the degree of surreptitiousness that accompanies the behavior. Those patients who actively seek treatment appear to have less evidence of significant psychiatric disease than those who do not.

COMMON FEATURES OF PATIENTS WITH FACTITIOUS DISEASE

Although patients with factitious disease cannot be stereotyped there are recurrent descriptions which characterize many of these patients irrespective of the type of disease simulated. They tend to be female, usually below age 40, unmarried with conflicts and/or strong repressive mechanisms in regards to dependency, hostility, and sexuality. Their illness behavior is self-destructive, and there are themes of masochism running throughout their lives. They received little as children, were often unwanted and/or part of large sibships. In adult life many of them sought out careers associated with medicine but then through their self-inflicted diseases reversed the situation and entered the sick role. The one psychiatric diagnostic description appropriate for many of the patients is that of "borderline personality." One must keep in mind that despite their apparent cunning, they are fragile individuals predisposed to psychotic and/or suicidal episodes.

Some of these patients may be significantly depressed and the factitious disease behavior is a symptom of the depression. These depressed patients appear to have a better prognosis, with the institution of antidepressant therapy, than do the patients with borderline personality.

CONFRONTATION AND MANAGEMENT TECHNIQUES

The first step in attempting to establish a therapeutic relationship with patients who have factitious disease is to confront them with the fact that it is known what they are doing. This must be done prior to psychiatric consultation in order that the psychiatrist is not placed in the role of detective, thereby destroying a potentially useful relationship (Hollender and Hersh, 1970). Keeping in mind that the patient is indeed sick, psychologically if not physically, the patient can be approached with the tactic that the physician appreciates the fact that the patient must be very distressed. It must be acknowledged that the patient must be hurting very much in order to go to such lengths to seek medical care. A willingness to continue to work with the patient must be communicated in order to avoid feelings of rejection. In essence what is important is not to deny the patient's illness but rather to refine the patient's disease!

Despite the appealing simplicity of the above approach, unfortunately it is frequently not successful. There are three major directions that patients will take when confronted with the factitial nature of their disease (Abram and Hollender, 1974). (1) They may either deny or admit that it is factitial—refuse psychiatric consultation but then either stop or reduce the behavior which caused the disease; (2) they may deny the illness—refuse psychiatric consultation and then resume the same behavior with another physician or medical center; or (3) acknowledge the factitial nature of their illness and cooperate with the physicians in an effort to change behavior patterns. It is regrettable that the third option is probably the least frequently pursued— and as noted by Abram and Hollender, "Consequently the prognosis is often as poor as it is for the heroin addict who, despite an appalling cost, finds his way of life more appealing than any other."

ETHICAL ISSUES CONCERNING FACTITIOUS DISEASE

The diagnosis or suspicion of factitious disease almost inevitably raises several problems of an ethical nature. The first of these is the question as to how far should the physicians proceed in regards to invading the privacy of the patient. There have been recommendations that the patient's personal effects be searched in an effort to find paraphernalia which might confirm the factitious nature of the patient's problem (Cummings et al., 1974; Berkowitz et al., 1971). Over and beyond the question of a search is the fact that specific tests may be obtained, without the patient's knowledge, in order to establish the diagnosis of a factitious disease (Palumbo et al., 1969). Such tests may even include placing a radioactive substance into a patient (Kurlandsky et al., 1979) or into the drug that the patient is suspected of taking (Berkowitz et al., 1971). Such invasions of the patient's privacy or body could be regarded as inappropriate, unethical or even assaultive in view of the traditional doctor–patient relationship. To the contrary, it could be argued that the activity of the physician to establish a diagnosis of factitious illness is in the patient's best interest and by the patient's active seeking of medical care there is an implied consent for the physician to do all that is possible to treat the patient.

Another issue is that of confidentiality. What is the physician's responsibility to maintain professional confidentiality when the patient has sought the sick role under fraudulent circumstances. For example, can relatives, referring physicians, and insurance companies be informed as to the factitious etiology of the patient's complaints. A conference which addressed this specific problem yielded two opposing opinions (Ford and Abernethy, 1981). One view was that by violating the trust which characterizes the doctor–patient relationship the patient loses those privileges generally accorded the sick person. Another view is that the confidentiality of the doctor–patient relationship cannot be unilaterally determined by the physician; it is the patient not the physician who determines the relationship. If the physician is displeased with the terms of the relationship, then it is the responsibility of the physician to terminate the relationship.

Ready answers to these complex ethical questions cannot be offered. Each situation must be evaluated as to its unique circumstances and decisions need to be made after careful review of both sides of the issue. The resolution of the problem may be somewhat more clear when the patient is psychotic. An aggressive diagnostic–therapeutic stance can be rationalized on the grounds that the patient is not competent to make decisions and that in the patient's best interests a paternalistic relationship is necessary.

SUMMARY

The artificial production or simulation of a disease process is most likely much more frequent than is usually recognized. Some disease such as hypoglycemia or dermatitis are more easily simulated than others; a high index of suspicion should be maintained when the diagnosis is cloudy or the patient fails to respond to treatment as expected.

Phenomenologically the most common features of the patient who produces factitious symptoms are female sex, an age between teens and the forties, unmarried marital status, and an association with the medical profession such as nursing. There appear to be two major underlying psychiatric problems. The first which is less frequent and more treatable is that of an underlying depression. The second is that of borderline personality disorder. The latter is difficult to treat and requires a psychotherapeutic approach. Management of both types of patients frequently elicits significant ethical issues which have no ready solutions.

Factitious disease falls outside of the usual expectation of the physician; the patient overtly seeks treatment for a disease which is within the patient's control. The correct diagnosis, which may have been preceded by a lengthy and arduous evaluation process, often elicits anger in the physician. What is important to recognize is that the patient is indeed ill but that the disease needs to be redefined and a new treatment plan instituted. Unfortunately many of these patients would rather have the disease of their choice than accept psychiatric therapy.

REFERENCES

Abram, H.S., and Hollender, M.H. 1974. Factitious blood disease. South Med J 67:691–696.

Ackerman, A.B., Mosler, D.T., and Schwamm, H.A. 1966. Factitial Weber-Christian syndrome. JAMA 198:731–736.

Aduan, R.P., Fauci, A.S., Dale, D.C., et al. 1979. Factitious fever and self-induced infection. Ann Int Med 90:230–242.

Agle, D.P., Ratnoff, O.D., and Spring, G.K. 1970. The anticoagulent malingerer. Ann Intern Med 73:67–72.

Alberti, K.G.M.M., Oxbury, J.M., and Higgins, G. 1972. Factitious hypoglycemia: Chlorpropamide self-administration by a non-diabetic. Br Med J 1:87–88.

Barosi, G., Morandi, S., Cazzola, M., Ricevuti, G., and Ascari, E. 1978. Abnormal splenic uptake of red cells in long-lasting iron deficiency anemia due to self-induced bleeding (factitious anemia). Blut 37:75–82.

Berkowitz, S., Parrish, J.E., and Field, J.B. 1971. Factitious hypoglycemia: Why not diagnose before laparotomy? Am J Med 51:669–674.

Beumont, P.J.V., George, G.C.W., and Smart, D.E. 1976. 'Dieters' and 'vomiters and purgers' in anorexia nervosa. Psychol Med 6:617–622.

Brandenburg, R.O., Jr., Gutnik, L.M., Nelson, R.G., Abboud, C.F., Edis, A.J., and Sheps S.G. 1979. Factitial epinephrine-only secreting pheochromocytoma. Ann Intern Med 90:795–796.

Burman, K.D., Cunningham, E.G., Klachko, D.M., Bazzouri, W.E., and Burns, T.W. 1973. Factitious hypoglycemia. Am J Med Sci 266:23–30.

Cummings, J.H. 1974. Progress report: Laxative abuse. Gut 15:758–766.

Cummings, J.H., Sladen, G.E., James, O.F.W., et al. 1974. Laxative-induced diarrhea: A continuing clinical problem. Br Med J 1:537–541.

Curran, J.O. 1973. Hysterical dermatisis factitia. Am J Dis Child 125:564–567.

Daily, W.J.R., Coles, J.M., and Creger, W.P. 1963. Factitious anemia. Ann Intern Med 58:533–538.

Duncan, G.G., Jensen, W., and Eberly, R.J. 1961. Factitious hypoglycemia due to chlorpropamide. JAMA 175:904–906.

Ellenbogen, C., and Nord, B.M. 1972. Freshly voided urine temperature: A test for factitial fever (letter). JAMA 219:912.

Fairburn, C.G. 1980. Self-induced vomiting. J Psychosomat Med 24:193–197.

Fisher, B.K., and Pearce, K.I. 1974. Neurotic excoriations: A personality evaluation. Cutis 14:251–254.

Ford, C.V., and Abernethy, V. 1981. Factitious illness: A multidisciplinary consideration of ethical issues. Gen Hosp Psychiatry 3:329–336.

Gorman, C.A., Wahner, H.W., and Tauxe, W.N. 1970. Metabolic malingerers. Am J Med 48:708–714.

Hale, V., and Evseichick, O. 1943. Fraudulent fever. Am J Nurs 43:992–994.

Hawkings, J.R., Jones, K.S., Sim, M., and Tibbetts, R.W. 1956. Deliberate disability. Br Med J 1:361–367.

Herzberg, J. 1977. Self excoriation by young women. Am J Psychiatry 134:320–321.

Herzberg, J.H., and Wolff, S.M. 1972. Chronic factitious fever in puberty and adolescence: A diagnostic challenge to the family physician. Psychiatry Med 3:205–212.

Hollender, M.H., and Abram, H.S. 1973. Dermatisis factitia. South Med J 6:1279–1285.

Hollender, M.H., and Hersh, S.P. 1970. Impossible consultation made possible. Arch Gen Psychiatry 23:343–345.

Jordan, R.M., Kammer, H., and Riddle, M.R. 1977. Sulfonylurea-induced factitious hypoglycemia: A growing problem. Arch Intern Med 137:390–393.

Keane, W.M., Atkins, J.P., Perlstein, D.A., Gluckman, S.J., Faludi, G., Harris, J. 1981. Factitious parotid tumor. Otolaryngol Head Neck Surg 89:406–408.

Kramer, P., and Pope, C.E. 1964. Factitious diarrhea induced by phenophthalein. Arch Int Med 114:634–636.

Kurlandsky, L., Lufoff, J.Y., Zinkham, W.H., Brody, J.P., and Kessler, R.W. 1979. Munchausen syndrome by proxy: Definition of factitious bleeding in an infant by ^{51}Cr labeling of erythrocytes. Pediatrics 63:228–231.

Lyell, A. 1972. Dermatitis artefacta and self-inflicted disease. Scot Med J 17:187–196.

Moore, G.L., McBurney, P.L., and Service, F.J. 1973. Self-induced hypoglycemia: A review of psychiatric aspects and report of 3 cases. Psychiatry Med 4:301–311.

Murray, H.W. 1979. Factitious fever updated—Editorial. Arch Int Med 139:739–740.

Palmer, P.L. 1979. The dietary chaos syndrome, a useful new term? Br J Med Psychol 52:187–190.

Palumbo, P.J., Molnar, G.D., Taylor, W.F., Moxness, K.E., and Tauxe, W.N. 1969. Insulin antibody binding in diabetes mellitus and factitious hypoglycemia. Mayo Clin Proc 44:725–737.

Petersdorf, R.G., and Bennett, I.L., Jr. 1957. Factitious fever. Ann Intern Med 46:1039–1062.

Ramos, E., Hall-Craggs, M., and Demers, L.M. 1980. Surreptitious habitual vomiting simulating Bartter's syndrome. JAMA 242:1070–1072.

Ratnoff, O.D. 1980. The psychogenic purpuras: A review of autoerythrocyte sensitization, autosensitization to DNA, "hysterical" and factitial bleeding and the religious stigmata. Semin Hematol 17:192–213.

Rich, C.L. 1978. Self-induced vomiting: Psychiatric considerations. JAMA 239:2688–2689.

Rose, E., Sanders, T.P., Webb, W.L., and Hinest, R.C. 1969. Occult factitial thyrotoxicosis. Ann Intern Med 71:309–315.

Rosenthal, R.H., Webb, W.L., and Wruble, L.D. 1980. Diagnosis and management of persistent psychogenic vomiting. Psychosomatics 21:722–730.

Rumans, L.W., and Vosti, K.L. 1978. Factitious and fraudulent fever. Am J Med 65:745–755.

Service, F.J., and Palumbo, P.J. 1974. Factitial hypoglycemia: Three cases diagnosed on the basis of insulin antibodies. Arch Intern Med 134:336–340.

Service, F.J., Rubenstein, A.H., and Horwitz, D.L. 1975. C-peptide analysis in diagnosis of factitial hypoglycemia in an insulin-dependent diabetic. Mayo Clin Proc 50:697–701.

Shafer, N., and Shafer, R. 1980. Factitious disease including Munchausen's syndrome. NY State J Med 80:594–604.

Sneed, R.C., and Bell, R.F. 1976. The dauphin of Munchausen: Factitious passage of renal stones in a child. Pediatrics 58:127–130.

Tattersall, M.H.N., Hill, R.S., Tagoe, A.B., and Lewis, S.M. 1972. Factitious anemia. Br Med J 2:691–692.

Veldhuis, J.D., Bardin, C.W., and Demers, L.M. 1979. Metabolic mimicry of Bartter's syndrome by covert vomiting. Am J Med 66:361–363.

Victor, R.G. 1972. Self-induced phlebotomy as cause of factitious illness. Am J Psychother 26:425–431.

Waisman, M. 1965. Pickers, pluckers and imposters. Postgrad Med 38:620–630.

Walfish, P.G., Kashyap, R.J., and Greenstein, S. 1975. Sulfonglurea-induced factitious hypoglycemia in a non-diabetic nurse. Can Med J 112:71–72.

Websters Third New International Dictionary. 1961. Springfield, Mass: G. & C. Merriam.

Wolff, H.P., Vecsei, P., Kruck, F., Roscher, S., Brown, J.J., Dusterdieck, G.O., Lever, A.F., and Robertson, J.I.S. 1968. Psychiatric disturbance leading to potassium depletion, sodium depletion, raised plasma-resin concentration and secondary hyperaldosteronism. Lancet 1:257–261.

Zaidens, S.H. 1951. Self-inflicted dermatoses and their psychodynamics. J Nerv Ment Dis 113:395–404.

10

THE MUNCHAUSEN SYNDROME

A previously undefined syndrome, consisting of the deliberate seeking of repetitive hospitalization through the use of simulated disease and the association with fantastic storytelling, was initially described by Asher in 1951. He dedicated this syndrome to the memory of Baron von Munchausen, a legendary storyteller of 18th-century Germany. Subsequent to the delight-fully whimsical paper of Asher there has been a remarkable interest in this comparatively rare disorder. Despite objections that the eponym is in-appropriate, because it does not accurately describe the patients, the name has continued, probably because of its whimsical nature. Alternative names for the syndrome such as peregrinating problem patients (Chapman, 1953), hospital hoboes (Clark and Melnick, 1958), and hospital addiction (Barker, 1962) have not found acceptance. Case reports of Munchausen syndrome have come from all over the world and the yearly number of published articles concerning the Munchausen syndrome progressively increases. To the present time several hundred cases have been reported, some multiple times, and one patient has been immortalized by the publication of an "epic poem" detailing his history (Bean, 1959). Periodic review articles have attempted to summarize various aspects of the pertinent literature (Ford, 1973; Ireland et al., 1967; Pankrantz, 1981; Stern, 1980) but by 1982 the number of articles available would make a comprehensive review a Herculean task.

The question might be legitimately raised as to whether the amount of attention generated is appropriate, considering the rarity and apparent resistance to treatment of the disorder. It would appear that phyisicians are fascinated by these patients whose life goals revolve around their attempts to deceive. In addition to the published accounts of their often incredible exploits (and their almost unbelievable tolerance for uncomfortable medical procedures) the patients frequently serve as the subjects for comic relief in otherwise more tedious grand rounds schedules.

In a more serious vein, these patients are unhappy people desperately attempting to bolster their low self-esteem. Because their behavior is so dramatic and because it represents the extreme of a continuum of somatization behavior careful study of their psychological characteristics is worthwhile. Their behavior, and the underlying psychodynamics, often demonstrates, in bold relief, that which may be more subtle in other patients whose somatizing behavior is less extreme. Munchausen syndrome therefore may serve to teach us about abnormal illness behavior in general.

THE HISTORY OF THE MUNCHAUSEN STORIES

Asher dedicated the syndrome to the memory of Hieronymous Carl Friedrich von Munchausen (1720–1797), a retired German cavalry officer widely known as an entertaining raconteur. However, the name of Baron von Munchausen would have been most probably lost in history had it not been for Ruldolph Eric Raspe (1737–1794). Raspe, a highly intelligent, well-educated man was born in Hanover. He obtained a position as a curator for a royal museum but embezzled from the museum and was forced to flee Germany for the Netherlands. He later landed in England where he used his skills as a geologist before falling upon hard times. The motivation underlying the writing of the Munchausen stories is unknown. Apparently it was not for financial gain and they were originally published anonymously as a pseudoautobiography, *The Singular Travels, Campaigns and Adventures of Baron von Munchausen* (Raspe, 1948). The stories may have represented anger at a society which had rejected the author, but Raspe's biographer regards the stories as an exaggerated projection of himself (Carswell, 1950). Although it is unlikely that Raspe had any intimate contact with the Baron, it is certain that he at least knew of him because they were both from the same area, Hanover-Cassel.

Notwithstanding the circumstances surrounding their creation the Munchausen stories, fantastic and satirical, proved to be very popular. They constitute one of the most successful books ever written, and there have been numerous editions and multiple translations in the nearly 200 years since the first publication in London in 1785. An early translation into German caused Baron Munchausen considerable grief. He felt himself to be humiliated, and his privacy was lost as flocks of sightseers trespassed onto his estate in an effort to get a glimpse of him. He died a morose and embittered recluse, the innocent victim of another man's capriciousness (Sakula, 1978).

The irony of this history is that the syndrome is named for Baron Munchausen, a respected and honorable man whose tall tales were intended only as entertainment for friends. In fact the real scoundrel, whose antisocial behavior and peregrination was in many respects compatible with the "Munchausen" patients, was Raspe.

ILLUSTRATIVE CASE HISTORIES

Before proceeding to a review of the medical literature concerning Munchausen syndrome the following clinical histories will serve as an introduction to this unusual syndrome.

Comparatively few patients with Munchausen syndrome have been studied extensively, an understandable situation considering the nature of the syndrome. Even the information provided about those cases reported in detail must be questioned to some degree because of the patients' tendency to prevaricate. Family members may not be entirely truthful, and therefore information obtained from these supplemental sources may also be questionable. The two cases presented below were selected because opportunities were available to follow them over time, and there was reason to believe that the stories had reasonable validity. Case 1 was seen by myself over a period of years and has been reported previously (Ford, 1973); supplemental information was obtained from the patient's mother. Case 2 has been reported several times (Allegre et al., 1976; Bender, 1979; Justus and Kitchens, 1976; Justus et al., 1980); the last report was quite detailed and believed to be reliable because the patient had a terminal illness and wanted to make a "deathbed confession" (Justus et al., 1980).

CASE 1. A 24-year-old Jewish male was seen in psychiatric consultation at the request of the surgery service. He had been hospitalized for several days for symptoms originally believed to be due to a bowel obstruction; however, all laboratory and radiologic examinations had been normal. He had told the surgeons that the scars on his abdomen were due to an operation for a perforated peptic ulcer and subsequent complications.

Information originally offered to the consultant was that the patient felt "depressed" because of a recent layoff from his job, his inability to get another job because of his illness, and the subsequent repossession of his new car. He also stated that he had been taking pentazocine because of "regional enteritis" and was on probation by the court because of the forgery of a prescription for the drug, allegedly because he could not afford to see a physician.

The patient was referred to the psychiatric outpatient department but kept only two visits. In the months following he had three admissions to the hospital for acute symptoms. Once he gave a history of having Mediterranean fever, another time he claimed a history of porphyria, and the third time he was evaluated for a foreign body granuloma. Fevers in the emergency room disappeared when he was admitted to the ward, and on one occasion hematuria was shown to be due to self-inflicted trauma to the urethra.

Following his fourth admission to the hospital, he agreed to a transfer to the inpatient psychiatric service, and he was hospitalized there for two months. Records from other hospitals were obtained, and his mother was interviewed.

Past history indicated that the patient was an only child. He was born with a congenital ankylosis of the jaw which led to feeding problems and, later, a speech defect which provoked teasing from other children. The patient's father was described as a kind, indulgent, ineffective man who was often at home because of ill health and abdominal complaints. Meanwhile, the much more aggressive mother pursued a business career. At age eight, because of bizarre school behavior aimed at attracting attention, the patient was placed in a home for emotionally disturbed children. His father died shortly thereafter, and after the funeral the patient was returned to the state institution while the mother continued her career in another state. He was placed in a foster home at age 15 and engaged in acting-out behavior throughout his adolescence. After barely graduating from high school, he entered college but was soon dismissed for academic failure.

The patient then moved in with his mother, and they established a "love–hate" relationship. The mother provided for his material needs but constantly criticized him. At one time, she requested that the physicians "permanently commit" him to a state hospital. The mother's occupation involved traveling, and each time she left town the patient would feel "unbearable loneliness and fear." These separations served as precipitants for the "Munchausen" behavior. He was hospitalized at many hospitals where he told tall tales such as being an Israeli war veteran. He frequently flew to other cities and on two separate occasions had commercial airlines make unscheduled landings, with ambulances waiting, because of his acute abdominal symptoms.

Psychological testing obtained during his psychiatric hospitalization demonstrated superior intelligence and creativity in an immature, passive, ineffectual personality. There was no evidence of psychosis. The clinical diagnostic impression was that of a borderline personality. Past medical records indicated at least two prior psychiatric hospitalizations. At one psychiatric hospital, he had been diagnosed as an inadequate personality, and at the other he had been diagnosed as a pseudoneurotic schizophrenic, although it was stated that there was no firm evidence of a thought disorder.

During the patient's admission to our psychiatric unit, he managed to constantly stay in center stage. He once fractured a wrist in recreation therapy and, on another occasion, made a suicide gesture by taking an overdose of medication. He played various roles complete with costumes, such as a successful young businessman, "Joe College," or as a member of the country club set. Each role was complete with the appropriate mannerisms, and he stated that when he assumed different identities he could almost believe them himself at times.

Efforts to establish a working psychotherapeutic relationship with this patient were unsuccessful. He could not tolerate a close relationship, and acting-out behavior was prominent. He failed to keep regular outpatient visits after discharge. When seen again years later, he offered the information that he had continued to make trips on airliners to other cities where he would manipulate physicians into performing surgical operations. In the interim, he had had all of his teeth pulled, and, on examination,he had a classical "road map abdomen."

CASE 2. A 46-year-old divorced man with a well-established diagnosis of Munchausen syndrome allowed himself to be hospitalized and studied psychiatrically for a period of 10 weeks (Justus et al., 1980). Because of a diagnosis of chronic myelogenous leukemia, he realized that he had a shortened survival time and was anxious to "come clean" and relate his history. He cooperated in the obtaining of old medical records (which totaled 33 pounds) and permitted psychological testing.

The patient was born into a deprived home situation. The mother was a barbituate addict, and the father was an uneducated man who was extremely harsh in his interactions with the patient. At age 7 the patient was caught while setting fire to a building and was sent to a state school. While in the school he was hospitalized twice. Later in life he recalled the warmth and tenderness while sick as being a very positive experience.

He was returned home to the care of his parents when he reached adolescence, but his mother soon died of an overdose. He was then cared for by an overbearing, often irrational, grandmother. He left home as soon as possible and had a brief common-law marriage which ended when his wife died of leukemia. He then enlisted in the service and became a medical corpsman. To escape an unpleasant duty station he feigned appendicitis and had an operation. Later he began to use meperidine and he was eventually medically discharged from the service as unfit for duty "by reason of psychopathic personality without psychosis." He then married a woman pregnant by another man. Life was apparently stable for the next 5 years while he worked as an emergency room orderly and as a first aid man for a construction firm.

When the patient was jilted by his wife, he attempted suicide by narcotics. Because of his illicit possession of the narcotics, he was prosecuted and sent to prison for several years. After release on parole, he manipulated a return to the prison for four additional years. During his second prison stay, he developed new techniques to simulate conditions which required a general anesthesia. He described general anesthesia as an erotic and pleasurable experience.

Following the patient's second release from prison, he spent the next several years in international travel interspersed with drug, legal, and amatory problems. During the period leading up to his extended hospitalization for evaluation, the patient traveled incessantly, repetitively using ingenious ploys to obtain hospitalization and narcotics. At times he would impersonate physicians. He had developed chronic myelogenous leukemia but would not accept this diagnosis and instead insisted that he had leukocytosis secondary to filariasis, which he had reportedly contracted in the Orient. He had a total of almost 400 hospitalizations which involved all geographical areas of the United States. During hospitalizations he told a wide variety of untrue stories such as being a commander in the Persian Navy or being the sole survivor of a secret helicopter accident behind enemy lines during the Korean War.

Psychological testing indicated an IQ of 137, and the MMPI was suggestive of acute emotional distress. He appeared to be markedly depressed and anxious and to lack sufficient coping skills to deal with those feelings.

Toward the end of the reported hospitalization (Justus et al., 1980), the patient set up a situation where he knew he would once again be rejected, and he then left the hospital. No doubt there will be subsequent published reports of his history when he resurfaces someplace new.

Comment. Each of these case histories illustrates a chaotic childhood, early experience with disease and/or death, institutionalization during childhood, antisocial behavior, an emphasis on deceiving people, and compulsive traveling with repetitive hospitalizations during adult life, Neither patient was judged to be psychotic, yet the behavior of each was, to say the least, bizarre. The following review of the literature will further detail the phenomenology of the syndrome, proposed etiologies, and suggestions for strategies of management.

DIAGNOSTIC CRITERIA

The original description of the Munchausen syndrome by Asher (1951) defined three major characteristics of these patients, malingered or simulated diseases, pseudologia fantastica (pathological lying), and peregrination (traveling). These features have persisted as the major criteria for the syndrome, although there have been no official diagnostic criteria, and the most recent edition of the American Psychiatric Association's Diagnostic and Statistical Manual III (DSM III) lists only "chronic factitial disorder" (1980).

Many of the reported cases of patients who have been called "Munchausen" do not meet the tripartite diagnostic criteria listed above. It would appear that the Munchausen behavior is a continuum and only the more extreme cases have the features of grandiosity with pseudologic fantastica, the wide travels and the dramatic presentation of a simulated rare disease. It has been appropriately noted by Chertok (1972) that study of both the classic cases and variants of the syndrome are equally helpful in the attempt to understand the complex issues of malingering and factitious illness.

It must also be noted that these patients often have genuine diseases and/or "hard" physical findings which facilitate their capacity for dramatic presentations in hospital emergency rooms. At times these diseases can be life-threatening and require active medical intervention (Justus et al., 1980). In his original description Asher (1951) was quick to point out that the patient's stories were a "... matrix of fantasy and falsehood in which fragments of complete truth are surprisingly imbedded." Similarly he noted that not all of the patients' symptoms are entirely false and the "... patients are often quite ill although their illness is shrouded by duplicity and distortion."

No one underlying psychiatric diagnosis typifies the Munchausen patient. Among those diagnoses which have been assigned to these patients are schizophrenia and various types of personality disorders, including sociopathic (psychopathic), inadequate, hysterical, and borderline. The borderline personality description appears to be particularly apt for most of these patients (Nadelson, 1979). The borderline personality is often associated with a history of chaotic, inconsistent childhood. It can be described by the characteristics of low ego strength, poorly modulated emotional responses, high charged conflict interpersonal relationships, and on occasion brief reactive psychotic episodes. (The diagnostic criteria for the borderline personality disorder are included in Chapter 9.)

A useful suggestion has been made by Ries (1980) that the diagnostic system used by DSM-III is particularly useful in describing patients who have Munchausen syndrome characteristics. This diagnostic system employs 5 separate axes which include I, the diagnosis of a specific psychiatric disorder, e.g., chronic factitious disorder; II, developmental or personality characteristics which may have influenced the psychiatric disorder, e.g., borderline personality; III, the presence of important concurrent physical conditions which are relevant to understanding the patient, e.g., pseudo-seizures and congenital nystagmus; IV, psychosocial stresses, e.g., separation from husband; and V, the highest level of adaptive functioning during the previous year, e.g., poor, no employment, and very limited interpersonal relationships.

THE PHENOMENOLOGY OF MUNCHAUSEN SYNDROME

Demographic Features and Incidence

The majority of case reports describing the Munchausen syndrome have been from Great Britain and the United States, although patients from many other countries have also been described. Most of the patients who have been reported have been white, but at least two black men with Munchausen syndrome have also been reported (Jones et al., 1978; Puzzuoli, 1978).

The sex ratio is that there are approximately twice as many men as women (Pankratz, 1981). The age distribution has been from childhood to over 60 years of age. Average ages as computed by Pankratz (1981) are approximately 40 for men and approximately 30 for women. Patients have frequently worked in the medical care area in some capacity, most frequently as nurses, laboratory technicians, or orderlies. They are most often described as very intelligent and clever, although their work histories are not compatible with their apparent talents (see below). The exact incidence is unknown, but several hundred cases have been described in the literature. The Psychiatric Consultation Service of Vanderbilt Hospital (585 beds) sees, on the average, approximately two patients with this diagnosis per year.

Presenting Symptoms

The Munchausen patient typically presents to the emergency rooms of hospitals (often large teaching hospitals) with dramatic symptoms in their need for immediate attention (e.g., symptoms compatible with myocardial infarction) or which are inclined to stimulate the interest and curiosity of the physician, such as those symptoms which might suggest acute intermittent porphyria. Usually the visit to the emergency room is made at those times, such as evenings or weekends, when access to senior staff and medical records may be more difficult. Once established upon the ward, the Munchausen patient usually becomes the "star patient" or "fascinoma" and thereby obtains a disproportionate amount of the health care team's time. The stories that these patients tell make them more interesting and also serve to achieve a greater sense of involvement with the staff. For example, one patient might give a history of fighting in the Israeli war for independence, being captured and tortured by the Arabs (Ford, 1973), and another may tell of being a foreign university president on his way back to his country (Jones et al., 1978). The stories and their variations are often chosen with an almost uncanny capacity to interest and engage the caretakers, and the patients play their roles remarkably well.

Discovery of the factitious nature of the complaint may occur when (1) diagnostic tests are all negative and sophisticated laboratory techniques establish that the complaints are not medically possible, or (2) when a visiting physician or house officer recognizes the patient from a prior admission at another hospital. When the hoax is eventually discovered and confrontation takes place, the patients often refuse psychiatric evaluation, react with indignity or anger, sign out of the hospital against medical advice (AMA) and/or frequently threaten to sue the hospital and physicians because of the "unfair" accusations.

Following discharge, the patient then disappears only to resurface, usually with another name, at another hospital. Because of the speed of air travel, the patient may be admitted within a few hours to another hospital hundreds or thousands of miles away (Justus et al., 1980). The peregrination of these patients may be extreme with their making numerous trips crisscrossing the country. Over a "career" the number of hospitalizations may total 400 or more (Justus et al., 1980; von Maur et al., 1973). This traveling serves to help disguise the patient's behavior, but it should also be noted that compulsive traveling has been associated with underlying depression (Stengel, 1939).

The different symptoms patients use to gain admission to hospitals are notable for their ingenuity. The patients may also incorporate an incidental but genuine physical finding in order to be even more convincing. For example, one patient used congenital nystagmus as a finding which made his symptoms and complaints of head trauma an indication for acute hospitalization (Ford, 1982). The original symptom groups of Asher (1951), the acute abdominal type, the hemorrhagic type and the neurologic type, have been greatly expanded by these resourceful impersonators. At the present time, essentially every subspecialty journal has recorded at least one patient who has simulated illness in that field. Diseases which have been simulated or factitially produced include, in addition to the original groups, hyperpyrexia and fevers of unknown origin (Ferguson and Maki, 1978; Ford, 1973;

Michaels et al., 1964), chest pain suggestion of acute myocardial infarction (Bagan, 1962; Bursten, 1965; Cavenar et al., 1980; Mayer, 1978; Puzzuoli, 1978), tuberculosis (Griffith, 1961), caisson disease (Kemp and Munro, 1969), acute allergic emergencies (Hendrix et al., 1981) filariasis (Justus et al., 180), porphyria (Williams, 1961), hypercalcemia (Frame et al., 1981), septic arthritis (Paperny et al., 1980), and trophoblastic disease (Board and Hammond, 1980).

One symptom complex, that referrable to kidney stones, appears to be a particularly popular choice of these patients (Atkinson and Earll, 1974, Carrodus and Earlom, 1971; Jones et al., 1978; Laudadio et al., 1979; Sharon and Diamond, 1974; Sneed and Bell, 1976). Perhaps this is because the pain of renal calculi has a classic, easily recognized pattern, is known to be severe, requires acute treatment, and it is relatively easy to produce apparently objective findings (e.g., hematuris and actual stones). I have seen two different patients who simulated the acute distress of a kidney stone using the settings of being aboard transcontinental airliners to create unusually dramatic productions. In each instance, the airliner made an emergency unscheduled landing, with ambulance waiting, in order that the "patient" could be rushed to a hospital!

In general there is no apparent symbolic significance to the choice of the simulated disease, and different symptoms and organ systems have been used by the same patient at different times (Ford, 1973; Yassa, 1978). However, as a rule the patient develops a "routine" and will present with similar symptoms and offer a similar history at the various hospitals which he visits. A typical patient is the man reported by von Maur and colleages (1973). The *modus operandi* of this man is to appear at hospital emergency rooms with complaints of epigastric pain and hematemesis or with seizures (he has an abnormal EEG). At the time of the report, this man had been hospitalized 423 times and had received at least 102 upper GI series.

Although the Munchausen patient typically uses physical symptoms to gain admission to hospitals, there have also been situations where these patients have presented with a variety of psychiatric symptoms (Cheng and Hummel, 1978; Gelenberg, 1977; Snowdon et al., 1978). One subgroup of these patients is that of feigned bereavement; they have just lost a close relative by death and are depressed. This history, as can be imagined, elicits considerable sympathy.

Another very interesting symptomatic presentation is a recent report of a man with "pseudo-Munchausen syndrome" (Gurwith and Langston, 1980). This man presented himself to a hospital complaining that he suffered from Munchausen syndrome and demanding admission. He claimed that he had mimicked medical conditions and had received surgical operations, chemotherapy for simulated cancer, and ECT for pretended depression. Scars on his abdomen proved to be superficial discolorations that could be removed by soap and water. Contact with other physicians, whom he claimed had treated him in the past, yielded the information that he was unknown to them. The physicians did not give in to his hints that they should search his room but instead confronted him with the factitious nature of his Munchausen syndrome. The patient left the hospital AMA with his physicians opining that his pseudo-self-abuse to be a more desirable psychologic adaptive mechanism than the genuine self-abuse of true factitious disease.

Childhood Histories of Munchausen Patients

Detailed, accurate past histories are difficult to obtain in these prevaricating patients. However, information frequently offered or obtained from auxillary sources, is that the patients had markedly emotionally deprived childhoods. One frequently hears that the patient was physically abused or otherwise mistreated (Barker, 1962; Bursten, 1965; Cramer et al., 1971; Ford, 1973; Friedmann and Weinstein, 1976; George and Cheatham, 1965; Justus et al., 1980; Ries, 1980), one or both parents had serious illnesses or died (Bursten, 1965; Cheng and Hummel, 1978; Cramer et al., 1971; Ford, 1973; Friedmann and Weinstein, 1976; George and Cheatham, 1965; Hale, 1966; Justus et al., 1980; Sapira, 1981; Steinbeck, 1961; Stone, 1977), institutionalization in orphanages or other settings such as reform school was required (Barker, 1962; Bursten, 1965; Cramer et al., 1971; Ford, 1973; Friedmann and Weinstein, 1976; George and Cheatham, 1965; Justus et al., 1980; Ries, 1980), and that there was reported delinquency or bizarre behavioral patterns (Barker, 1962; Bursten, 1965; Ford, 1973; George and Cheatham, 1965; Hale, 1966; Hoyer, 1959; Justus et al., 1980; Stone, 1977; Wimberly, 1981). Frequently someone in the medical profession served as an important relationship during childhood (Cramer et al., 1971).

In summary the childhoods of these patients are characterized by chaotic life situations often associated with disease or physical abuse.

Adult Adjustment

Despite their self-reported exploits and grandiose self-descriptions, these patients have on the whole failed to have made a mature adult adjustment. Work histories are poor, but if the patient worked at all, it is likely that it has been in some area of health services such as nursing or as a medical corpsman (Blackwell, 1965; Cramer et al., 1971; Ford, 1973; Frame et al., 1981; Hoyer, 1959; Justus et al., 1980; Nadelson, 1979; Wise and Shuttleworth, 1978). Marriages, if existent at all, have been brief and/or turbulent (Ford, 1973; Justus et al., 1980; Stone, 1977). The patients have frequently had legal difficulties particularly in the area of narcotics offenses (Ananth, 1977; Barker, 1962; Blackwell, 1965; Chugh, 1966; Cramer et al., 1971; Ford, 1973; Friedmann and Weinstein, 1976; Justus et al., 1980; Steinbeck, 1961; Wimberly, 1981) and may have been imprisoned (Justus et al., 1980; Wimberly, 1981). A history of one or more psychiatric hospitalizations is common as well as a history of suicidal attempts (Barker, 1962; Blackwell, 1965; Bursten, 1965; Cheng and Hummel, 1978; Cramer et al., 1971; Ford, 1973; George and Cheatham, 1965; Hale, 1966; Hoyer, 1959; Justus et al., 1980; Stone, 1977).

In summary, a pattern of repetitive maladjustive behavior has characterized these patients' adult lives.

ETIOLOGIC EXPLANATIONS FOR THE MUNCHAUSEN SYNDROME

In their efforts to understand what appears on the surface to be incomprehensible behavior many authors have speculated as to the conscious and unconscious motives of these patients' self-destructive behavior. A critical review of the various motivations which have been proposed includes the following.

A Desire for Free Board and Lodging

This most obvious explanation may be the least probable. Although board and room may be obtained in the bargain, the price, in terms of painful procedures, seems rather high. In addition, most derelicts have little difficulty obtaining more comfortable accommodations at organizations such as the Salvation Army. However, in a more abstract way, a hospital may come to symbolize home and the nurturing nurses as mothers (Justus et al., 1980).

An Effort to Escape from the Police and/or Incarceration

It is more understandable why someone might subject themselves to hospitalization to avoid jail, but there is little evidence that this is a common motivation. Some reports, however, suggest that in individual cases this may be a significant etiologic factor (Ananth, 1977; Bursten, 1965; Friedmann and Weinstein, 1976; Vail, 1962).

Narcotic Addiction

Malingering symptoms in order to obtain access to narcotics is an apparently reasonable explanation for the syndrome. Although withdrawal symptoms have not been described in these patients, with the possible exception of the case reported by Puzzuoli (1978), Mendel (1974) has stressed that a large number of these patients have been narcotic users, and he believes that the Munchausen behavior should be considered a syndrome of drug abuse. However, my personal experience does not support the idea that these patients on the whole are addicts. Rather their surreptitious efforts to obtain narcotics may be motivated more by their need to deceive physicians than the end result, namely, the narcotics themselves.

A Desire to Be the Center of Attention

This explanation described in the initial report by Asher (1951) suggested that patients may be engaged in a reversal of the "Walter Mitty" syndrome. Instead of playing the dramatic role of the surgeon, they submit to the equally dramatic role of the patient. Asher does not speculate as to whether this may be conscious or unconscious motivation. Certainly the patients have the ability to manipulate staff in such a manner that they either become the "star" patient or the focus of anxious concern.

Organic Brain Disorders

Organic brain dysfunction has been postulated to be the cause of the Munchausen behavior in at least some patients (Ireland et al., 1967; Pankratz, 1981). The patient reported by Pankratz had evidence of severe problems with perceptual organization despite adequate verbal intelligence. Although some patients on careful testing may demonstrate a defect in cognitive functioning, which might explain one aspect of behavior (e.g., pseudologia fantastica), it seems unlikely that brain dysfunction would be etiologic for all aspects of the behavior (which is often extremely clever) in most patients.

Psychodynamic Explanations

A variety of different unconscious factors have been suggested to explain the Munchausen behavior. Spiro (1967) has emphasized the masochistic aspects of the syndrome and has employed the concepts of Berliner (1947) and Menaker (1953) to understand these patients. According to Spiro the hospital serves the dual role of providing for dependency needs while also representing a place of fear and pain, analogous to the patient's childhood situation where the parents (or surrogates) mixed love with beatings. Bursten (1965), who as also stressed the masochistic themes of the syndrome, sees the Munchausen patient as creating a reversal where aggressive impulses once directed outward are "given" to another person (the physician) and then redirected toward the patient.

Prior relationships to physicians in these patients' histories have been stressed by Cramer et al. (1971), and this finding has been confirmed in many other case reports, both in a history of personal relationships and as evidenced by the patients' efforts to seek employment in areas of health service. These authors suggest that physicians are selected objects with whom love and anger are acted out. The Munchausen patients attempt to identify with physicians whom they idealize; when the identification with the active role breaks down they revert to the passive patient role.

Explanations employing counterphobic mechanisms have also been offered to explain the syndrome. It has been suggested that the Munchausen patient seeks out that which he fears the most (Bursten, 1965). By "playing" sick he rises above his fear of illness and death and obtains mastery of the situation. Thus castration anxiety is defended against by the seeking of repeated operations (Cramer et al., 1971).

The person who offers a false identity, simulates illness, and presents himself to a physician is imposturing the role of a patient. Thus those psychodynamics employed to understand other impostors may be of use in an attempt to understand the Munchausen patient. Imposture as a significant factor in the psychodynamics of these patients has been postulated by a number of authors (Bursten, 1965; Cramer et al., 1971; Ford, 1973; Spiro, 1967). Imposture has been interpreted as an attempt to reduce conflict between the imposter's exaggerated ego ideals and the devalued guilt-laden part of his ego (Deutsch, 1955). Persons who have failed to establish a sense of self-identity may use imposture as an effort to "create" an identity (Greenacre, 1958). Deutsch's (1955) description of the "as if" personality (i.e., highly plastic and suggestible with emptiness and lack of individuality) seems to be a particularly apt description of many of the Munchausen patients.

Imposture as an attempt to mastering prior trauma has also been suggested (Grinker, 1961; Spiro, 1967), and Ford (1973) has suggested that the imposture serves to master current feelings of helplessness in response to separation anxiety. Consistent with the latter hypothesis is the opinion of Conrad (1975) that imposters have a fear of "genital inadequacy" and that the imposture is an attempt to avoid exposure.

A Synthesis of the Various Etiologic Explanations

It is probable that there is no single explanation which serves to explain the motivations, both conscious and unconscious, of the Munchausen patients. Rather, it seems reasonable to assume that for any particular patient there may be a number of different motivations which may even vary from time to time. However, there appears to be some general themes recurrent in the behavioral patterns of most patients which can be summarized as follows.

Although the secondary gains of hospitalization (i.e., room and board, procurement of narcotics) may be contributing factors to the behavior of Munchausen patients, it appears much more probable that a serious psychiatric disorder underlies this syndrome. Such a disorder is best described in terms of character pathology. These patients have minimal ego strengths and an inability to deal with relative minor stresses. Diagnostically, they are best termed inadequate or "borderline" personalities. The choice of illness simulation as a response to stress is probably tied to prior experience in their lives with illness, physicians, and/or institutions. It seems reasonable to regard the syndrome as a defense against overwhelming anxiety and/or psychotic decompensation. Masochistic themes which are prominent in some patients are related to a devalued sense of self in addition to simply being the price paid for obtaining the goal of being the "star" patient.

Indeed these are no ordinary patients. In the process of defending against their fears of impotence, they become important persons commanding the attention of "physician-parents" yet at the same time able to feel superior because they have rendered the physician impotent by virtue of having deceived them.

TREATMENT AND MANAGEMENT

Almost all attempts to treat patients with the Munchausen syndrome have been unsuccessful. This is not surprising considering the paradoxical situation of trying to establish a therapeutic relationship with a patient whose symptoms are predicated upon deceit of the physician. Most physicians who have attempted treatment with these patients have found that the patient may accept help for a while but then terminates treatment by leaving the hospital against medical advice or simply disappearing from either inpatient or outpatient treatment. This is probably related to the observation that despite the fact that through their symptoms these patients seek close relationships with physicians (or other members of the health professions) when in the treatment setting they find the intimacy for which they sought too frightening and must flee it (Ford, 1973; Gelenberg, 1977).

Early reports of the syndrome emphasized the need to recognize the patients and prevent their abuse of hospital facilities. The patients were viewed primarily as miscreants who were exploiting hospitals and the medical profession for the purpose of obtaining free lodging and/or narcotics. Methods to deal with this type of patient consisted of suggestions to publish blacklists or circulate descriptions in order to create a "rogues gallery" (Birch, 1951; Williams, 1951). Published letters to the editors of various medical journals served to alert other physicians and hospitals. More recently, "informational letters" have been used to warn of "professional" patients "working" in an area (Mayer, 1978). With increased experience with the syndrome it has been recognized that the syndrome cannot be explained by secondary gain alone and that these patients have serious psychiatric disorders.

An initial problem in approaching these patients from a psychotherapeutic stance is how to confront them with the physician's knowledge that the illness is factitious or simulated. Hollender and Hersh (1970) state that it is best that the referring physician make the confrontation in order that the consulting psychiatrist can serve as an ally of the patient instead of being regarded as an inquisitor or detective. The approach described by Wise and Shuttleworth (1978) appears to be the most useful technique. They describe confronting the patient with her behavior and telling her that the doctors recognize the patient's need to emphasize her distress and then offer help of a psychiatric nature.

Direct confrontation of the patient should be approached with caution. I have previously hypothesized that the syndrome may serve as a defense against psychotic decompensation (Ford, 1973). To frontally attack the defense might precipitate a psychotic reaction or an increase in factitial behavior. Even if, as a consequence of confrontation, the patient merely signs out against medical advice he is likely to immediately reseek admission at another hospital and thereby start the cycle over again.

Using the techniques of an emphasis on the therapeutic relationship, with little attention to the acquisition of insight, Fras and Coughlin (1971) reported success with seven-month follow-up in the patient with severe factitial renal disease. At least one episode of factitial behavior followed an effort to confront her with her contributions to her behavior.

In a situation where a mother had simulated disease in her four children it was noted that during a year of supportive therapy there were no further hospitalizations of her children (Black, 1981). I have also reported a case where the patient remained asymptomatic with nonconfrontative support treatment but disappeared when there was an effort to make the therapy more intensive (Ford, 1982).

In contradiction to the conservative treatment strategy suggested above, Stone (1977) expresses the opinion that treatment to be successful "... will only come about through timely vigorous and repeated confrontation about the true nature of the patient's illness and about his vengeful exploitative and antisocial attitudes." However, Stone recognizes the risky nature of this course and feels it should be reserved for hospitalized patients who possess sufficient strengths to make a more mature adaptation possible. In the case reported by him, the patient, after vigorous confrontation, left treatment angry but was later able to request help and restarted therapy with another therapist. The follow-up period for this patient was only 10 months but optimism was expressed in regard to continued remission of symptoms.

An article by Jamieson and colleagues (1979) reported a therapeutic technique which combines the two treatment strategies described above. This involved two psychotherapists. One therapist acted in the capacity of being a confronter, while the other therapist, who was seen separately and at a different time, acted in a much more supportive manner. This treatment plan appeared to work for several months until the patient left town and was lost to follow-up.

There has been only one case of a reported successful treatment of Munchausen syndrome and it was associated with the several unique circumstances (Yassa, 1978). In this particular case, the patient was evidently legally committed in a psychiatric hospital from which she would elope and then seek admission to other hospitals with simulated physical disease. The patient was treated over a three-year period of time with a combination of supportive psychotherapy and behavioral modification. During this time she was rehabilitated to the extent where she was able to leave the hospital and obtain employment. It must be noted that while the treatment plan described is reasonable and well considered, the legal environment of most localities would not permit the extended involuntary hospitalizations required to pursue such a program.

In summary, one must conclude that treatment attempts with these patients have not been encouraging. A few isolated patients have been helped, at least transiently, but the overwhelming majority of patients have rejected efforts to treat them. At the present level of our understanding, it seems most important to quickly recognize these patients in order that they can be spared unnecessary dangerous diagnostic and surgical procedures and the concurrent financial burden that is imposed upon hospitals by them (Mayer, 1978; Sale and Kalucy, 1978). They must be approached with a therapeutic posture which appreciates the severe pathologic extent of their underlying psychiatric disorder(s). Nadelson (1979) has cautioned against excessive zeal in the therapy of these patients and has noted the potential negative effects of psychiatric treatment. If psychiatric treatment is undertake the most effective method is likely to be psychotherapy with those modifications required for treatment of the borderline personality (Stone, 1977). Psychiatric hospitalization may be required for the acute situation after the patient has been confronted with the factitious nature of his/her disease.

MUNCHAUSEN BY PROXY

A particular malignant form of Munchausen behavior is the use of one's children to provide a dramatic entry into the health care system. This has been called *Munchausen by proxy* and the original description of this syndrome (Meadow, 1977) has been followed by numerous reports from England and the United States. This variant of the Munchausen syndrome involves the simulation or actual production of factitious disease in children by their mothers. Symptoms which have been produced include reports of factitial bleeding (Kurlandsky et al., 1979; Lee, 1979; Meadow, 1977) hematuria (Outwater et al., 1981), the surreptitious administration of drugs or toxins (Black, 1981; Fleisher and Ament, 1977; Rogers et al., 1976) and neurological symptoms (Verity et al., 1979). At least one child has died as a consequence of this production of factitious disease and the syndrome has been appropriately called a form of child abuse (Rogers et al., 1976).

The motivation which underlies this variant of the Munchausen syndrome is apparently the opportunity to play the role of the highly involved caring parent; these mothers behave as "good" mothers in the hospital setting and are able to elicit sympathetic interest and involvement from the hospital staff (Meadow, 1977). In one situation, where a mother produced factitial bleeding in her twin infants, it was noted that she was suspected of having abused a child by a prior marriage. It was hypothesized that this mother felt overwhelmed by the demands of her infant children and the simulation of disease in them was her method of finding relief from the children without showing her inadequacy (Lee, 1979).

It has also been noted that some of these women who create factitious illness in their children also engage in the Munchausen behavior of simulating disease themselves at other times (Black, 1981; Less, 1979; Verity et al., 1979).

CONCLUSIONS AND SUMMARY

The Munchausen syndrome is a fascinating collection of symptoms involving simulation of disease, pathologic lying, and wandering. It is an extreme form of abnormal illness behavior which has now been reported as occurring in many geographic locations. Explanations for this perplexing behavior have varied but appear to be much more complex than the simple seeking of room and bed. In recent years the syndrome has been increasingly viewed as a psychological defense strategy. These patients have severe ego deficits and employ the Munchausen symptoms to defend against severe anxiety and/or psychosis.

Treatment is extremely difficult because of the patients' need to deceive and their discomfort with intimacy. Long-term psychiatric hospitalization combined with a psychotherapeutic approach is most probably the ideal treatment approach but unfortunately is often neither a practical alternative nor is it likely to be accepted by the patient. From a more realistic standpoint the major goal of "management" should be early recognition of these patients in order to prevent undue danger to them from potentially dangerous diagnostic procedures and surgical operations. A nonthreatening supportive relationship is useful in that it may reduce the patients need to engage in the Munchausen behavior but such treatment is not curative.

REFERENCES

Allegra, D., Woodward, J., and Chandler, J. 1976. Munchausen as physician and patient. Ann Intern Med 85:262–263.

American Psychiatric Association. 1980. Factitious disorders. In *Diagnostic and Statistical Manual of Mental Disorders*, 3rd edition. Washington, D.C.: APA, pp 285–290.

Ananth, J. 1977. Munchausen syndrome: Problematic diagnosis. N Y State J Med 77:115–117.

Asher, R. 1951. Munchausen syndrome. Lancet 1:339–341.

Atkinson, R.L., and Earll, J.M. 1974. Munchausen syndrome with renal stones. JAMA 230:89.

Bagan, M. 1962. Munchausen's syndrome: A case and review of the literature. Boston Med Q 13:113–119.

Barker, J.C. 1962. The syndrome of hospital addiction (Munchausen's syndrome). J Ment Sci 108:167–182.

Bean, W.B. 1959. The Munchausen syndrome. Perspect Biol Med 2:247–253.

Bender, A.S. 1979. Itinerant patient with hematologic abnormalities. Ann Intern Med 90:444.

Berliner, B. 1947. On some psychodynamics of masochism. Psychoanal Q 16:459–471.

Birch, C.A. 1951. Munchausen's syndrome. Lancet 1:412.

Black, D. 1981. The extended Munchausen syndrome: A family case. Br J Psychiatry 38:466–469.

Blackwell, P. 1965. Munchausen at Guys. Guys Hosp Rep 114:257–277.

Board, J.A., and Hammond, C.B. 1980. Factitious trophoblastic disease: Munchausen's mole. South Med J 73:831–832.

Bursten, B. 1965. On Munchausen's syndrome. Arch Gen Psychiatry 13:261–268.

Carrodus, A.L., and Earlom, M.S.S. 1971. Haematuria as a feature of the Munchausen syndrome: Report of a case. Aust New Zeal J Surg 40:365–367.

Carswell, J. 1950. The Romantic Rogue. New York: Dutton.

Cavenar, J.O., Maltbie, A.A., Hillard, J.R., Worchel, B.J., and O'Shanick, G.J. 1980. Cardiac presentation of Munchausen's syndrome. Psychosomatics 31:946–948.

Chapman, J. 1953. Peregrinating problem patients: Munchausen's syndrome. JAMA 165:927–933.

Cheng, L., and Hummel, L. 1978. The Munchausen syndrome as a psychiatric condition. Br J Psychiatry 133:20–21.

Chertok, L. 1972. Mania operativa: Surgical addiction. Psychiatry Med 3:105–118.

Chugh, K.S. 1966. Haemorrhagica histrionica: The bleeding Munchausen syndrome. J Indian Med Assoc 46:90–93.

Clark, E., and Melnick, S.C. 1958. The Munchausen syndrome or the problem of hospital hoboes. Amer J Med 25:6–12.

Conrad, S.W. 1975. Imposture as a defense. In Tactics and Techniques in Psychoanalytic Therapy, vol. II, Countertransference. Giovacchini, P.L., ed. New York: Jason Aronson, pp 413–426.

Cramer, B., Gershberg, M.R., and Stern, M. 1971. Munchausen syndrome: Its relationship to malingering, hysteria and the physician–patient relationship. Arch Gen Psychiatry 24:573–578.

Deutsch, H. 1955. The imposter: Contribution to ego psychology of a type of psychopath. Psychoanal Q 24:483–505.

Ferguson, E.E., and Maki, D.G. 1978. A baffling hyperpyrexia. Hosp Pract 13:111–124.

Fleisher, D., and Ament, M.E. 1977. Diarrhea, red diapers and child abuse. Clin Pediatr 17:820–824.

Ford, C.V. 1973. The Munchausen syndrome: A report of four new cases and a review of psychodynamic considerations. Psychiatry Med 4:31–45.

Ford, C.V. 1982. Munchausen syndrome. In *Extraordinary Disorders of Human Behavior*. Friedmann, C.T.H., and Faquet, R., eds. New York: Plenun, pp 15–27.

Frame, B., Jackson, G.M., Kleerekoper, M., Rao, D.S., DeLorenzo, A.S.D., and Garcia, M. 1981. Acute severe hypercalcemia a la Munchausen. Amer J Med 70:316–319.

Fras, I., and Coughlin, B.E. 1971. The treatment of factitious disease. Psychosomatics 12:117–122.

Friedmann, C.T.H., and Weinstein, M.H. 1976. Munchausen's syndrome: Report of a case. Am Surgeon 42:611–614.

Gelenberg, A.J. 1977. Munchausen's syndrome with a psychiatric presentation. Dis Nerv Syst 38:378–380.

George, M.D., and Cheatham, J.S. 1965. Munchausen's syndrome: A case report and a brief discussion. J Iowa Med Society 60:20–22.

Greenacre, P. 1958. The imposter. Psychoanal Q 27:359–380.

Griffith, A.H. 1961. A case of pulmonary tuberculosis with 'Munchausen syndrome'. Tubercle, Lond 42:512–515.

Grinker, R.R., Jr. 1961. Imposture as a form of mastery. Arch Gen Psychiatry 5:449–452.

Gurwith, M., and Langston, C. 1980. Factitious Munchausen syndrome. N Engl J Med 302:1483–1484.

Hale, P. 1966. The background of a "Munchausen" patient (hospital addict). Postgrad Med J 42:791–793.

Hendrix, S., Sale, S., Zeiss, C.R., Utley, J., and Patterson, R. 1981. Factitious hymenoptera allergic emergency: A report of a new variant of Munchausen's syndrome. J Allergy Clin Immunol 67:8–13.

Hollender, M.H., and Hersh, S.P. 1970. Impossible consultation made possible. Arch Gen Psychiatry 23:343–345.

Hoyer, T.V. 1959. Pseudologia fantastica. Psychiat Q 33:203–220.

Ireland, P., Sapira, J.D., and Templeton, B. 1967. Munchausen's syndrome: Review and report of an additional case. Amer J Med 43:579–592.

Jamieson, R., McKee, E., and Roback, H. 1979. Munchausen's syndrome: An unusual case. Amer J Psychother 23:616–621.

Jones, W.A., Cooper, T.P., and Kiviat, M.D. 1978. Munchausen syndrome presenting as urolithiasis. West J Med 128:185–188.

Justus, P.G., and Kitchens, C.S. 1976. Secondary leukemia with Munchausen filiarisis. Ann Intern Med 85:685.

Justus, P.G., Kreutziger, S.S., and Kitchens, C.S. 1980. Probing the dynamics of Munchausen's syndrome: Detailed analysis of a case. Ann Intern Med 93:120–127.

Kemp, J.S., and Munro, J.G. 1969. Munchausen's syndrome simulating caisson disease. Br J Indust Med 26:81–83.

Kurlandsky, L., Lukoff, J.Y., Zinkham, W.H., Brody, J.P., and Kessler, R.W. 1979. Munchausen syndrome by proxy: Definition of factitious bleeding in an infant by ^{51}Cr labeling of erythrocytes. Pediatrics 63:228–231.

Laudadio, C., Eickenberg, H.V., and Amin, M. 1979. Factitious illness in urology: Munchausen's syndrome. J Ky Med Assoc 75:234–236.

Lee, D.A. 1979. Munchausen syndrome by proxy in twins. Arch Dis Child 54:646–647.

Mayer, N. 1978. The baron revisited: A case report. JACEP 1:276–278.

Meadow, R. 1977. Munchausen syndrome by proxy: The hinterland of child abuse. Lancet 1:343–345.

Menaker, E. 1953. Masochism: A defense reaction of the ego. Psychoanal Q 22:205–220.

Mendel, J.G. 1974. Munchausen's syndrome: A syndrome of drug dependence. Compr Psychiatry 15:69–72.

Michaels, A.D., Domino, E.G., and Moore, R.A. 1964. The case of the feverish imposter: A psychiatric and neurologic puzzle. J Neuropsychiat 5:213–220.

Nadelson, T. 1979. The Munchausen spectrum. Gen Hosp Psychiatry 1:11–17.

Outwater, K.M., Lipnick, R.N., Luban, N.L.C., Raversroft, K., and Ruley, E.J. 1981. Factitious hematuria: Diagnosis by minor blood group typing. J Pediatr 98:95–97.

Pankratz, L. 1981. A review of the Munchausen syndrome. Clin Psychology Rev 1:65–78.

Paperny, D., Hicks, R., and Hammar, S.L. 1980. Munchausen syndrome. Am J Dis Child 134:794–795.

Puzzuoli, G. 1978. Munchausen's syndrome: A case report. West Va Med J 74:12–13.

Raspe, R.E. 1948. *Singular Travels, Campaigns and Adventures of Baron Munchausen.* London: Cresset Press.

Ries, R.K. 1980. DSM III: Differential diagnosis of Munchausen's syndrome. J Nerv and Ment Dis 168:629–632.

Rogers, D. Tripp, J., Bentouim, A., Robinson, A., Berry, D., and Goulding R. 1976. Non-accidental poisoning: An extended syndrome of child abuse. Br Med J 2:793–796.

Sakula, A. 1978. Munchausen: Fact and fiction. J R Coll Physicians Lond 12:286–292.

Sale, I., and Kalucy, R. 1978. Munchausen syndrome. Med J Aust 2:523–525.

Sapira, J.D. 1981. Munchausen's syndrome and the technologic imperative. South Med J 74:193–196.

Sharon, E., and Diamond, H.S. 1974. Factitious uric acid and urolithiasis as a feature of the Munchausen syndrome. Mt. Sinai J Med 41:696–698.

Sneed, R.C., and Bell, R.F., 1976. The dauphin of Munchausen: Factitious passage of renal stones in a child. Pediatrics 58:127–130.

Snowdon, J., Solomons, R., and Druce, H. 1978. Feigned bereavement: Twelve cases. Br J Psychiatry 133:15–19.

Spiro, H. 1967. Chronic factitious illness. Arch Gen Psychiatry 18:569–580.

Steinbeck, A.W. 1961. Hemorrhagica histrionica—The bleeding Munchausen syndrome. Med J Aust 1:451–456.

Stengel, E. 1939. Studies on the psychopathology of compulsive wandering. Br J Med Psychol 18:250–254.

Stern, T.A. 1980. Munchausen's syndrome revisited. Psychosomatics 21:329–336.

Stone, M.H. 1977. Factitious illness: Psychological findings and treatment recommendations. Bull Menninger Clin 41:239–254.

Vail, D.J. 1962. Munchausen returns. Psychiat Q 36:317–324.

Verity, C.M., Winckworth, C., Burman, D., Stevens, D., and White, R.J. 1979. Polle syndrome: Children of Munchausen. Br Med J 2:422–423.

von Maur, K., Wasson, K.R., DeFord, J.W., and Caranasos, G.J. 1973. Munchausen's syndrome: A thirty-year history of peregrination *par excellence*. South Med J 66:629–632.

Williams, B. 1951. Munchausen's syndrome. Lancet 1:527.

Williams, C.B. 1961. Peripatetic pseudoporphyria. N Engl J Med 264:924–927.

Wimberly, T. 1981. The making of a Munchausen. Br J Med Psychol 54:121–129.

Wise, G.R., and Shuttleworth, E.C. 1978. Munchausen's disorder: A case of a factitious neurological emergency. J Clin Psychiatry 39:353–355.

Yassa, R. 1978. Munchausen's syndrome: A successfully treated case. Psychosomatics 19:242–243.

11

DISABILITY SYNDROMES

Following an injury or acute illness most workers return to work within a relatively short period of time and consistent with medical judgments that they are no longer disabled. However, they are notable and often dramatic exceptions. These patients who have apparently made a medical recovery but continue to complain of disability are of considerable concern to the employers and insurance carriers who may be faced not only with the significant medical expenses but in addition may be responsible for payment of ongoing salary or disability benefits. These patients with various disability syndromes are frustrating to physicians, for despite outward appearances of seeking medical care in order to get well, their covert intentions may be to seek justification to remain in the sick role.

There have been a variety of terms used to describe the type of patient who continues to claim disability following an accident despite apparent medical recovery. These include traumatic neurosis, compensation neurosis, accident neurosis, and disability neurosis. Some of the terms are pejorative and imply etiology, while others are less specific and merely descriptive. Unfortunately these diagnostic labels have been used inconsistently among the various authors who have been interested in the subject of disability. This chapter will attempt to develop more precise descriptions and definitions of the various syndromes of psychological etiology which may lead to disability, but which are attributed to physical causes by the patient. Because many of these disability syndromes follow trauma the emphasis will be on reactions and recovery to physical injury, particularly industrial and automobile accidents. It must be stressed, however, that many of the syndromes described can also occur with medical illness.

Before proceeding to the various disability syndromes it is important to review psychological antecedents and reactions to accidents and trauma.

Concepts of secondary gain will also be considered because it is so often evoked as an important factor in disability syndromes.

PSYCHOLOGICAL ASPECTS OF ACCIDENTS AND TRAUMA

On close examination of the psychological aspects of an accident it becomes increasingly apparent that they are far more complex than is obvious at first glance. In fact one can speak of an "anatomy of an accident" where multiple components interact to determine the eventual psychological meaning and outcome for the individual involved. These various components can be roughly divided into four major categories: (1) antecedents to the accident, including issues such as "accident proneness" and lifelong coping style(s) of the patient; (2) psychological factors related directly to characteristics of the accident itself, i.e., degree of unexpectedness, type of injury and culpability for the accident; (3) response of the individual to the trauma, i.e., anxiety, depression or denial; and (4) response of the environment to the injured person, i.e., issues such as presence of secondary gains, reactions of employees, and family members. Each of these preceding psychological aspects of accidents will influence the eventual adjustments that the victim will have to make in his/her life, both intrapsychic and in relationship to the environment.

Antecedent Factors

Accident Proneness. Popularized by Flanders Dunbar in the 1940s "accident proneness" (or accident habit) has become a household word. It appears clear that some people are more prone to accidents than others and it appears reasonable to postulate that unconscious psychological factors play a major role in determining susceptibility to accidents.

Dunbar (1947) found that fracture patients were 14 times more likely to have had disabling accidents than other hospitalized patients. The fracture patients averaged 4 accidents per person while the nonfracture patients averaged only 0.3 accidents per person. She found in the life pattern of the accident prone that there was usually an extreme resentment of authority, often unconscious, and that authority could be represented by a large number of parties such as parents, spouses, or employers. Froggatt and Smiley (1964) reviewed accident statistics and concluded that, although accidents do not occur in a random distribution, "accident proneness" varies over time rather than being a permanent characteristic of an individual.

Hirschfield and Behan (Hirschfield and Behan, 1963, 1966; Behan and Hirschfield, 1963) have conceptualized an explanation which may account for a significant number of "accidents." They hypothesize that a person who is experiencing life stress and subsequent disabling emotional responses may find that disability due to psychological causes is socially unacceptable. An accident serves to transform psychological disability into a somatic disability and therefore an unacceptable disability into an acceptable disability. These authors report that they have investigated a large number of accidents and find psychological antecedents to the accident in the vast majority of cases.

Another type of accident proneness is that which has been reported to be associated with automobile accidents. Investigation of fatal accidents frequently reveals that the driver "at fault" had recently had an emotional upsetting experience such as a fight with a spouse (Conger et al., 1959; Selzer et al., 1968). Such an experience may lead to alcohol consumption and/or increased impulsivity with decreased attention. Similar situations in regard to industrial accidents can be readily postulated. More recently Stuart and Brown (1981) have found that life stress (as measured by life change units) in college students is statistically correlated with accidents at a very significant level.

Personal Coping Mechanisms. Each person develops individualized methods of coping with stress. As a consequence the emotional responses to trauma are likely to be different among patients with similar injuries. These responses will vary not only in the acute phase but will also influence the course of convalescence and the return to normal activities. Illustrations of potential responses to injury would be infantilelike behavior from a passive-dependent person or impulsive hostile acting-out toward nursing staff from a sociopathic person. During convalescence persons with counterdependent defenses and a need to deny illness may attempt to return to work prematurely, while those who are passive-aggressive may procrastinate as long as possible before returning to an active and responsible role in society.

Psychological Factors Related Directly to an Accident

Just as each person is unique and because of antecedent factors may respond differently to a personal injury there are aspects of the injury itself with will also influence the responses of the victim.

The Degree of Unsuspectedness. While no accident is expected per se there are varying degrees to which the injured person had anticipated the event. For example, a professional football player will be taken less by surprise if he suffers a knee injury than would a person hit by a car in a crosswalk while crossing the street. There is evidence that the degree of unexpectedness is associated with a higher incidence of posttraumatic neurotic symptoms. Braverman (1977) has found that beginners or inexperienced skiers had fewer posttraumatic psychological symptoms than did experienced skiers who did not anticipate injury. He also found a similar situation in industrial accidents in that the more experienced workers for whom accidents were rare also had increased psychological symptoms as opposed to less-experienced workers for whom accidents were more common.

Temporal Relationship to Other Life Events. In the study cited just above it was also noted that accidents seemed to cluster at times just before a vacation or occur just before the end of a vacation. This finding is interesting because of a long-standing belief of military personnel that death or injury is most likely to occur on the last patrol or last mission before rotation off combat duty.

Type of Injury Sustained. Reactions to trauma may vary because of the meaning to the person of the type of injury sustained. For example, a burn may be of different significance or meaning because of prior experience than would be a cutting or crush injury. Traumatic amputations are almost inevitably associated with a normal grief response and need for reorganization of the body image (Kolb, 1954). They may also be followed by phantom limb sensations, which may include severe chronic pain syndromes.

Part of the Body Injured. Some parts of the body have greater symbolic (and real) and psychic investment value than other parts. For example, a relatively minor injury on the face of a woman may evoke considerable anxiety but be relatively unnoticed in a husky laborer. Injuries to the genitals typically engender disproportionate anxiety as opposed to other parts of the body. For some individuals, because of special skills, such as pianists or professional skaters, injuries to the hands or feet may be of greater significance than to someone without such skills.

Culpability for the Injury. This is a particularly important psychological issue in trauma and one with which almost every victim struggles to some degree. Was the accident due to negligence on the part of the injured person, who must therefore accept and work through guilt for the consequences, or was it due to an error on the part of someone else? In the latter situation one may rage (and possibly take punitive action) for the injustice suffered. Even when no one is clearly at fault there is usually a reluctance to "accept fate" and human nature being what it is there is an effort to place culpability somewhere. "If only I had stayed at home with my sick child," "People that age should not be allowed on the highway!", or "The emergency room personnel were incompetent" are the types of statements heard very frequently.

The finding of fault for an accident has psychological uses for the victim who then uses this as a defense against feelings of impotence and helplessness. However, there are also legal and financial implications in the form of secondary gain which will be explored below in greater depth.

Responses of the Victim to Trauma

There are a number of psychologic responses to trauma. Many of these commonly follow characteristic patterns and must be considered as normal rather than pathologic. It is when there are marked deviations from the normal patterns that one should become concerned about a pathologic process that will require specific treatment. It must be noted that a failure to demonstrate the usual psychologic responses is, in itself, abnormal and should be viewed with clinical concern. A number of authors have described psychological reactions to trauma and, although terminology has varied, the descriptions of the clinical phenomena observed have been remarkably consistent (Mattsson, 1975; Schnaper, 1975; Schnaper and Cowley, 1976; Titchener, 1970; Weisz, 1973). The typical psychological processes following trauma are as follows.

Regression. Trauma, as with all serious somatic illness, is associated with psychological regression. The trauma victim behaves in a less mature fashion, often in a dependent and more childlike manner than was characterized by the premorbid personality. Feelings of helplessness are associated with expectations that others will assume care and responsibility. Although most accident victims will display regression to some degree a few will become markedly infantile with dependent demands and expectations far in excess of their apparent disability.

Anxiety. Unsure of what has happened and its implications for further dysfunction, pain, or implication for the continuation of life itself, the victim of trauma will experience anxiety to varying degrees. This may vary from abject terror with agitation and hyperventilation to another variant of extreme anxiety, namely, a "freeze state" where the patient appears unresponsive to stimuli or obeys commands in a "zombi"-like fashion. Anxiety associated with acute trauma usually remits fairly rapidly over a period of several hours. It can be managed by repetitive explanations to the patient of what is taking place in terms of medical procedures, etc., and quiet reassurance. The presence of close relatives or friends (if they are emotionally composed) often has a calming influence. Although the acute anxiety may remit, it is not unusual for it to recur periodically, occasionally to a disabling extent (see posttraumatic neurosis below).

Cognitive Distortions. Patients with severe trauma, as a consequence of the effects of severe anxiety, impaired physiology (e.g., electrolyte imbalance) and pharmacologic agents such as morphine, are prone to disorders in their thinking processes. Information may be misinterpreted or distorted; often patients may overhear partial conversations of health care team members who mistakenly assume that the patient is unconscious. Particularly, if there is a period of unconsciousness, the patient may use fantasy to fill in the amnesia. Transient beliefs that one has been kidnapped or is being held prisoner are common.

Denial. Most persons experiencing significant injury or illness as a part of the normal grief responses will, to a varying length of time, deny the seriousness of the injury. This denial takes different forms, such as an essential denial that injury has occurred at all, minimization of its extent, or the expression of confidence that it will be transitory. For example, a man experiencing a traumatic paraplegia may insist that he will "walk again." To the extent that denial does not interfere with effective medical treatment, and serves to protect the psyche from overwhelming anxiety, it is a normal and necessary ego defense mechanism.

Grief. Once denial has been discarded there is an almost inevitable feeling of grief as the losses suffered by the accident victim must be worked through and accepted. These losses, at a concrete level, may include loss of bodily function, cosmetic deformity, or actual loss of a body part. At a more abstract level the losses include a transient or permanent loss of activities which are gratifying, financial liabilities, and perhaps, as important as all the above, the loss of a feeling of personal omnipotence. The victim of an accident often develops an acute awareness of the fragility of life and feeling of help-lessness which accompanies the realization that the body is vulnerable to destruction and inevitable death.

Anger. Accidents are rarely just. The victim reacts to the injustice he has suffered with anger and rages "Why me?" The anger is frequently displaced from abstract causes to more direct objects. Employers and physicians are common objects of the anger. "I would never have lost the leg if the surgeon had been competent!" Anger because it serves as a defense against de-pression may last a prolonged period of time and have many secondary repercussions such as repeated litigation. Unfortunately it may also interfere with optional medical care.

Response of the Social System to the Accident Victim

Accidents do not occur in an interpersonal vacuum. Following an accident there are not only the psychological responses of the individual who experienced the trauma but also a wide ripple effect involving those who provide care for the victim or who are related by family or friendship. The following list of social relationships which impact on the accident situation is representative but not exclusive. Nor are the examples of potential responses by any means overly inclusive.

Spouse and Family. In a healthy marriage and family situation the wife (or husband) and children are supportive and appropriately encouraging for the disabled person to return to activities as soon as is medically feasible. However, there are different and more pathologic responses. A wife fearful of loss of financial security may angrily or passively-aggressively deal with a husband who she feels is depriving her of her share. Such attitudes may increase guilt or depression, facilitate inappropriate denial and complicate convalescence. At the other extreme of behavior a wife may be overly solicitous and encourage regression. An illustrative situation is where the wife has felt dominated and the accident is seen as a way of "turning the tables." Reluctant to allow a restoration of the old relationship she encourages her husband to remain in the sick role while she assumes the dominant role in the marriage.

Employer. An injured or disabled employee represents a financial threat to an employer. If the accident was work-related then the employer may be liable for damages as well as having to pay the salary of an unproductive worker over an undetermined length of time. There is ripe potential for an adversarial relationship. The employer may immediately engage in actions which negate or minimize culpability for the accident (e.g., establishing evidence that the employee was disregarding established safety rules) or attempt to minimize the injury. Such actions of course are in the self-interest and may be prudent insofar as they are honest. Unfortunately this is not always so, and I have personal acquaintance with a situation where an employer directed an industrial physician to reclassify third-degree burns of the hand, and therefore disabling, as first-degree burns (nondisabling). Although such regrettable actions do occur it must be stressed that many more englightened employers demonstrate both emotional and financial support to injured employees.

Physicians. The initial responses of the physician are important factors in determining the subsequent behavior of the patient during his convalescence. If the physician is employed by the company for which the patient works, then there is a potential conflict of interest as the physician may become the agent of the company (this raises important ethical issues, see above). Chambers (1963) notes that this problem can be minimized if the company physician remains aware of the fact that the patient did not choose him and that rapport must be cultivated rather than be taken for granted. Irrespective of the relationship with the employer, the physician who initially evaluates and treats the patient can, by his manner, be oversolicitous to relatively minor injuries, thereby conveying a sense of greater damage and concern than is warranted. On the contrary, the physician may be contemptuous or disinterested, thereby setting the stage for a potential adversarial relationship between the patient and subsequent physicians who may be involved in the medical care.

M.H. Miller (1961) notes that many " ... cases of continuing medical incapacity, despite medical recovery, seem to occur in settings where the doctor and patient don't like each other too well, and perhaps haven't from the beginning."

Union Stewards/Attorneys. These two groups of individuals are lumped together because they are third parties who, while ostensibly representing the patient's best interest, also have a vested interest in the outcome of an injury. Too often the interest expressed is to encourage the patient to maximize injuries (Keiser, 1968). The union steward may see an injury as something to use against the employer in terms of bargining power and the patient's attorney will be trying to obtain the largest settlement possible (thereby increasing the legal fee). Such messages that it is better to be ill can be powerful disincentives to get well. Keiser (1968) reports that some attorneys may "coach" patients as to how to react to certain tests or overtly discourage patients from getting well too fast. As noted by Miller (1959) counsel of this type helps promote an adversarial relationship rather than the cooperative relationship characteristic of the doctor–patient relationship. Such misguided efforts to do the best possible for the client can result in a "compensation neurosis" which " ... can last a lifetime and can result in a loss which considerably overshadows the gain with litigation."

THE ISSUE OF SECONDARY GAIN

Secondary gains are considered to be those benefits which accrue to a person as a result of illnesses. There are a variety of different benefits that one might obtain from an illness or injury. The "sick role" releases one from usual responsibilities such as school or work. Injuries are often compensable and salaries and/or damages may be paid for disabilities. There are also psychological gains such as increased attention, concern, or pity. An injury may be used as a rationalization for a failure to live up to one's personal goals or the expectations of others. For example, an injury to an athlete may be used to rationalize a performance which is less than expected.

The concept of the secondary nature of such benefits from an illness is clear when the person involved suffers an injury which was clearly not caused by himself/herself, e.g., hit in a crosswalk by an automobile. The issue of the "secondary" nature of the benefits becomes much less clear when the accident was the result of victim's own negligence and is essentially opaque when consideration is given to certain psychiatric disorders such as "conversion-hysteria" or malingering. In the case of conversion reactions the assumption is usually made that the conversion symptom represents the symbolic comprise of a conflict within the unconscious of the affected person. For example, an angry impulse to strike out, which is in conflict with personal convictions that anger is wrong, could result in a conversion reaction manifested by the paralysis of an arm. The patient unaware of the unconscious etiology of the symptom regards it as evidence of being sick. In this situation relief from the unconscious conflict concerning anger would be regarded as the primary aim and benefits such as increased concern from a spouse and/or relief of responsibilities from work would be regarded as secondary gain.

Secondary gain becomes an issue of concern at any time that the patient's symptom is assumed to be of psychogenic etiology, and the patient stands to gain by having such a symptom. This is very frequently the case in disability syndromes. With a lack of objective evidence to presume continuing medical reasons for disability then a paramount problem arises as to whether the patient is suffering from a genuine psychiatric disability or is merely trying to defraud employers, insurance companies, and others to obtain special privileges and financial benefits.

Why a person should be motivated, either consciously or unconsciously, to claim physical disability in order to obtain certain benefits can by no means be answered in a simple manner. It has been noted by Martin (1974) that the secondary gains are also associated with "secondary losses" which include loss of respect and attention from those in helping roles and the loss of community approval with social stigma and guilt inherent in the role of being chronically disabled. Martin views some patients' willingness to accept secondary gain as a means of not having to deal with a basic inadequacy in coping skills. The patient would rather attribute his behavior to greed than face his inadequacies, and family and physicians can similarly attribute patients' symptoms to the same sources rather than face the real issues. Although these patients may be successful in obtaining benefits, the quality of their lives is actually poor and the trade-off of symptoms for benefits appears to be an unsatisfactory alternative to the previous quality of life (Ford, 1978). Certainly more must be involved for many of these patients besides "ripping off" the system. Yet, merely to say that the patient has basic inadequacies or consciously manipulates the system to cover a more severe underlying psychiatric disorder may once again beg the question of the significance of secondary gain.

Among the factors which must be considered in regard to secondary gains, particularly compensation, are (1) the actual cost to employers, insurance companies, and the government—irrespective of the possibility of underlying psychiatric illness the cost can be quite considerable as indicated by detailed case reports (Robertson, 1978); (2) the cost in terms of morale of other workers (and/or associated military personnel)—the knowledge, or at least the suspicion, that others have exploited employers and insurance companies may have a very deleterious effect upon those who do accept their responsibilities, leading to attitudes such as "Everyone else does it so I might as well do the same"; and (3) the adverse effect upon the disabled individual. As noted above the life of the disabled person is not the "bed of roses" that some may imagine it to be. The continuation of secondary gains, may serve to perpetuate the perception of illness and disability and therefore not be in the best interests of the patient, even though there may be a desperate attempt to maintain the sick role. Despite the fact that it may sound like a value judgment reflecting the "work ethic," I can honestly say that I have never seen a person with a psychologically determined disability syndrome who was not pervasively unhappy.

That the presence of secondary gain, at least in the form of disability payments, acts as a disincentive to rehabilitation cannot be seriously challenged. Belter and colleagues (1979) found that disabled social security beneficiaries were significantly less likely to be rehabilitated when they were compared to nonbeneficiaries with a similar extent of physical disability. Similarly Krusen and Ford (1958) noted that of patients treated for back injuries, those patients who expected to receive compensation continued to have significantly more symptoms than those who did not expect to financially benefit from their injuries. The severity of the injury was not the determining factor as both groups were very similar as to the length and requirement for hospitalization. Although the number of physical therapy treatments per se was not related to improvement, the group anticipating compensation did receive a significantly greater number of treatments. The authors concluded that response to therapy was less determined by the nature of the injury than the basic personality of the patient. Women who expected to receive compensation had the worst response to treatment; only 54.2% showed improvement at the time of discharge. This finding was consistent with the work of Belter et al. (1979) who noted that women may be in more conflict as to whether to return to work than are men. Women receiving disability payments can often continue to function as homemakers and thereby "kill two birds with one stone."

Fowler and colleagues (1979) compared psychiatric patients who were considering compensation claims for the Veterans Administration to patients not considering such claims. They found that those considering claims had histories of a lower frequency of employment, a lower annual income, and a higher frequency of fights, juvenile court appearances, and felony convictions. Compensation claim patients also had an increased frequency of headaches, anxiety attacks, conversion reactions, ideas of persecution, and gustatory disturbances. The authors noted that the symptom profile was consistent with antisocial personality characteristics as well as certain features of paranoid and borderline personalities.

In summary, secondary gain is a real phenomenon that affects the recovery rate for a significant number of accident victims. Not surprisingly those who have less in the way of marketable skills, those who have the most to gain by not working, or those who have personality traits consistent with sociopathy are the persons most likely to capitalize upon a compensable injury.

DIFFERENTIAL DIAGNOSIS OF DISABILITY SYNDROMES

As is obvious from the above descriptions of psychological antecedents and reactions to an accident, compounded by the issue of secondary gain, there are many places in which a disability syndrome may find its origin. Too often the various disability syndromes are lumped together with a term such as accident neurosis; however, this is a conceptually poor idea in regard to both prevention and treatment. The reasons why a person may become disabled are highly varied and a treatment approach effective for one type of disorder may reinforce the symptoms in another disorder. The following discussion of disability disorders attempts to not only distinguish the different syndromes but to indicate the degree of treatability, and when information is available, the type of specific treatment interventions which may be the most effective.

Depression

A depressed mood following physical injury is normal and its absence may be regarded as pathologic. There are three major syndrome-complexes in reference to depression which may occur.

Grief Reaction. The accident victim must, as a normal process, work through the loss(es) that have been suffered. Included may be loss of body parts, change in body image due to scars, the loss of prior activities which were gratifying, the potential loss of a job, financial reverses and so forth. This list of real losses can obviously be extended. In addition frequently seen is the more abstract loss of a feeling of personal omnipotence and immortality. Thus the accident may precipitate an existential crisis as the victim struggles to integrate the losses and to concurrently explore a new meaning of life; profound religious experiences and "conversions" may occur in this situation. A life-threatening injury can, in some circumstances, serve as the precipitant for emotional and personal growth (Titchener, 1970).

As with a any grief reaction, such as with the death of a close relative, the loss must be mourned and worked through with a redirection of the psychic energy previously invested in the lost object. The physician can assist in this by encouraging the patient to talk about the loss and providing reassurance that grief is a normal and necessary part of the recovery process. With the progression of time the patient should be encouraged to redirect his energies into new activities.

Reactive Depression. Reactive ("neurotic") depression can be considered an extension of normal grief in the pathologic direction. The person with a reactive depression is reacting to a loss but in an inappropriate or exaggerated manner. Such a response is determined by prior events in the person's life and the characterologic features of the individual. Persons with prior personal injuries or disease during childhood, or with close relatives who have suffered injuries or died prematurely, may respond in an exaggerated manner as the unresolved conflicts and emotions of the previous experience are once again activated. Persons with a strong sense of responsibility and pervasive feelings of guilt concerning other aspects of their lives may respond to an accident with profound guilt that they have caused themselves or others damage. Such expressions of guilt may be inappropriate and symptomatic of the patient's depression.

Patients with a neurotically determined depression will benefit from more intensive and insight-oriented psychotherapy as compared to the supportive psychotherapy indicated in the adjunctive therapy of grief reactions. One must be prepared to deal with issues that go beyond the traumatic experience itself and to explore it in relationship to childhood experiences and character structure. Therefore many of these patients will benefit from a psychiatric referral.

Endogenous Depression. Endogenous depression (unipolar and bipolar major affective disorder) may be precipitated by the strong emotional and/or physiologic responses engendered by the traumatic event. Not infrequently the endogenous depression may have preceded and/or have been responsible for the accident. This can occur through the reduced concentration and general self-destructive or nihilistic attitudes which frequently accompany severe depression. It is of utmost importance to recognize and institute treatment as soon as feasible for the patient who has a major affective disorder. Severe depression many interfere with the recovery process in regard to such important factors as the patient's motivation and cooperation and probably even at a basic physiologic level.

Symptoms typical of an endogenous depression include sleep disturbance, usually with early morning awakening, poor appetite, depressed mood, and psychomotor retardation. An apathetic patient making little in the way of an effort to get well should suggest the possibility of an endogenous depression. Diagnosis is facilitated by a history of previous mood disorders (either depression or hypomanic episodes) or a family history which includes affective disorders or alcoholism.

Treatment should be instituted promptly in patients with a major affective disorder because, as mentioned, it may interfere with other aspects of convalescence. Unfortunately most of the antidepressant medications have a delay of 1–3 weeks before a clinical response can be detected. One must remain alert to the possibility of suicide and take appropriate precautions for those patients determined to be at high risk. Tricyclic antidepressant medications are probably the drugs of choice, although in some situations the monoamine oxidase inhibitors or electroconvulsive therapy may be indicated. The type of drug chosen and dosage will be largely determined by the physiologic status of the patient.

Posttraumatic Neurosis

The term posttraumatic neurosis is frequently used to describe any type of psychiatric syndrome following trauma. However, as used here the term implies a specific syndrome, which has been described multiple times, although with a variety of diagnostic terms, i.e., combat fatigue, gross stress reaction, and posttraumatic stress disorder (Laughlin, 1954a, 1954b; Modlin, 1967; Horowitz et al., 1980). The most important components of this syndrome are the trauma itself and the role of anxiety. The trauma is defined as injury or the very real threat of physical injury. Anxiety, in its various manifestations, is the primary symptom in this disorder, and it is directly related to the trauma itself. Following the trauma, which may be variable in the extent of somatic injuries, but which was generally a terrifying experience, the patient develops symptoms of chronic anxiety manifested by a vague dread of increased vulnerability and an anticipation of danger. Symptoms may include an increased sensitivity to noise, headaches, and dizziness. The chronic anxiety is punctuated by periodic episodes of superimposed acute anxiety manifested by an increased startle reaction, tremor, and increased muscle tension. Palpitations and diaphoresis may occur when the patient is placed in situations which bring to mind the original traumatic situation. Sleep is frequently disturbed and repetitive nightmares which reenact the trauma are common. Additional symptoms often present also include irritability and impaired memory and concentration despite the lack of objective evidence of brain dysfunction. Loss of sexual interests and social withdrawal are frequently accompanying symptoms and these symptoms in particular portend a poor prognosis (Modlin, 1967). The person with a posttraumatic neurosis tends to withdraw interest from external objects and events and instead becomes preoccupied with his own behavior and feelings rather than the environment (Keiser, 1968). Symptoms generally will abate in a gradual manner over a period of weeks to months after the trauma, but in some persons they may continue in a severe and disabling extent for a prolonged period of time.

An important variable in producing the syndrome is the degree of unexpectability associated with the accident and trauma. The less the accident was anticipated, the greater the probability of developing a posttraumatic neurosis, and the more likely the symptoms will be severe (Braverman, 1977). A second important variable is the degree of terror that the accident provokes and as mentioned above this may be more important than the extent of injuries sustained. For example, certain types of accidents may be associated with great fright despite the little in the way of injury.

Examples are an automobile falling into deep water with the successful escape of the victim, or an escape from a burning crashed airliner with only minimal injuries suffered.

The trauma and stress experienced may also be chronic and repetitive as exemplified by the German concentration camps of World War II. Neiderland (1968) has described a survivor who had symptoms characteristic of the posttraumatic syndrome persisting for many years after rescue from a concentration camp. Similarly posttraumatic stress disorders are now being recognized in veterans of the Viet Nam war. The various syndromes secondary to the unique stresses of war or persecution are beyond the scope of this book and the reader is referred to other sources (Ostwald and Bittner, 1968; Friedman, 1981; Warmes, 1972).

What is at issue with the posttraumatic neurosis is the feeling of individual that his/her ordered and predictable environment has changed and in a fearful manner threatening life and body integrity. The stress at least temporarily has overwhelmed the coping abilities of the invididual and the ego defensive mechanisms are unable to repress the resultant anxiety. The entire personality may need to reorganize as a means of incorporating the meaning of the trauma it has experienced (Keiser, 1968; Crocq, 1974).

Premorbid personality characteristics are by no means the sole determinants of the syndrome, and it has been pointed out by Rappaport (1968) that when stress is sufficient no person is immune from developing psychological neurotic syndromes. In fact, the work of Modlin (1967) suggests that those persons with posttraumatic syndromes, whom he evaluated at the Menninger Clinic, could be viewed as having fewer neurotic conflicts than the general population. These patients were described as being very typical of lower and lower middle class middle Americans. It was hypothesized that because of their rather stereotyped cultural background there was a lack of flexibility in their psychological defenses. Therefore, they reacted to trauma with fairly direct anxiety rather than binding the anxiety with previously learned neurotic defenses such as obsessions.

The treatment of individuals with posttraumatic neurosis involves helping them achieve some type of ego mastery over the traumatic event. This frequently can be obtained by supportively listening to the patient repititiously recount his experiences and relive the emotions experienced. This procedure helps to desensitize the traumatic experience. This cathartic approach can be promoted in individual therapy, sometimes with amobarbital narcosis as an adjunctive technique or in a group therapy setting (Laughlin, 1954b; Bloch and Bloch, 1972). The transient use of sedatives or minor tranquilizers may be useful. This allows the extremely anxious patient to calm sufficiently in order to cooperate with psychotherapy. The type of psychotherapy indicated can frequently be effectively provided by a primary care physician. In some ways this may be preferable in order to avoid the concept that the posttraumatic neurosis represents a psychiatric disease. In fact the patient can, and should, be told in a supportive manner that the symptoms are normal and will abate with time and treatment.

The following case history is illustrative of the posttraumatic syndrome.

In an ironical situation a 28-year-old surgery resident, who was assigned to an emergency room rotation, was out driving with his wife when suddenly and unexpectedly their car was hit by another car driven by a drunk driver. The crash was severe and both the resident and his wife were rendered transiently unconscious. Upon recovering consciousness the physician recalls waiting, with terror, while ambulance personnel apparently ignored him and his wife while rushing the other driver to the hospital. Meanwhile he felt helpless and humiliated as a crowd gathered to observe the accident, but no one offered any assistance. Another ambulance arrived, and he was finally transported to a hospital emergency room (other than that where he was employed).

On arrival at the emergency room he was frightened and bewildered by the fact that little information was made available to him concerning his wife (who had not suffered severe injuries). Emergency room personnel did not introduce themselves. His anxiety, manifested by severe trembling, received only the response of covering him with a blanket. There was little sympathy offered and an assumption made (inaccurate) that he understood all procedures which were performed. He became preoccupied with a favorite tweed jacket that he was wearing and became angry when it was unceremoniously cut from him (an example of displacement). A fracture to the humerus was reduced, causing great pain to the patient, with the callous statement that because of the head injury a general anesthesia and/or analgesics were contraindicated. A request for a plastic surgeon to suture lacerations on the chest were met with derisive comments that he must think himself to be a movie star. The feelings of helplessness and humiliation continued and, although there was a passive acceptance of the treatment offered, it was at the cost of considerable anxiety and subsequent anger.

Following a brief hospitalization the physician/patient was released home. Sleep was disturbed for several weeks because of severe nightmares which revolved around themes of automobile and airplane crashes. He refused sleeping medication for fear that his spleen might rupture while he was asleep and he would die. Appetite decreased and there was a severe startle reaction to even the sound of a refrigerator door being slammed closed. Headaches and dizziness persisted for a month. Other behavioral changes included an expectation that he would be cared for, despite the fact that physically he remained capable of doing at least light work. He repetitively told the story of the accident and his treatment to anyone who would listen. There were marked expressions of anger at the person who caused the accident, the treatment received at the hospital, and at the service chief who wanted him to return to work. An attorney was contacted and plans were made to sue not only the drunk driver but also the hospital emergency room.

With the aid of supportive psychotherapy symptoms abated over a period of weeks and he returned to work after 2 months of disability, actually not an unreasonable period of time. Nightmares and the startle reaction faded gradually and were almost completely gone after 6 months. Plans to sue the drunk driver continued but the suit against the emergency room physicians was dropped, although considerable anger remained.

An interesting outcome was a change in behavior toward emergency room patients whom the resident himself treated. He demonstrated increased attention and concern making sure that he introduced himself and explained all procedures in detail. His increase concern was frequently acknowledged by patients who would return after recovery to thank him for his care, often bearing presents to concretely express appreciation. He noted that receiving this positive feedback from patients was a distinct change from before his accident.

The Hypochondriacal Neuroses

Following an accident (or acute illness resulting in a period of disability) a small percentage of persons, following apparent medical recovery, will remain preoccupied with somatic symptoms. Typically these patients have numerous somatic symptoms, often fitting no well-defined medical syndromes, for which they insistently seek medical care. The symptoms are attributed by the patient to the accident even when no direct relationship is apparent. The patient "doctor shops" going from one physician to another seeking a diagnosis, rejecting each explanation that nothing is wrong, and seizing upon any minor finding or transiently abnormal laboratory result as evidence to substantiate illness. This typical hypochondriacal behavior, well known to all physicians, appears to have been unleashed by the accident suffered by the patient. This form of abnormal illness behavior can be divided into two major syndromes described below.

Primary Hypochondriasis. In primary hypochondriasis we are dealing with a long-standing lifestyle (see Chapter 6). The patient has always been hypochondriacal and has sought medical treatment extensively in the past with little or no objective evidence of disease. The condition usually has its onset in childhood or adolescence followed by a seemingly endless string of physical complaints, visits to various physicians and numerous therapeutic trials of medications, many of which caused side reactions. However, hypochondriasis by no means confers upon the patient an immunity from illness or accidents and when such occur they become rapidly incorporated into the patient's lifestyle and are used to justify prior illness behavior. The patient may minimize the previous medical history, now that there is an acute objective symptom or injury, and the physician (particularly if he has been called in to deal with the new problem) is focused upon only the acute problem. As a consequence a detailed history prior to the accident may not be available to the physician who subsequently responds to each complaint of the patient as if it were a possible complication of the trauma. The repetitive workups serve to reinforce the patient's symptoms and the primary problem, existing before the accident, not only continues but is intensified. Doctor shopping may occur to an even greater extent than previously because medical bills are being paid by third-party payers who are financially liable for the accident.

Treatment of this condition is, at best, difficult as all who have seen the moral righteousness of a truly sick hypochondriac can testify. It is essential that the underlying lifestyle be identified as soon as is possible and that the principles employed in the treatment of the primary hypochondriac be instituted as soon as possible. These include a supportive relationship, frequent visits to the physicians which are not predicated on the development of new symptoms and diagnostic studies and treatment initiated by objective evidence of disease rather than by subjective complaints.

The "Humpty Dumpty" Syndrome. The "Humpty Dumpty" syndrome is the eponym offered by me (Ford, 1978) to a constellation of symptoms originally described by Nemiah (1963). In this syndrome, following an accident or acute illness, the patient demonstrates the characteristic behavior of hypochondriasis, complete with perceived disability, despite the history of not being hypochondriacal in the past. To the contrary, the history indicates that the patient was an extremely hard working, conscientious, and responsible person. The background history frequently indicates that in childhood the patient, often because of death or illness of a parent, was thrust into a position of early responsibility. Work started early and frequently schooling was prematurely terminated. Early marriage and family financial responsibilities often required the patient to work overtime or at more than one job. It is hypothesized that such an individual has dealt with dependency needs through reaction formation and that an accident provides for overgratification of these previously repressed dependent wishes. The fragile characterologic defenses crumble and the patient behaves in such a manner as to provide for a continuation of having the dependency needs gratified. Unfortunately the price paid is very high: The patients are usually chronically depressed, marital problems are common, and finances almost always more of a problem than before.

Important factors which also accompany this syndrome are that the patient, who is frequently a member of a minority group, is not well educated, has little job flexibility, and is beginning to notice the effect of age upon his employment capabilities. Therefore, disability payments also contribute some important secondary gain features to the overall picture.

Treatment of the Humpty Dumpty syndrome must be basically prophylactic in nature. Once well established the symptoms are as refractory to
favorable modification as is the reconstitution of "Humpty Dumpty" himself. The physician must be aware of the particular constellation of psychodynamic factors which may make a person susceptible to this syndrome. A
return to work, even modified work, as soon as possible must be arranged.
The employer can be a very helpful and perhaps a vital adjunctive agent in
the rehabilitation. Positive statements from the employer as to the value of
the employee and willingness to make alterations in the work schedule, etc.,
may salvage a valuable employee and prevent considerable human misery.

The following case history is illustrative of the Humpty Dumpty
syndrome.

A 43-year-old Latin-American man had been disabled for five years at the
time he was initially seen for psychiatric consultation. While at work he had
been hit by an automobile and suffered a fracture of his left leg. Despite his
numerous and vague complaints, resulting in repetitive medical and orthopedic consultations, the only objective finding was that the injured leg was
three-eights of an inch shorter than the other. Financial settlement of his
claims via litigation did not alter his symptoms. He felt that the amount of
money was unsatisfactory and that the company doctor had attempted to
return him to work prematurely, thereby aggravating the original injury.

The patient's personal history was regarded to be of considerable significance. He was born into the family of a strict, hardworking but poor
farmer in the southwestern United States. His father died when he was eight,
and two years later his mother became bedridden with a chronic disease.
With his mother's illness, he began working half-time in order to help
support her, and three years later at the age of 13 he dropped out of school in
order to work full time. The patient married at age 22 and fathered eight
children. In order to support his large family he worked long hours at a
factory (averaging over 70 hours per week) and to further support his income
periodically worked evenings as a musician. He reported that he had gone
for periods as long as six months without taking a day off work.

Of importance and consistent with the formulations of Hirschfield and
Behan (1966), he admitted that he had been experiencing increasing
nervousness and sleeplessness just prior to the accident, and he himself
questioned whether the accident could have been avoided if he had been
more careful.

The patient was followed in supportive psychotherapy and given a trial of
tricyclic antidepressant therapy. However, his symptoms remained refractory
to these attempted therapeutic interventions. Despite his avowed "macho"
statements that he was the head of the household, his wife reported that it
had been necessary for her to assume the responsibility for the family. She
also indicated significant sexual problems in the marriage since the injury.

Compensation Neurosis

The term compensation neurosis is frequently, and inappropriately, used to describe any situation where financial compensation may result from an accident. As used here the term will apply to situations where it can be determined that issues related to compensation are the *major* factors in either producing or perpetuating the patient's claim of disability. It is assumed by the use of the term "neurosis" that the process is to some extent unconscious and results from some aspect of psychic conflict. This is distinct from malingering (discussed below), which presumes a conscious falsification of symptoms.

There are two major forms of compensation neurosis. Each is to a large extent determined by the underlying motivation of the individual rather than by the presenting symptoms.

Compensation as a Solution to Social Inadequacy. This straightforward syndrome may occur when a person of limited social capabilities and employment skills experiences a compensable accident. The prospect of payment, through permanent and regular disability payments, reduces the prospects of having to continually work at menial jobs. Disability payments may be as much, if not more with associated benefits, then the patient's earning capabilities. As important, if not more so than the compensation, are the associated solutions to psychic conflict. The patient can rationalize the inadequacy as being not due to inherent problems but instead to the accident and the subsequent disability suffered. Instead of perceiving oneself as a social misfit the role of a sick person can be assumed without suffering intrapsychic guilt or social stigma. An ancillary syndrome is that of the working wife/mother who suffers an accident. The prospect of compensation and assuming the role of disabled person may resolve the conflict that she has about working outside of the home.

Basically this form of compensation neurosis is a societal problem more than it is a medical problem. The physician can best serve the patient and the needs of society by providing concerned care, taking care to reinforce symptoms as little as possible, but not engaging in unnecessary diagnostic treatment procedures and by accurately reporting medical opinions to involved parties. It may be necessary to work closely with public agencies, particularly those associated with rehabilitation and vocational training.

The "Justice Neurosis". This term derived from the German medical literature (Ramsay, 1939) concisely describes the motivation and conflict inherent in a number of disability situations. The crux of this syndrome is that the accident victim feels that he has experienced an injustice and, that for the scales to be balanced, someone must pay! Not infrequently it is not the actual compensation which is desired but rather the public acknowledgment of the injustice by the judicial assessment of damages.

Patients who seek redress of their grievances through litigation can be remarkably persistent in their pursuit of justice. The distress which they cause physicians, employers, insurance companies, and other persons may be considerable and the harrassment caused by these patients may also be very time-consuming to the parties involved. The physician will find that in addition to the time occupied with provision of medical services, time is also required to deal with the multiple agents involved with these patients (attorneys, insurance claim officers, etc.). Defensive medicine becomes the "game plan" and the doctor–patient relationship is unsatisfactory for both parties.

Patients with a "justice neurosis" may have a history consistent with that of paranoid personality or of prior litigation. They may be chronically unhappy persons looking for someone, or something, onto whom they can focus their displeasure. They often have suffered numerous injustices in the past for which they could seek no satisfaction. With a discernible cause for their misery they can attack this with the fury which has built up over the years, perhaps even decades, of ill-fortune and mistreatment.

Despite these potential predisposing factors the fact remains that usually the patient has indeed suffered an injustice and may have been treated shabbily or with little sensitivity in regard to his injury. As a consequence someone *will* have to *pay*. Too often this could have been avoided thus preventing considerable emotional distress to all, not the least of whom the patient himself.

Where did things go wrong? If we reinvestigate the anatomy of an accident we find that there are numerous places where the seed of future litigation could be implanted. The employment conditions or personnel policies at work could lead to chronic feelings of resentment. The employer's immediate response to the accident may have been anger rather than concern, or there may have been implications by the employer or the company doctor that the patient was not really injured when first evaluated. All of these potential personal slights may lead to intense feelings of anger which fester with time. There are many other potential causes for anger: a drunk driver who caused the accident; the indifference of emergency room staff to pain; the boredom of the consulting physician; penurious attitudes of insurance companies; the implication of malingering. The list is almost endless.

One must keep in mind the basic psychological responses to trauma and how these can go awry. In brief review, the person involved in an accident experiences a transient regression. Defenses are less mature and differentiated: there is an expectation that one will be actively cared for. Then there is a loss of a sense of omnipotence (omnipotence as used here does not imply a grandiose or infantile quality but rather a healthy psychological status where one feels in control of one's life) and concurrently a feeling of increased vulnerability. Narcissism prevails and there is an increased preoccupation with the body. Failure to appreciate these basic responses may result in narcissistic injury to the accident victim. Angry, goal-directed prosecution of one's grievances can be seen as a means of regaining a sense of mastery over the traumatic experience and restoring one's sense of omnipotence.

Treatment of these patients with "justice neurosis" is by no means easy. By the time that the physician becomes aware of the problem there may already be an adversarial relationship. As with the other disability syndromes, prevention is the important issue, for after set in motion they are difficult to modify favorably. In treating the patient with an injury, or who later presents as a disability syndrome, it is essential to take a complete history with special attention to the details of the accident and the responses of various persons to it. The recounting, to an authority figure, of the experience and of the perceived misjustices may have cathartic value and lessen the emotional intensity. One must remain objective and affectually neutral insofar as possible in order not to become drawn into the patient's intense pursuit of justice nor to lose sight of the fact that the patient may very well be entitled to fair compensation for the suffering and losses which have been sustained.

Malingering

In recent years most authors who have written about malingering have been inclined to view it from a psychodynamic viewpoint and to explain the symptom in terms of unconscious motivations. Although such formulations may well be accurate interpretations of psychic phenomenon, the fact remains that a certain number of patients consciously deceive physicians and others such as insurance claim agents, by deliberately simulating diseases or symptoms which they do not have. When malingering results in compensation then a fraud has been perpetrated. Yet despite the fact that many physicians believe that malingering after an injury is not uncommon I am unaware of any case of malingering which has been prosecuted in a court of law. Chambers (1963) reports that malingering was present in 3 of 17 cases of disability neurosis which he evaluated.

Why is the diagnosis of malingering made so infrequently? Perhaps because it is actually an accusation rather than a diagnosis (Szasz, 1956). The training and professional orientation of a physician is that of helper rather than that of a policeman. The physician may resist making a diagnosis of malingering because of fear of "missing something" yet paradoxically with another patient be willing to undertake a dangerous operation with even less certainty of the diagnosis. Fear of malpractice suit or actual attacks by the patient (Parker, 1979) may also make the physician reluctant to accuse the patient of malingering. As a consequence the medical system is "easy pickings" for the con artist or sociopathic personality who sees money potentially available with very little risk. As has been pointed out by Robertson (1978) each physician may have a different part of the story and conflictual medical testimony in court tends to protect the malingerer. Robertson suggests that the medical evidence be examined by independent physicians prior to trial. Such a committee of experts could better advise the judge than the independent testimony of individual physicians.

Physicians must be bold enough to state that they can find no evidence of medical-psychiatric disease. At that point responsibility for prosecution belongs to those who have a financial interest at stake. Despite this appeal to intellectual honesty, it is only fair to provide some concurrent words of caution. Malingering can in itself be a persons's defense against the awareness of an even more severe illness. This complex situation was illustrated by the case history reported in Chapter 8.

Malingering is a complex problem, but after carefully considering all of the available medical history and findings, the physician should not be reluctant to state that he can find no evidence of physical or psychiatric disease to explain the patients symptoms.

Other Psychiatric Diagnoses

To detail all of the possible psychiatric sequelae of trauma and their resultant disability would be, in fact, to include all of the contents of the psychiatric diagnostic manual. What has preceded is a description of the syndromes more frequently related to the specific issue of disability following trauma. It must be recognized that each individual is unique and the anatomy of each accident different. Individuals may also respond to the stress of trauma with such diverse disorders as schizophrenia, dissociative reactions, hysterical conversion reactions, or phobias.

The following brief self-explanatory case reported by Berger (1975) illustrates a phobic response: A masonry worker was standing on a scaffold 25 stories above ground level when it gave way. He dangled by his safety belt for 5 hours before being rescued. When he returned to work two weeks later he was totally incapable of working at any level above that of the first floor. At any height above that he would be overcome with panic.

GENERAL PRINCIPLES IN THE MANAGEMENT OF DISABILITY SYNDROMES

Prevention and Initial Evaluation

Effective management of the patient with a disability syndrome occurs before the patient has been identified as such. Preventive measures are far more effective than attempts to treat these syndromes once they have been established. It may appear trite to say that all trauma victims require conscientious, considerate, and empathetic attention to their emotional needs as to their somatic injuries. However, it is an unfortunate fact that many of the interpersonal contacts between emergency room personnel and trauma victims are devoid of any human warmth. It cannot be emphasized too strongly that every victim of physical trauma suffers an emotional trauma concurrently. The net result is psychological regression and the victims' employment of more immature defenses. Patients are therefore at increased risk for further narcissistic injury and as mentioned above, many disability syndromes have their origins in an initial physician (or nurse) contact which has gone awry (M.H. Miller, 1961).

The preservation of life and limb, or course, takes precedence over obtaining a meaningful psychosocial history. But once the patient is medically stable, then it is essential to obtain a detailed account of the accident, which includes antecendent factors as well as details as to how the accident occurred. Subsequent management of the patient will to some extent be dependent upon identifying and then utilizing the patient's coping mechanisms. In addition to the utilitarian benefit of the factual information obtained, the process of history-taking serves to increase the quality of the relationship between physician and patient. Convinced of the physician's genuine interest, the patient is more likely to cooperate with treatment and rehabilitation plans.

Accurate Diagnosis

If preventive measures are not effective and a disability syndrome does emerge, then it is incumbent upon the physician to establish a diagnosis of the specific type of disorder and to make therapeutic interventions as rapidly as possible. Some of the potential interventions for one type of disorder may be contraindicated for another. Therefore all patients who fail to get well on a schedule consistent with medical expectations should not be regarded, for example, as "compensation neurotics."

The diagnosis of a major affective disorder should elicit a vigorous treatment plan, which may include antidepressant medications or psychiatric hospitalization. A premature return to work may result in another accident. To the contrary, a person with marked counterdependent defenses (the Humpty Dumpty syndrome) should be returned to work, even partial work, as soon as possible. Patients with primary hypochondriasis should be quickly identified in order that unnecessary medical procedures will not reinforce their somatization patterns. However, the patient with numerous physical complaints may be suffering from a posttraumatic neurosis, and these patients should receive supportive psychotherapy and in some situations sedatives or minor tranquilizers.

Important information to obtain, in order to arrive at an accurate diagnosis, includes the premorbid history and the presence or absence of specific symptoms which are reflected of depression or anxiety. In regard to depression and anxiety, particularly important are sleep disturbance, presence or absence of nightmares, appetite, sexual libido, tachycardia or palpitations, and diapheresis. Also important to ascertain are (1) the degree and focus of the patient's anger, and (2) the patient's realistic expectations for continued employment, e.g., is this a manual laborer who with age was becoming a marginal worker before the accident?

Return to Work and Rehabilitation

In general, the injured worker should be encouraged to work as soon as possible even if the return entails shorter hours or less strenuous duties. Resumption of the usual adult role will help reduce the ever-present dangers toward regression. However, a premature return to work which results in a failure should be avoided because it may reinforce the feelings of inadequacy and disability. From a realistic view the physician's efforts in this regard may be less effective than he/she desires. As stated by H. Miller (1961), in reference to the activities of attorneys and union officials, "The conscientious doctor who tries to keep his patient at work despite a minor injury is pitting himself single-handed against powerful social and economic forces all of which press in the opposite direction. It seems certain that effective prevention would demand far-reaching social readjustments rather than purely medical measures."

The focus, at least in the United States, has been upon financial compensation (see below) rather than upon rehabilitation for persons who have suffered injuries (Ross, 1977). This places the emphasis upon the degree of reduced function. Because disease is emphasized over health, the patient's view of himself becomes that of a person who is sick, and as a consequence the patient will behave as a person with an illness. However limited rehabilitation services may be, it is important for the physician (or through social services consultation) to explore the availability of these programs. The rehabilitation program may be the most important part of treatment. Although it may sound like sermonizing, a patient can be told that, despite the fact that disability payments may preclude the financial necessity for working, the patient would probably feel better and be less depressed if a return to work could be arranged. Patients can be praised for such efforts while acknowledging increased discomfort or other problems associated with a return to work.

The Issue of Compensation

Similar to the situation with rehabilitation, the issue of compensation is largely out of the hands of the physicians. Compensation is a complex problem involving the legal, economic, and political sectors of society in addition to medicine. The major role of the physician may be to facilitate decision-making by the patient in such a manner as to create as little adverse psychological effect as possible.

Most authors have been inclined to regard lump-sum payments as contributing less to prolonged disability syndromes than do indefinite period payments contingent upon the continuation of disability (Pokorny and Moore, 1953). It has also been urged that compensation claims be settled as quickly as possible (Miller, 1959; Ross, 1977) because as litigation stretches out the patient's symptoms progressively become more deeply entrenched and less modifiable to a favorable outcome. Preoccupation with the issue of obtaining financial rewards for sickness may bear with it the high cost of a lengthy, unhappy and impaired quality of life hardly justified by the meager compensation received. The paradox in the compensation issue has been highlighted by Ellard (1970), "... it is proper that injured men should be compensated and predictable that sometimes compensation may injure them further."

SUMMARY

Every serious illness or accident involves not only physical damage but also emotional trauma. The accident victim must heal from both injuries. Recovery from the emotional injuries is determined by a number of different factors, such as coping skills developed before the injury, the nature of the injury, and the response of the social system, including health care personnel, to the accident victim. Within the process of recovery there are many opportunities for the development of abnormal or aberrant illness behaviors. At times the healing process goes awry and the patient remains emotionally disabled. At other times the person, perhaps encouraged by others, finds that the sick role to be more appealing than health.

All persons are at risk for psychological adjustment problems following severe trauma. Persons who appear to be at higher risk for disability syndromes include those with a previous history of somatizing behavior, those who had marginal coping abilities or ongoing psychological problems at the time of the accident and those whose lifestyle was previously characterized by counterdependent behavior.

A variety of societal and economic forces contribute to the development of disability syndromes and therefore all of these syndromes cannot be prevented or necessarily successfully treated. However, preventative management techniques and timely recognition will reduce the incidence and severity of these disorders.

REFERENCES

Behan, R.C., and Hirschfield, A.H. 1963. The accident process II: Toward more rational treatment of industrial injuries. JAMA 186:303–306.

Belter, S.R., Fine, P.R., Simison, D., *et al*. 1979. Disability benefits as disincentives to rehabilitation. Milbank Mem Fund Q/Health and Society 57:412–427.

Berger, J.C. 1975. Some psychological aspects of industrial injury. Ill Med J 147:364–365.

Bloch, G.R., and Bloch, N.H. 1972. Traumatic and post-traumatic neuroses. Industrial Med 41:5–8.

Braverman, M.D. 1977. Validity of psychotraumatic reactions. J Forensic Sci 22:654–662.

Chambers, W.N. 1963. Emotional factors complicating industrial injuries. J Occup Med 5:568–574.

Conger, J.J., Gaskill, H.S., Glad, D.D., et al. 1959. Psychological and psychophysiologic factors in motor vehicle accidents. JAMA 169:1581–1587.

Crocq, L 1974. Stress et névrose traumatique. Psychologie Médicale 6:1493–1531.

Dunbar, F. 1947. *Mind and Body*. New York: Random House, pp 96–111.

Ellard, J. 1970. Psychological reactions to compensable injury. Med J Aust 2:349–355.

Ford, C.V. 1978. A type of disability neurosis: The "Humpty Dumpty Syndrome." Int J Psychiatry Med 8:285–294.

Fowler, R.C., Liskow, B.I., VonValkenburg, C., et al. 1979. Symptoms in veterans considering compensation claims. J Clin Psychiatry 40:65–71.

Friedman,M.J. 1981. Post-Vietnam syndrome: Recognition and management. Psychosomatics 22:931–943.

Froggatt, P., and Smiley, J.A. 1964. The concept of accident proneness: A review. Br J Indust Med 21:1–12.

Hirschfield, A.H., and Behan, R.C. 1963. The accident process I: Etiological considerations of industrial injuries. JAMA 186:193–199.

Hirschfield, A.H., and Behan, R.C. 1966. The accident process III Disability: Acceptable and unacceptable. JAMA 197:85–89.

Horowitz, M.J., Wilner, N. Kaltreider, N., and Alvarez, W. 1980. Signs and symptoms of post traumatic stress disorder. Arch Gen Psychiatry 37:85–92.

Keiser, L 1968. *The Traumatic Neurosis*. Philadelphia: Lippincott.

Kolb, L.C. 1954. *The Painful Phantom, Psychology, Physiology and Treatment*. Springfield, Ill.: Charles C. Thomas.

Krusen, E.M., and Ford, D.E. 1958. Compensation factor in low back injuries. JAMA 166:1128–1133.

Laughlin, H.P. 1954a. The neurosis following trauma: Part I. Med Ann D.C. 23:492–502.

Laughlin, H.P. 1954b. The neuroses following trauma: Part II. Med Ann D.C. 23:567–580.

Martin, R.D. 1974. Secondary gain, everybody's rationalization. J Occup Med 16:800–801.

Mattsson, E.I. 1975. Psychological aspects of severe physical injury and its treatment. J Trauma 15:217–234.

Miller, H. 1961. Accident neurosis: Lecture 2. Br Med J 1:992–998.

Miller, M.H. 1959. The compensation neurosis: J Forensic Sci 4:159–166.

Miller, M.H. 1961. Continuing incapacity despite "medical recovery." JAMA 176:205–207.

Modlin, H.C. 1967. The postaccident anxiety syndrome: Psychosocial aspects. Am J Psychiatry 123:1008–1012.

Neiderland, W.G. 1968. Clinical observations on the "survivor syndrome." Internat J Psychoanal 49:313–315.

Nemiah, J.C. 1963. Psychological complications in industrial injuries. Arch Environ Health 1:481–486.

Ostwald, P., and Bittner, E. 1968. Life adjustment after severe persecution. Am J Psychiatry 124:1393–1400.

Parker, N. 1979. Malingering: A dangerous diagnosis. Med J Aust 1:568–569.

Pokorny, A.D., and Moore, F.J. 1953. Neuroses and compensation: Psychiatric disorders following injury or stress in compensable situations. Arch Indus Hyg and Occup Med 8:547–563.

Ramsay, J. 1939. Nervous disorder after injury: Review of 400 cases. Br Med J 2:385–390.

Rappaport, E.A. 1968. Beyond traumatic neurosis. Int J Psycho-Anal 49:719–731.

Robertson, A.J. 1978. Malingering, occupational medicine and the law. Lancet 2:828–831.

Ross, W.D. 1977. How to get a neurotic worker back on the job successfully. Occup Health Safety 46:20–23.

Selzer, M.L. Rogers, J.E., and Kern, S. 1968. Fatal accidents: The role of psychopathology, social stress and acute disturbance. Am J Psychiatry 124:1028–1036.

Schnaper, N. 1975. The psychological implications of severe trauma: Emotional sequelae to unconsciousness. J Trauma 15:94–98.

Schnaper, N., and Cowley, R.A. 1976. Overview: Psychiatric sequelae to multiple trauma. Am J Psychiatry 133:883–890.

Stuart, J.C., and Brown, B.M. 1981. The relationship of stress and coping ability to incidence of diseases and accidents. J Psychosom Res 25:255–260.

Szasz, T.S. 1956. Malingering: "diagnosis" or social condemnation. Arch Neurol Psychiatry 195:432–443.

Titchener, J.L. 1970. Management of study of psychological response to trauma. J Trauma 10:974–980.

Warmes, H. 1972. The traumatic syndrome. Canad Psychiat Assoc J 17:391–396.

Weisz, G.M. 1973. Psyche-trauma-psyche: Surgeons' observations of psychiatric conditions in trauma patients. Isr Ann Psychiatry 11:91–98.

12

PHYSICIANS:
THE OTHER HALF
OF THE DOCTOR–PATIENT RELATIONSHIP

Balint (1957) has cogently observed that the prescription that the patient often requires is that of the drug "doctor." This incisive formulation allows us to conceive of the doctor–patient relationship as an active treatment modality which can be investigated much as any other therapeutic agent. The doctor–patient relationship is of particular importance with the somatizing disorders because it is precisely the wish to have a relationship with the physician for which the patient, motivated either consciously or unconsciously, strives. It goes almost without saying that the relationship between the patient and his physician is of utmost importance in all forms of illness. The lessons learned in treatment of the somatizing patient can be effectively used for patients who have varying degrees of organic disease accompanying the illness with which they present.

Before prescribing the drug "doctor" we must look carefully at its properties. Because our drug is an alive and dynamic force instead of a chemical, rather than define physical properties such as solubility, we will look at the personal characteristics of the physician. Of special importance are the psychological aspects of how the physician behaves and the determinants, often unconsciously motivated, of decision-making and communications, including nonverbal behavior, to the patient. Again an analogy can be drawn to a chemical drug and the parallel is to the study of pharmacologic action. We must also assume that if a drug has the potency to effect a beneficial change then, not being inert, it must also have the power to cause adverse reactions. Indeed, as with potent pharmacologic agents, the drug doctor can cause both remarkably beneficial changes as well as serious untoward reactions of a negative nature (Strupp et al., 1977).

In order to fully understand the doctor–patient relationship it is necessary to examine both sides of it. This chapter focuses upon the specific qualities of physicians. The preceding chapters have focused upon the different types of somatizing patients and the following chapter will be directed to specific aspects of the doctor–patient relationship.

SOCIETAL EXPECTATIONS OF PHYSICIANS

Physicians occupy a unique position of high prestige within our society. It is often assumed that a doctor is in some way different or superior to other members of the citizenry. "The physician, then, is seen by society as a heroic, God-like person—a super-intelligent, self-sacrificing, moral, trustworthy, perfect, reliable individual who has leadership abilities that are sacrificially presented to society for its use" (Wilson and Larson, 1981).

There is often disbelief, shock, or disillusionment when a physician is found to have psychiatric problems or to engage in illegal or unorthodox behavior. For example, the wife of a physician consulted me concerning her husband's apparently irrational attitude toward sexual behavior. She broke into the middle of her story with the exclamation, "I just don't understand why. He's a doctor!" As will be discussed later these societal expectations may place an additional burden upon the physician who feels that he must live up to an ideal, no matter how unrealistic it may be or how great the strain.

Similar to the "role" in society for sick persons proposed by Parsons (1951) there is also a proposed role for physicians. This role consists of the obligations for the physician to remain affectively neutral (nonjudgmental) in dealings with patients, to do everything possible to effect the patient getting well as quickly as is possible, and to put the interests of the patient above personal interests. The proposed rights of the physician include a degree of power (or control) over another person (the patient) not generally accepted outside of medicine and the right, outside of usual business practices, to determine fair compensation for services.

In summary, societal expectations for physicians are that they are high-minded altruistic persons who are admired, often idealized, and in whom is placed an unusual degree of trust and power. It comes as a rude shock to many persons to learn that physicians are not only human but for a variety of reasons may experience and demonstrate a greater than average amount of emotional distress and/or unorthodox behavior (Waring, 1974).

PSYCHOLOGICAL CHARACTERISTICS OF PHYSICIANS

Before proceeding to an examination of various psychological characteristics of physicians it is important to note several facts. First, much of the information that we have available concerning the psychic makeup of doctors is derived from the study of those who become psychiatrically ill or those who for one reason or another sought psychotherapy or psychoanalysis in order to achieve a greater understanding of themselves. It is not logical to extrapolate these findings, obtained from a minority of physicians, to all who practice medicine. Obviously many of the descriptions offered below do not fit many, perhaps most, physicians. Also, an important area where comparatively little information is available is that in regard to women physicians. In the past most physicians have been male and therefore almost all reports describing physicians have focused upon male physicians. Psychological descriptions of male physicians may not hold true for women physicians.

However, despite the above cautions, we must keep in mind the fact that medical schools in the United States and Canada are remarkably stereotyped. Courses required for admission are very similar and admission committees of different schools look for the same or very similar qualities in those students whom they accept. Curricula from school to school are so alike that few students encounter any scholastic difficulties in transferring to different medical schools. It is remarkable how little difference there is among the various medical schools and training hospitals. This is evidenced by the widely accepted practice of trainees transferring to different institutions for postgraduate residency training after graduation. The process of medical socialization is such that graduates of most programs have similar attitudes and similar slang, even when institutions are separated by thousands of miles.

As a consequence of this stereotyped training process, and socialization into the medical profession most physicians are more alike than they are different. Therefore it follows that those characteristics found in the more seriously disturbed members of the profession may indeed be present in a somewhat less exaggerated extent in many other physicians.

The Psychodynamics of Physicianhood

Psychodynamics is a term used to describe those operations of the psyche which are primarily unconscious. Included are the various ego defense mechanisms utilized by the individual and those prior life experiences, largely forgotten or repressed, which continue to influence emotions and behavior. The motivation to enter medicine, behavior related to the practice of medicine and emotional responses to the events inherent in the practice of medicine are all influenced by psychodynamic factors.

The motivation to choose medicine as a career may not be as simple as those glib answers provided on medical school application forms or offered in interviews. The most common reason to enter medicine given by medical school applicants is to blend an interest in science with a compassionate desire to help sick people (Golloway, 1981). In more candid moments, applicants may talk of a wish to improve their socioeconomic status or hopes of an occupation associated with personal prestige. These consciously stated reasons for entering medicine, while genuine, often serve as a screen for more powerful unconscious motivations.

The more covert and unconscious reasons for wishing to become a physician are hypothesized to revolve around early childhood experiences. Many physicians have had experience with disease and/or death in childhood (Abram, 1978; Golloway, 1981; Menninger, 1959). Either they, or a family member, were sick. The physician was seen as a powerful individual, often more powerful than the parents and other family members who were forced to stand around helplessly. The physician-to-be frequently developed a fear of disease and/or death and this fear was defended against by the mechanism of *reaction formation*. The formulation being, "I am not afraid of disease because I can conquer it."

Other unconscious motivations to enter medicine include efforts to resolve other types of childhood conflicts (McLaughlin, 1961; Nunberg, 1938; Simmel, 1926). Medicine can be a way of channeling natural aggressive instinct, via sublimation, into socially accepted and altruistic activities: the surgeon who cuts is also healing. Feelings of powerlessness in relationship to the father are mastered by identification with a more powerful figure, the doctor. Feelings of insufficient care from the mother are mastered by the transformation of these longings to the statement, " I do not need to be taken care of. I take care of others!" Thus both paternal and maternal elements are incorporated into the psychological makeup of the physician. The need for omnipotence and omniscience are prominent as defenses against feelings of helplessness and inadequacy, in regard to the dangers of disease and death, and as a way to master the competition with a powerful father.

A prospective study of college students which compared those who became physicians to those students who entered another profession indicated and those who entered medicine, especially areas of primary care, had childhoods which were more troubled than the comparison group. It was also observed that the physicians made prominent use of the ego mechanisms of hypochondriasis, reaction formation and altruism (Vaillant et al., 1972).

An investigation that directly observed physicians practicing medicine found evidence to support the psychodynamic formulations of earlier psychoanalysts (Zabarenko et al., 1970). The physicians were observed to have a need for omnipotence and used the admiration of their patients to gratify that need. The investigators observed that the physicians were often counterphobic about disease, such as often ignoring basic principles of antisepsis. The physicians were also observed to often exhibit a bimodal behavior pattern which suggested an alteration between the incorporated maternal and paternal identities. For example, an acute problem might elicit an authoritative response (paternalistic), while treatment of a chronic disease, or of children, might elicit maternal qualities.

The following clinical vignette demonstrates some of the psychodynamic characteristics frequently seen in physicians.

A young physician was admitted to a hospital comatose after a serious suicide attempt from an overdose of barbituates. The apparent precipitant was a rejection from his girlfriend. Seen subsequently in psychotherapy, the physician's life and the suicide motivation emerged as far more complex than initially appreciated. He had been raised in a series of foster homes because his chronically ill and complaining mother had neither the inclination nor the ability to care for him. She had already chased the father away. As soon as he was able he left his home state to enroll in a college situated in another state. A brilliant student, he supported himself through college and medical school by using scholarships and working part time. He took a perverse delight in relating to the therapist that he had withheld from his mother the knowledge that he was now a doctor!

The despair that the young physician had experienced on the breakup of his relationship with his girlfriend was actually caused by the fact that this breakup severed his relationship with his girlfriend's mother, a warm, loving person, who had become his surrogate mother.

The patient supported himself through freelance medical work, not liking to be tied to one job. He worked at the same clinic one day a week and reported that each day that he was scheduled to work there he would become very "depressed." It was in a low-income area and he would see each patient for as short a time as possible, trying to end the day quickly so that he could return home. He was able to express extreme guilt for his behavior, stating that the patients needed far more than his capability to give to them. Their needs stimulated memories of his own deprived background and his own feelings that he wanted someone to care for him.

With psychotherapy the physician-patient gained greater understanding of himself, improved his relationships with others, including reestablishing a cautious relationship with his mother. He decided that in the best interest of himself and patients that he would be better suited to a specialty requiring minimum patient contact. A follow-up of serveral years indicated he was pleased with his new specialty and satisified with his life.

In summary, the psychodynamic characteristics of many physicians are typified by the use of reaction formation as a predominant ego mechanism. Feelings of personal vulnerability are defended against by the seeking of omnipotence and omniscience and feelings of deprivation are transformed into the care of others. Anger and hurt are denied, sublimated, and transformed into socially accepted (and admired) altruism.

Psychological Characteristics of Medical Students and Postgraduate Trainees

The above description of psychodynamic features of physicians suggests that certain psychological characteristics and psychiatric problems in medical students predate their entry into medical school.

Indeed, studies of medical students indicate that they are not, psychologically speaking, a random selection of the general population. Lief and coworkers (1960) found that obsessive-compulsive personalities were prevalent in medical students and commented that this personality type either was more motivated toward medicine or more likely to be selected by the medical school. The results of another investigation of "normal" first-year medical students (Schlageter and Rosenthal, 1962) concurred that obsessive-compulsive personality types were the most common and that the students most commonly used the ego mechanisms of repression, isolation, productivity, and achievement, traits well suited to the task before them.

A study which compared medical students to "normals" of similar age found that the medical students were very bright and demonstrated more heterogeneity both socially and psychologically. Psychopathology was much more marked in the medical student group with half of the medical students exhibiting significant psychopathology as opposed to 6% of the "normal" controls (Golden et al., 1967). Pitts and colleagues (1961) studied the incidence of psychopathology in medical students. They found that 15% of their study group were psychiatrically ill, with affective disorders being the most common diagnosis. Of note was the fact that 35% of the total group of 40 subjects had a positive family history of psychiatric illness, mostly affective disorders or alcoholism.

Despite this increased frequency of affective disorders the incidence of suicide in male medicine students appears to be comparable to that of males of similar age in the general population. The female medical student suicide rate is comparable to that of the male medical student rate but three to four times higher than that of their female agemates in the general populations. Most suicides occur during the second and third years of medical school (Pepitone-Arreola-Rockwell et al., 1981).

When psychiatric counseling is made available for medical students, it is utilized at a fairly high rate. At one medical school, 13% of all enrolled medical students request and receive psychological counseling each year. This rate might be even higher except for the fact that "medical students tend to regard emotional conflict as a sign of weakness and inadequacy and have the fantasy that a physician is an omnipotent individual who takes care of others but should not need help himself" (Adsett, 1968). At another institution, a study of emotional problems in randomly selected medical students indicated that almost 70% expressed a desire for psychiatric consultation for definitive emotional problems (Woods et al., 1966). "Medical students disease" (see Chapter 2) may be the symptomatic presentation of some of those medical students who are in emotional distress.

One of the most important areas of psychological conflict experienced by medical students is that of sexuality. Woods and Natterson (1967) (Woods, 1972) have found that sexual conflicts in medical students are surprisingly frequent. They reported that over half the students whom they studied reported significant anxiety over some aspect of sexuality. Anxiety was related to issues such as conflicts concerning masturbation or fears of being a latent homosexual. Highly aberrant sexuality was rare, and the vast majority of students exhibited behavior which was described as inhibited. This constriction of emotional expression is consistent with the obsessive-compulsive personality frequently described in medical students.

Another characteristic of medical students which I have frequently observed is that of a lack of general social and interpersonal skills. Such deficiencies can be explained by the fact that while other undergraduate students were socializing, the future medical student was more involved with academic activities. An alternative explanation is that because of discomfort with social and sexual activities the would-be medical student used academic activities as a socially approved method of avoiding confrontation with important developmental issues such as dating or other interpersonal relationships (Brent and Brent, 1978).

The first year of postgraduate training (the internship year) is very stressful. It is a period of testing out one's newly established identity as a physician, accepting new and awesome responsibilities and a time of great physical demands and sleep deprivation. Approximately 30% of all interns develop symptoms of a major depression of severe emotional distress, although many of these disorders go untreated (Ford, 1981; Valko and Clayton, 1975). The reasons for this high incidence of psychiatric problems appear to be related to predisposing factors discussed above and the great external stresses, particularly sleep deprivation, placed upon the young doctor. The incidence of psychological distress in physicians in training is lower after the first postgraduate year but remains significantly high (Ford, 1981).

One of the most important psychological changes which occurs during the process of medical education is that of a change of attitudes toward sick persons. The applicant to medical school who professed an altruistic interest in helping patients has by the end of his internship become a hardened, cynical house officer whose relationship with patients has become adversarial rather than nuturing. Patients are called "turkeys" or "gomers," and an admission to one's clinical service becomes a "hit." A prospective research study found that, during a pediatric internship year, the young physician's attitudes changed, and they began to consider psychosocial factors and the doctor–patient relationship less important in treating patients (Werner and Korsch, 1979).

The demands of medical training are great and young physicians must sacrifice their own needs for those of patients. Interns and residents often receive little support or sympathy from hospital programs who put service needs first. That psychological problems occur is not surprising but perhaps the most damaging aspect of postgraduate medical education is its effect upon young physicians' attitudes toward patients. Habit patterns are established to the effect that time is of the essence and must be spent only with acutely and seriously ill patients. Patients who are looking for a dependent relationship are angrily rejected because the interns' own dependent needs have been deprived. It is little wonder that the somatizing patient becomes recognized as an enemy rather than someone ill, in need of help.

Psychiatric Illness in Physicians

It is a sobering fact, and contrary to the physician's wish for omnipotence, that psychiatric illness appears to be more common in physicians than in the general public. The evidence for this somewhat startling statistic comes from several different sources. Reports of private psychiatric hospitals from different geographical locations indicate that ratio of physicians to non-physicians admitted as patients to the hospital greatly exceeds the ratio of physicians to the general population. The ratios vary from 1/37 to 1/82 and compare to a ratio in the overall population of about one physician per 500 people (a'Brook et al., 1967; Duffy and Litin, 1964; Pearson and Strecker, 1960; Vincent et al., 1969). These figures are more impressive when one considers that physicians are reluctant to be psychiatrically hospitalized because of fears of what such an action might mean to their careers.

Physicians are also more likely to seek outpatient psychiatric treatment. A prospective study compared college students who become physicians with those who did not. On follow-up the physicians were more likely to have sought psychotherapy (34% vs 19%) and to have used psychotropic medications (36% vs 22%) (Vaillant et al., 1972). In a comprehensive study of psychiatric illness in British Columbia (Watterson, 1976) the overall incidence in physicians was found to be 1.27% per year (approximately 1 in 78 physicians).

The nature of the psychiatric problems experienced by physicians appears to largely fall into two major groups, affective disorders and addictions (Jones, 1977; Pearson, 1982). Addiction will be discussed in a separate section below.

That depression is common among physicians is not unexpected, considering the high incidence which has already been noted in medical students and hospital house officers. The net effect of this high prevalence of depression within the medical profession is a notably high loss of physicians via suicide. The various studies of physician suicide indicate that in the United States over 100 physicians kill themselves each year, enough to require the graduating class of an average size medical school to replace them (Ross, 1975). There are many epidemiologic problems in studying suicide rates, but one detailed computerized study demonstrated that physicians and dentists are twice as likely to suicide than are members of the general population (Rose and Rosow, 1973). The actual number may be greater because suicides may be hidden by a variety of different means. Accidents, which are common in physicians (Thomas, 1976), may also represent latent suicide intent.

Despite some reports to the contrary there is no convincing evidence that either the physician's specialty (e.g., psychiatry) or gender influences the risk of suicide (Rose and Rosow, 1973). Those demographic factors which do appear to influence the risk of suicide in physicians are old age and a divorced status. Both of these factors appear to increase the risk for suicide in physicians more so than they do for the general population.

Interestingly and ironically, it is the physician's therapeutic agents— drugs—which are used most commonly as a means of suicide. That this is not simply a question of drug availability is shown by the fact that dentists and pharmacists (whose suicide rates are similar) do not have the same propensity for using this means of suicide.

The prodromal signs or symptoms of physicians who have killed themselves are those which largely reflected the presence of *depression*. Behavior changes which have been retrospectively recognized include differences in the conduct of medical practice, increasing indecisiveness, disorganization, and a hurried existence. Premorbid symptoms have also included self-doubt about ordinary medical procedures and extensive tension when confronted with difficult diagnostic problems. Still other features noted in physicians who eventually suicide include long hours with no outside interests or time for family life or vacation, the use of denial or rationalization, an inordinate need for prestige and power, poorly controlled hostility and aggression, and substance abuse (Ross, 1975).

Prevention of suicide in physicians involves education of the entire profession, and medical families, as to the risk and as to signs and symptoms which can be recognized in a colleague. When a colleague (or spouse) is identified as being depressed, or otherwise impaired, a supportive "closing of the ranks" is necessary in order to get the person into treatment. It has been suggested that the physician's "best friend" be chosen as the one to confront the impaired physician and to suggest therapeutic help (Pearson, 1982). This must be accomplished with sensitivity because an abrupt or angry confrontation may destroy the physician's last remaining vestiges of self-esteem and may be an acute precipitant to a successful suicide (Sargent et al., 1977).

Addictive Substance Abuse in Physicians

Addiction is a major problem in the medical profession; estimations have suggested a rate of addiction of 30–100 times that of the general population (Modlin and Montes, 1964). However, there are major differences between the "street addict" and the addicted physician. The latter is likely to be married, older, and started to use drugs at an age when the street addict has already "burned out" (Roeske, 1981). Physicians also tend to use drugs in a pure form and rarely overdose as opposed to use of impure substances and the frequent "O.D.s" of street addicts. The physician addict generally maintains respectability and is not associated with other addicts or the criminal members of society. The prognosis for treatment of the physician addict is considered to be good as compared to the poor prognosis for the street addict (Roeske, 1981).

There are several factors associated with addictions in physicians. The most obvious is that of the ready accessibility of drugs. Other factors include underlying personality factors which predispose to addiction and life stress situations which make the use of drugs very attractive, e.g., fatigue or illness which interfere with the continuation of medical practice.

Modlin and Montes (1964) studied a group of addicted physicians who had been hospitalized at the Menninger Clinic. They found frequently recurring themes in the personal histories and personalities of the physicians. Marked problems in the childhood homes were common. There was no one specific constellation, but descriptions of fathers included such features as stern and depriving, volatile and flamboyant, passive and indifferent, or irritable and withdrawn. Descriptions of the physician-addicts' mothers included such terms as extremely nervous, pushing, demanding, dominating, perfectionistic, ambitious, harsh, hypochondriacal, and depressive. In general the physician-addicts had intense feelings of both dependency and resentment toward their mothers. The married lives of the physician-addicts were "uniformly full of discord and misunderstandings." They were demanding and dependent upon their wives without being able to reciprocate in providing love to either the wife or to their children, with whom they were often in direct competition for the wife's love and attention. The large majority of marriages had been characterized by sexual problems which became worse after the physician's addictions.

According to Modlin and Montes the most common age for the onset of addiction in their physician patients was between age 35 and 40. The initial use of drugs (which in the great majority of cases was meperidine, possibly mixed with other types of drugs) was because of the need to deal with problems of overwork, fatigue, and physical illness. These men had difficulty saying "no" to the various demands placed upon them, yet felt very unsatisfied by their medical practices. The interpretation offered as to why these physicians become addicted revolved around the men's failures to receive the hoped for gratification of underlying dependent needs from either marriage or medical practice; inability to grow into and achieve satisfaction from the role of a parent; and/or the development of chronic physical or somatized illness. Until the age of 35 to 40 the physician had looked forward to gaining a "future paradise" but once training was completed and medical practice failed to bring the anticipated emotional rewards, disillusionment set in.

A recent report (Johnson and Connelly, 1981) of the treatment of addicted physicians from the same center, the Menninger Clinic, found that addicted physicians tended to fall into two major classes. Those over 40 years of age were more likely to exhibit organic brain impairment and depression, while those under the age of 40 were very similar to those physician-addicts previously described by Modlin and Montes. The more recent study also commented upon the finding that many of the addicted physicians had come from a background of a lower socioeconomic status than that which they enjoyed as physicians. This change from a lower class or lower middle class status to an upper middle class status was suggested to be an additional stress leading to an increased propensity to the use of addictive substances.

Although addiction to a narcotic, stimulant, or barbituate is dramatic and therefore may attract more attention than addiction to a mundane substance such as ethanol, the overall problem of alcoholism in the medical profession is likely to be of a greater magnitude. One estimate is that between 13,600 and 22,600 physicians in the United States are alcoholic or will become so (Bissell and Jones, 1976). Physicians who use addictive drugs may also abuse alcohol and vice-versa as the pattern or addiction continues, albeit with different substances at different times (Modlin and Montes, 1964).

The incidence of alcoholism among physicians does not appear to be greater than that of the general population but about 2–3% of all physicians per year have disciplinary action taken against them by their state licensing boards because of alcohol-related problems (AMA council of Mental Health 1973). It would be reasonable to suspect that the actual incidence be higher, but exact figures are difficult, if not impossible, to obtain. One well-designed prospective study of Johns Hopkins University medical students indicated that at 10 and 20 years following medical school graduation less than 1% of the 1117 graduates were known to have had personal or professional problems with alcohol (Thomas et al., 1980).

Irrespective of the actual incidence of alcoholism in the medical profession, the effect of ethanol addiction to the affected physician is great indeed in terms of health problems, social disability (including incarceration), decreased effectiveness as a physician, and on occasion the loss of a medical license or operating privileges.

That the alcoholic physician is not considered to be an inadequate or borderline physician initially is shown by the facts that a disproportionate number report a high standing in their medical school classes (Bissel and Jones, 1976) and that medical school faculty are by no means exempt from alcoholism (Spickard and Billings, 1981).

An interesting and important finding in a study of recovered alcoholic physicians was that one third of the subjects reported that they had never been admonished for their alcohol abuse by anyone in the medical profession. These formerly alcoholic physicians also complained that those physicians responsible for their care had frequently never dealt with the alcoholism directly (Bissell and Jones, 1976). It would appear that physicians are very uncomfortable in dealing with a colleague's abuse of alcohol and tend to handle it by denial, as does the alcoholic physician himself.

Treatment of the physician for alcoholism appears to have a more favorable prognosis than for the general population. A recent study indicates that one year after discharge from an inpatient treatment center for alcoholism, 75% of the physicians treated remained abstinent from alcohol (Kliner et al., 1980) as opposed to a 61% abstinence rate for nonphysicians.

The Physician's Marriage

Marital problems appear to be very common among physicians. A paradox observed by Trainer (1981) is that physicians are regarded as fine "catches" and many a young woman considers marrying a physician as a triumph.

Medical marriages are stable. The end in divorce less frequently than most other groups of white-collar professionals according to a study of California divorce statistics (Rose and Rosow, 1972). The divorce rates for white male physicians are the lowest. Divorce rates are approximately 40% higher for women physicians than for male physicians, and black physicians have a divorce rate 70% higher than their white colleagues. But, it has been noted that a lower divorce rate is not necessarily reflective of higher quality marriages (Haar, 1973). A physician may be reluctant to divorce because of an exaggerated need to maintain his idealized public image, and his wife may desire to maintain her special social status as "the doctor's wife." Also it is important that divorce can be financially disastrous to an upper middle class family and avoided for that reason.

Evidence that medical marriages are less than satisfying comes from several sources. In a prospective study of men selected in college for "soundness," those who were later to become physicians reported a higher frequency of poor marriages or divorces than did their Ivy League college classmates who did not go to medical school (Vaillant et al., 1972). Another source of information concerning medical marriages comes from observations made by psychiatrists who work with physicians and/or their wives. It is a clinical impression that physician's wives present in disproportionately large numbers as psychiatric patients (Miles et al., 1975).

Wives who are seen in psychiatric treatment often complain that their husbands are too undemonstrative, stilted or cold, domineering (or, conversely, dependent or passive), stern, compulsive, and perfectionistic, and not fulfilling their responsibilities as husbands and fathers (Evans, 1965). The relationship has been described by Evans as being "hostile-dependent." He also noted that these physicians wives also frequently described their mothers as domineering, distant, or rejecting! The wives' most frequent psychiatric diagnosis was that of a passive-aggressive personality and their "good" premorbid adjustments had been more apparent than real. With marriages these women had reestablished with their husbands the same type of relationship they had experienced with their mothers; and both were unsatisfying! Other authors (Goldberg, 1975; Miles et al., 1975) have made similar observations to the effect that the basic marital pattern of the physician's marriage is one where a dependent histrionic woman, with an inordinate need for affection and nurturing, marries an emotionally detached man. The fact that he is a physician and therefore perceived to be a very caring person may have much to do with her choice. Conversely the qualities of the woman, her dramatic flair with underlying dependency, may be very appealing to the physician. Thus some physicians have "married not partners but patients" (Vaillant et al., 1972). With the passage of time the wife becomes progressively more resentful that her dependent needs are not being met. Her resulting depression combined with pouting, or other expressions of anger, causes further withdrawal from her physician-husband. He becomes more emotionally detached and more immersed in his work. Therefore, the long hours worked by the physician may not be the cause, but rather the response to an unhappy marriage. These responses of physician and wife set up a vicious circle, and problems may escalate to where the wife eventually is seen in psychiatric treatment: suicidal, depressed, addicted, or a combination of all three.

Supplementing the above formulations are the observations of Robinson (1978), the husband of a physician who described a grief syndrome which occurs in medical school when the married medical student begins the clinical years and is away from home much of the time. The nonstudent spouse manifests protest, despair, and then *detachment*. This type of response may explain why when the physician wishes to cut back on his duties and establish a warmer family life, he may discover that he does not have a close relationship with either his wife or children (Vincent, 1969).

Another characteristic of physicians which complicates marriage is that in their day-to-day work they are not used to conflict; rather they are directive and "orders" are rarely questioned. As a consequence the physician may possess fewer skills in working out interpersonal conflicts at home (Lewis, 1965).

Sexual problems in the medical marriage are frequently reported (Evans, 1965; Lewis, 1965; Modlin and Montes, 1964). One report indicated that less than 20% of a group of psychiatric patients who were physicians' wives reported a satisfactory sexual adjustment in their marriages (Evans, 1965). Similarly Lewis (1965) found that sexual conflicts in the marriages of the physicians' wives whom he treated were twice as frequent as in a control series of non-physicians' wives also receiving treatment (64% vs 32%). It is also my clinical impression, based on the treatment of a number of physicians and/or their wives, that sexual problems are more prevalent in the medical marriage than with other psychotherapy patients. These problems usually fit into the area of decreased sexual interest rather than that of perversion or severe sexual dysfunction.

Contrary to the oft-used rationalization of hard work and fatigue it would appear that the sexual difficulties in the medical marriage have a more basic etiology. As noted above, medical students have an unusually high incidence of concerns about issues of sexuality and relatively little overall sexual experience prior to entering medical school. The women who marry physicians are often looking for a parent than a mature heterosexual relationship. With such a match, sexual difficulties would not be unanticipated.

Not all reports concerning the medical marriage are as pessimistic as the foregoing discussion. Although the work of Garvey and Tuason (1979) has some methodological problems (response bias and selection of the study sample), their data are very interesting and run contrary to many popular beliefs about physician marriages. These investigators found that their midwest physician respondents reported fewer divorces than the general population and that the quality of their marriages were rated as better than average. Having a wife who was considered to be extroverted was a factor related to an estimation of a good marriage. Of note, and contrary to popular belief, were findings which indicated that the amount of the wives' education, the number of hours worked by the physician and his specialty were not correlated with the estimation of the quality of the marriage.

Important to acknowledge is that, although the medical marriage does have some serious and unique problems which need to be worked through, there are also many strengths and the potential for establishing an excellent marriage (Marcus, 1980). Perhaps reflective of these potential strengths Goldberg (1975) has observed that the physicians and wives with whom he has worked in conjoint marital therapy have done "rather better" than other couples also seen in conjoint therapy.

THE STRESSES OF MEDICAL TRAINING AND PRACTICE

There are many unique and different stresses and strains that the physician must deal with (McCue, 1982; Roeske, 1981). These are in addition to those that any person experiences in the process of maturation and establishing oneself in a chosen profession. The preceding sections of this chapter have emphasized inherent psychological characteristics of the physician which complicate his professional and personal lives. To focus exclusively upon this aspect of the life of the physician would be unfair and a simplistic view of the complexities of becoming and being a physician.

A decision to enter medicine is almost always received with pleasure and rewards of praise from family and friends. Because of this positive response (my son, the doctor-to-be), rescinding the decision may not be easy for the premedical college student. Premedical studies do not prepare one for much in life besides medical school, and therefore there is a considerable investment in being accepted to medical school from both a practical and emotional aspect. The typical premedical student studies longer hours than other undergraduates. This is the initiation of a life of sacrifice and of delaying personal gratification, features that are likely to continue throughout a career. Anxiety remains high until the letter of acceptance to medical school arrives in the mail.

The first two years of medical school are marked by hard work and, for most students, the sobering realization that the competition is keen and many others are brighter or more competent. With the third year of medical school comes not only an increase in the time spent away from home but the almost terrifying initiation into life–death issues and the realization that mistakes may kill or permanently damage another living person.

The sigh of relief that accompanies medical school graduation signals only the briefest respite from the multiple demands of medicine. The internship and residency are too often characterized by excessive responsibility, long hours with sleep deprivation, and dealings with hospital administrators whose management techniques in regard to the house staff would look archaic to almost any modern business executive.

Somewhere in the frantic pace of medical education, which is also characterized by an unduly long dependence upon parents, thereby lengthening adolescence, most young doctors marry. Marriage often occurs after a hurried or inadequate courtship and frequently before other important developmental tasks have been accomplished. With marriage comes increasing responsibilities, financial and perhaps parenting.

When training, and sometimes military service, is completed the now not so young physician can begin medical practice. This beginning is often accompanied by an immense debt: loans for medical school and opening an office. Medical practice makes demands on time not only for patients but also managing the financial side of a medical practice, something not covered in medical education. A string of insurance salesmen and "financial advisors" beats a path to the door. Not uncommonly medical practice not only does not bring the expected emotional rewards but also does not prove to be as financially remunerative as was anticipated. As a consequence there is a feeling of being a failure and not infrequently he may be accused of same by his wife. The fear of a malpractice suit adds significant stress to the professional life of the physician. The effects of such a suit, even when it was not justified, may be devastating (Mawardi, 1979).

The accumulative effect of the various stresses (and many, if not most, physicians will immediately recognize the story as described) is to place great strain upon the physician. Personal needs, particularly underlying dependent needs are not met and ego defense mechanisms may falter. However, the very seeking of help, or wish to seek help, is in itself a strain upon many physicians. There is a feeling of a need to live up to the expectations of society in regard to being an "ideal," omnipotent, and ever-reliable person (De Sole et al., 1969). It is difficult to seek relief by accepting the sick role because one cannot abandon patients (and perhaps the next payment on the income tax shelter). As a consequence it is no surprise that some physicians become depressed or turn to addiction or suicide as a solution. Perhaps more importantly in regard to the themes of this book, there can be little doubt as to why there is little patience with dependent, somatizing, or depressed patients.

The Physician as Patient

Anecdotal reports and tradition suggest that the sick physician is a notoriously poor patient. However, there is relatively little information, collected in a systematic manner, to support the view that the physician is either a "good" or "problem" patient.

To what degree physicians (and their families) utilize medical services themselves is unknown. One study of house officers indicated that they were less likely to have made arrangements for their own medical care, or to have had routine physical examinations, than were a group of graduate students of similar age (Heller et al., 1967). Another survey indicated that physicians frequently use prescription drugs for their own minor ailments, but without consulting another physician (Cockerham et al., 1980). Contrasted with the foregoing is a statistical investigation which demonstrated that physicians and their spouses had at least as many, or more, surgical operations, depending upon the type of procedure, then did an age-matched control group of other professions. This suggests an increased utilization of medical/surgical services by physicians and their families (Bunker and Brown, 1974).

Physicians who are admitted to psychiatric hospitals leave the hospital AMA (against medical advice) much more frequently than do other patients (Jones, 1977; Modlin and Montes, 1964). However, it must be kept in mind that physicians who are knowledgeable of the medical system are much less likely to be intimidated by it.

From our knowledge of those psychodynamic factors which are frequently identified in physicians we can make several predictions of illness behavior. Physicians often use the ego mechanisms of hypochondriasis and reaction formation. We would therefore expect to see a push–pull phenomenon in regard to illness behavior: periods of overconcern with health alternating with periods of defending against fears of illness. This is illustrated by the following clinical vignette.

A young radiologist developed a palpable 1–2-cm nontender submandibular mass. He became severely anxious and urgently sought consultation from four different specialists, a hematologist, a pathologist, a general surgeon, and a head and neck surgeon. When the size of the mass spontaneously shrunk after a week he rationalized that it was an inflamed lymph node, and he did not bother to keep any of the return appointments to the various specialists he had seen.

Another psychological characteristic of physicians, oft noted, is their need for ominipotence. With a need to have a belief in one's own powers it is not surprising to learn that physicians often treat themselves or their families (as noted above).

Problems occur when the physician is sick and needs to becomes a patient because of (1) inherent psychological attitudes and defenses of the physician in regards to disease and the ambivalence of the physician to accept the sick role (Goldberg, 1975); and (2) inevitable changes which occur in the doctor–patient relationship when the physician is a patient. The latter situation, the doctor–doctor/patient relationship is discussed in the following chapter.

SUMMARY

Physicians, as a group, are typified by a number of psychological characteristics. Characteristics such as counterphobic defenses against a fear of disease and counterdependent behavior are important in motivating a person toward a medical career. Other features such as the obsessive-compulsive personality, and the capacity to inhibit personal gratification, appear to be well suited to the arduous training process and the rigors of patient responsibility. Thus it is those very characteristics which create the physician that result in some types of predictable personal and professional behavior. It is also these characteristics which lead to an increased incidence of certain types of psychiatric illness and/or psychological distress. Physicians appear to be prone to depression (with a resultant high suicide rate), addictions, and marital discord. This psychological morbidity is the result of predisposing personal characteristics and stress, engendered by the high demands of the profession and the unrealistic expectations of other persons.

Patients who have problems with interpersonal relationships, dependency, addictions, or somatization have the capacity to tap into the physician's intrapsychic conflicts in reference to the same issues. Thus the situation is rife with the potential for untoward therapeutic endeavors. A greater understanding of those characteristics of *being a physician* will result in a more effective utilization of the doctor–patient relationship as an important therapeutic force in the treatment of patients.

REFERENCES

Abram, H.S. 1978. Emotional aspects of heart disease: A personal narrative. Int J Psychiatry Med 8:225–233.

a'Brook, M.F., Hailstone, J.D., and McLauchlan, I.E.J. 1967. Psychiatric illness in the medical profession. Br J Psychiatry 113:1013–1023.

Adsett, C.A. 1968. Psychological health of medical students in relation to the medical education process. J Med Educ 43:728–734.

AMA Council on Mental Health. 1973. The sick physician: Impairment by psychiatric disorders, including alcoholism and drug dependence. JAMA 223:684–687.

Balint, M. 1957. *The Doctor, His Patient and the Illness.* New York: International Universities Press.

Bissell, L.H., and Jones, R.W. 1976. The alcoholic physician: A survey. Am J Psychiatry 133:1142–1146.

Brent, R.L. and Brent, L.H. 1978. Medicine: An excuse from living. Res Staff Physician 24(12):61–65.

Bunker, J.P., and Brown, B.W. 1974. The physician-patient as an informed consumer of surgical services. N Engl J Med 290:1051–1055.

Cockerham, W.C., Creditor, M.C., Creditor, U.K., and Imbrey, P.B. 1980. Minor ailments and illness behavior among physicians. Med Care 18:164–173.

DeSole, D.E., Singer, P., and Aronson, S. 1969. Suicide and role strain among physicians. Int J Soc Psychiatry 15:294–301.

Duffy, J.C., and Litin, E.M. 1964. Psychiatric morbidity of physicians. JAMA 189:989–992.

Evans, J.L. 1955. Psychiatric illness in the physician's wife. Am J Psychiatry 122:159–165.

Ford, C.V. 1981. The emotional distress of interns and residents. Presented at the 134th American Psychiatric Association Annual Meeting, New Orleans, May 15.

Garvey, M., and Tuason, V.B. 1979. Physician marriages. J Clin Psychiat:40-129-131.

Goldberg, M. 1975. Conjoint therapy of male physicians and their wives. Psychiatric Opinion 12(4):19–23.

Golden, J.S., Marchionne, A.M., and Silver, R.J. 1967. Fifty medical students: A comparison with "normals." J Med Educ 42:146–152.

Golloway, G. 1981. Are doctors different? Reflections on the psychodynamics of physicians. J Fla Med Assoc 68:281–284.

Haar, E. 1973. Commentary on "marital stability among physicians." Med Aspects Human Sexuality 1(June):78.

Heller, R.J., Robertson, L.S., and Alpert, J.J. 1967. Health care of house officers: A comparative study. New Engl J Med 277:907–910.

Johnson, R.P., and Connelly, J.C. 1981. Addicted physicians: A closer look. JAMA 245:253–257.

Jones, R.E. 1977. A study of 100 physician psychiatric inpatients. Am J Psychiatry 134:1119–1123.

Kliner, D.J., Spicer, J., and Barnett, P. 1980. Treatment outcome of alcoholic physicians. J Stud Alcohol 41:1217–1220.

Lewis, J.C. 1965. The doctor and his marriage. Tex State J Med 61:615–619.

Lief, H.I., Young, K., Spruiell, V., Lancaster, R., and Lief, V.F. 1960. A psychodynamic study of medical students and their adaptational problems: Preliminary report. J Med Educ 35:696–704.

Mawardi, B.H. 1979. Satisfactions, dissatisfactions and cause of stress in medical practice. JAMA 241:1483–1486.

McCue, J.D. 1982. The effects of stress on physicians and their medical practice. N Engl J Med 306:458–463.

McLaughlin, J.T. 1961. The analyst and the Hippocratic oath. J Am Psychoanal Assoc 9:106–123.

Marcus, I.M. 1980. Harmony vs discord in marriage: A view of physician's marriages. J La State Med Soc 132:173–178.

Menninger, K.A. 1959. Psychological factors in the choice of medicine as a profession. In A *Psychiatrist's World: Selected Papers*. Fall, B.H., ed. New York: Viking Press.

Miles, J.E., Krell, R., and Tsung-Yi, L. 1975. The doctor's wife: Mental illness and marital pattern. Int J Psychiatry Med 6:481–487.

Modlin, H.C., and Montes, A. 1964. Narcotics addiction in physicians. Am J Psychiatry 121:358–369.

Nunberg, H. 1938. Psychological interactions between physician and patient. Psychoanal Rev 25:297–308.

Parsons, T. 1951. *The Social System*. New York: Free Press.

Pearson, M.M. 1982. Psychiatric treatment of 250 physicians. Psychiatric Annals 12:194–206.

Pearson, M.M., and Strecker, E.A. 1960. Physicians as psychiatric patients: Private practice experience. Am J Psychiatry 116:915–919.

Pepitone-Arreola-Rockwell, F., Rockwell, D., and Core, N. 1981. Fifty-two medical student suicides. Am J Psychiatry 128:198–201.

Pitts, Jr., F., Winokur, G., and Stewart, M.A. 1961. Psychiatric syndromes, anxiety symptoms and responses to stress in medical students. Am J Psychiatry 118:333–340.

Robinson, D.O. 1978. The medical-student spouse syndrome: Grief reactions to the clinical years. Am J Psychiatry 135:972–974.

Roeske, N.C.A. 1981. Stress and the physician. Psychiatric Annals 11:245–258.

Rose, K.D., and Rosow, I. 1972. Marital stability among physicians. Calif Med 116:95–99.

Rose, K.D., and Rosow, I. 1973. Physicians who kill themselves. Arch Gen Psychiatry 29:800–805.

Ross, M. 1975. Physician suicide risk: Practical recognition. South Medical J 68:699–702.

Sargent, D.A., Jensen, V.W., Petty, T.A., and Raskin, H. 1977. Preventing physician suicide: The role of family, colleagues, and organized medicine. JAMA 237:143–145.

Schlageter, C.W., and Rosenthal, V. 1962. What are "normal" medical students like? J Medical Educ 37:19–27.

Simmel, E. 1926. The "doctor-game," illness and the profession of medicine. Int J Psychoanal 7:470–483.

Spickard, A., and Billings, F.T. 1981. Alcoholism in a medical-school faculty. N Engl J Med 305:1646–1648.

Strupp, H.H., Hadley, S.W., and Gomes-Schwartz, B. 1977. *Psychotherapy for Better or Worse: The Problem of Negative Results.* New York: Jason-Aronson.

Thomas, C.B. 1976. What becomes of medical students: The dark side. Johns Hopkins Med J 138:185–195.

Thomas, C.B., Santora, P.B., and Shaffer, J.W. 1980. Health of physicians in midlife in relation to use of alcohol: A prospective study of a cohort of former medical students. Johns Hopkins Med J 146:1–10.

Trainer, J.B. 1981. Is the medical marriage hazardous to your health? J Fla Med Assoc 68:261–264.

Vaillant, G.E., Sobowale, N.W., and McArthur, C. 1972. Some psychologic vulnerabilities of physicians. N Engl J Med 287:372–375.

Valko, R.J., and Clayton, P.J. 1975. Depression in the internship. Dis Nerv Syst 36:26–29.

Vincent, M.O. 1969. Doctor and Mrs.—Their mental health. Can Psychiatr Assoc J 14:509–515.

Vincent, M.O., Robinson, E.A., and Latt, L. 1969. Physicians as patients: Private psychiatric hospital experience. Can Med Assoc J 100:403–412.

Waring, E.M. 1974. Psychiatric illness in physicians: A review. Compre Psychiatry 15:519–530.

Watterson, D.J. 1976. Psychiatric illness in the medical profession: Incidence in relation to sex and field of practice. Can Med Assoc J 115:311–317.

Werner, E.R., and Korsch, B.M. 1979. Professionalization during pedatric internship: Attitudes, adaptation, and interpersonal skills. In *Becoming a Physician: Development of Values and Attitudes in Medicine.* Shapiro, E., and Lowenstein, L, eds. Cambridge, Mass.: Ballinger.

Wilson, W.P., and Larson, D.B. 1981. The physician and spouse: Physician know thyself and thy mate. No Carolina Med J 42:106–109.

Woods, S.M. 1972. Sexual problems of medical students. Medical Aspects Human Sexuality 6:66–85 passim.

Woods, S.M., Natterson, J., and Silverman, J. 1966. Medical student's disease: Hypochondriasis in medical education. J Medical Educ 41:785–790.

Woods, S.M., and Natterson, J. 1967. Sexual attitudes of medical students: Some implications for medical education. Am J Psychiatry 124:323–332.

Zabarenko, R.N., Zabarenko, L, and Pittenger, R.A. 1970. The psychodynamics of physicianhood. Psychiatry 323:102–118.

13

THE DOCTOR–PATIENT RELATIONSHIP

The "doctor–patient relationship" is a phrase used both within the medical profession and by the lay public. The term is frequently confused with "bedside manner," which then discounts it to the level of an individual personal style, such as the mannerisms of a "society doctor." However, the style of relating to the patient is only one small aspect of the doctor–patient relationship. It is more than something that is done to a patient by a physician, e.g., humanitarian concern from the physician (Hollender, 1958a). Rather, it is a dyadic social system influenced to a large degree by emotional factors (Henderson, 1935). It has been observed that the doctor–patient relationship was all that physicians had to offer patients until comparatively recently, and that it is what distinguishes human medicine from veterinary medicine (Houston, 1938).

The importance of the doctor–patient relationship is frequently alluded to, at times, as if some ritualistic veneration is demanded by an occasion such as medical school graduation. More frequently this potent therapeutic tool is neglected. A 1960 study of physicians, who had graduated eight years previously, indicated that they viewed the doctor–patient relationship to be the most inadequately taught of all the major areas of their studies (Gee, 1960). Although there have been efforts by some medical schools to rectify this deficiency it is my opinion that most medical graduates remain woefully ignorant of the potent effect, both positive and negative, that they exert upon patients. The reasons for this lie not only in the construction of the medical school curricula, which are heavily weighted toward the bioscientific model (see Chapter 2), but also in the innate characteristics of physicians themselves, who can be described as action oriented and defending themselves against many of the same anxieties experienced by their patients (see Chapter 12). For these reasons I believe it useful to conceive of the doctor–

patient relationship as an active and potent force which can be employed effectively with all patients but is essential in the treatment of the somatizing patient. To quote Findley (1953), "... the physician is a vastly more important institution than the drug store."

To continue with the analogy of the drug "doctor," which was introduced in the last chapter, let us explore the potency of this "drug," which is concretely demonstrated by the placebo effect.

THE PLACEBO EFFECT

It has been observed that until the latter portion of the 19th century the history of medical treatment was the history of the placebo (Shapiro, 1959). Patients were cut, cupped, purged, bled, and fed all types of bizarre materials, including such delicacies as powdered mummy, the moss scraped from the skulls of hanged criminals, and crocodile dung. Despite such ineffective, and perhaps even noxious "treatment," physicians did manage to help their patients and continued to be afforded a place of respect and honor within society. That many of the treatments offered had beneficial results can be attributed to the placebo effect, a frequently unappreciated but potent agent in the therapeutic armamentarium of the physician.

The placebo has been defined by Shapiro (1964) as any therapeutic procedure or component of any therapeutic procedure, which is given to have an effect on a patient, a symptom, syndrome, or disease but which is objectively without *specific* activity for the condition being treated. From this it follows that much of medicine continues to be based upon the placebo effect, although the various practitioners do not regard their specific treatments as placebos. It is an interesting observation that physicians often regard the treatments of other physicians as being placebos but have faith in the therapeutic efficacy of their own techniques (Shapiro, 1970). This apparent inconsistency can be at least partially explained by the fact that the potency of the placebo effect is directly related to the physician's personal faith in the treatment prescribed. The observation that "the doctor's attitude toward his treatment is an ingredient compounded into every prescription" is most apt (Shapiro, 1970).

Although placebos can be explained by a variety of hypothetical etiologic mechanisms such as suggestibility or hypnotizability, it is the belief of myself and others (Adler and Hammett, 1973; Findley, 1953; Houston, 1938; Shapiro, 1970) that the doctor–patient relationship plays an important, probably essential role. The effects are mediated through the facilitation of faith, hope, and expectation engendered through the patient's personal relationship and trust in his physician.

That placebos are indeed effective therapeutic agents is a well-established fact. Beecher (1955), reviewing a number of different studies, found an average significant effectiveness for placebos of about 35%. A more recent review by Evans (1981) confirmed Beecher's findings demonstrating an almost identical proportion of patients (36%) who demonstrate a significant placebo effect.

Interestingly placebos cannot only have beneficial therapeutic action but they may also have associated toxic effects. Adverse reactions such as dry mouth, nausea, headache, or drowsiness may be found in 9–25% of all subjects (Beecher, 1955). Placebos may induce objective changes in measurable physiologic parameters such as an increase in the number of circulating neutrophils and a decrease in eosinophils. These changes may occur despite the fact that the composition of the placebo can be a naturally occurring physiologic substance such as isotonic saline (Beecher, 1955).

Although it might be assumed that the more "suggestible" or less-intelligent persons are more responsive to placebos, the data do not bear this out (Beecher, 1955). According to Shapiro (1970) anxiety is the only consistent factor in the individual which has been identified as affecting the placebo response. The person is more likely to be a responder if anxious, but no other personality or demographic characteristic is predictive of a response. A placebo does appear to have greater efficacy in a stressful situation, such as early postoperative wound pain. The response is certainly not related to presence or absence of "genuine organic pain." Patients with pain known to be of an organic etiology (such as postoperative) frequently have pain relief with placebos. A corollary of this observation is that a placebo will *not* distinguish pain of organic etiology from psychogenic pain. Therefore a placebo for pain relief is of no diagnostic value despite the fact that house officers have repetitively used this time-honored but invalid method as a diagnostic test for "functional" disorders.

Although the power of placebos is often attributed to a change in the perception of the patient (but without organic changes) a recent investigation suggests that the placebo can effect objective changes in a person's experience of pain. Levine and colleagues (1978) have found that the administration of naloxone (an opiate antagonist) will block the analgesic effect of a placebo given to relieve pain after a tooth extraction. These authors hypothesize that administration of the placebo effects release of endorphins, which then affect pain perception, and that this effect can be blocked by binding opiate receptor sites with naloxone.

Other research which suggest mechanisms by which placebos may effect physiology is that increasing body of knowledge which demonstrates that psychosocial factors influence the immune system and that such influence is mediated through the hypothalamus (Stein et al., 1976).

CHARACTERISTICS OF THE PHYSICIAN–PATIENT RELATIONSHIP

Statements are frequently heard to the effect that the treatment of the patient's disease is a science and the care of the patient is an art. Associated with these attitudes are opinions to the effect that this art cannot be taught, it is either a "gift" or something acquired, in a process akin to osmosis, from being in the company of a great clinician. Engel (1981) eloquently refutes these statements and opines that a distinction between art and science is inappropriate for the treatment of disease and for patient care. He states that the doctor–patient relationship can and should be taught for there is a body of knowledge to be imparted. I share the opinion of Engel that the doctor–patient relationship is as teachable as any other topic which has been sanctified by being labeled as scientific. There are limitations of course; someone who is clumsy will never become a skillful surgeon, and one who is a misanthrope will never become a sensitive physician. Engel uses the nonverbal communications, which have evolved through phylogeny, as an example of knowledge that can be taught. The nonverbal behavior is of value in disclosing the patient's affective status. The following discussion emphasizes a different type of knowledge which can also be taught; several models of behavior and expectations between doctor and patient; and specific components of the relationship including issues such as communication and trust. Although these various components are obviously closely interrelated, and in clinical experience cannot be isolated one from another, each will be discussed individually for didactic purposes.

Models of the Doctor–Patient Relationship

In an important theoretical paper, Szasz and Hollender (1956) proposed that there are three general types of relationships between physicians and patients, and that these have their prototypes in different developmental stages of the relationship between parents and children. However, before proceeding to a discussion of these models, it is useful to review the theoretical concept that the doctor–patient relationship reenacts many aspects of the relationship between a parent and child, aspects which are based both in reality and in fantasy. Among the more articulate spokesmen of this view has been Nunberg (1938), and the following description is abstracted from his work.

Every sick or suffering person becomes anxious and looks to another person for support, protection, and consolation. For the child this is the parent, frequently the mother, but the adult in our disease-oriented culture generally turns to the physician. A sick person characteristically regresses, that is to say, becomes psychologically less mature. Children have a need to view their parents as omnipotent and omniscient and indeed, compared to the child's limited resources, the parents do have these qualities. The sick, and regressed, adult transfers those expectations and attitudes which were once held in regard to the parent to the physician; or to use the words of Wahl (1964) the physician stands *in loco parentis* (in place of parents).

Activity–Passivity Model. In this model of the doctor–patient relationship, the physician is the active and dominant participant. The prototype is that of the parent–infant relationship. The physician makes all decisions and deals with the patient as if he were unable to respond or to act. This type of relationship is demanded when the patient is anesthesized, in coma or immobilized by acute trauma. Most physicians (and patients) would consciously reject this model as unacceptable except under the circumstances listed above. Lewin (1946), however, has made a fascinating observation that the first "patient" for each physician is a cadaver. Lewin hypothesizes that the cadaver may have to come to be regarded as the ideal patient who is completely passive and unresistant and meets the psychological needs of the physician who needs complete control. What is suggested by this hypothesis is that some physicians may unconsiously prefer the activity–passivity model and slant their patient relationships and the nature of their medical practice in that direction.

Guidance-Cooperation Model. This model of physician–patient relationships continues to emphasize the dominant and controlling nature of the physician's role. The prototype is that of the parent–child relationship. The physician tells the patient what to do. It is of interest to note that in this respect the doctor writes "orders" in the hospital chart and "prescribes" what the patient is to ingest or what he is to do. The relationship is unequal in power, and the physician, with the presumption that his motives are altruistic, decides what is best for the patient. The patient is regarded as a "good" patient if he obeys his physician and a "bad" patient if he fails to follow orders. This model of the doctor–patient relationship is effectively used when the patient is seriously ill and/or regressed and the nature of the illness impairs the patient's judgment.

In real-life situations, the guidance–cooperation (paternalistic) model is the most prevalent model operative in the practice of medicine today. Many physicians have resented any encroachments into their power, decrying informed consent as the turning of the responsibility of medical care over to attorneys, and patients' efforts to become better-informed have been derided as consumerism. The physicians' (and medical students') endorsement of this paternalistic view of medical practice was highlighted in a study completed by Ort and colleagues (1964) who found that the affiliative relationship with patients which physicians most enjoy is one in which the physician remains in control. Conversely, patients have looked to their physicians to make decisions for them, often not wanting more information about their treatment alternatives and making statements such as, "You make the decision. You're the doctor."

Mutual Participation Model. This model of the doctor–patient relationship is predicated upon the philosophical view that equality among adults is a desirable value. It emphasizes a partnership in the management of the patient's illness, for which the physician acts as a consultant, and therapeutic decisions are joint decisions. The prototype of this model is the relationship between two adults. This particular model of physician–patient interactions is favored by the patient who wishes (or needs) to maintain control over his life and body. It is well-suited for the management of chronic diseases such as diabetes, where in time the patient may learn as much about the disease as the physician. It is also appropriate, and perhaps necessary, when there are considerable intellectual, educational, and experiential similarities between physician and patient.

However, as mentioned in the preceding discussion concerning the guidance–cooperation model, many physicians are uncomfortable in assuming the mutual participation type of medical care, because they feel that they are abdicating their responsibility. Many patients are also reluctant to assume an equal partnership with the physician; to do so is to at least partially renounce one's magical expectations of medicine! Others, because of age, mental deficiency, poor education or severe character disorders, may be unable to realistically employ this model of medical care.

Each of the above models is appropriate for some circumstances, sometimes for the same patient with the same disease. For example, a patient with diabetes mellitus may present in ketoacidotic coma requiring the activity–passivity model, respond to treatment but require in-hospital treatment for associated infection (utilizing the guidance–cooperation model), and then benefit from a long-term relationship where decisions regarding the management of the diabetic are mutually determined (the mutual participation model).

Each model may also be better-suited for different types of patients and their expectations of medical care. The skillful and perceptive physician has the capacity to assess the psychological needs of patients and make necessary adjustments in relationship to them. Physicians who are less flexible often have practices which are notably stereotyped in terms of the type of patient who is attracted to the physician's personal characteristics.

Components of the Doctor–Patient Relationship

The preceding discussion of the different models of the doctor–patient relationship focused upon the style of the interaction in regard to issues of control and decision-making. As important as this issue may be, there is far more to the interaction between a physician and the patient than a struggle for control. Henderson (1935) has emphasized the greater importance of the emotional components, as opposed to the cognitive and logical components, of a social system such as the doctor–patient dyad. I agree with that observation, and the following discussion of various aspects of the doctor–patient relationship will focus primarily on the affects (emotional feelings), which are generated by this intense relationship. In the absence of such feelings, one might as well be working as an automobile mechanic.

A number of specific qualities of the doctor–patient relationship are frequently mentioned by experienced clinicians (Carson, 1977; Comfort, 1978; Houston, 1938; Peabody, 1927; Pickering, 1978; Tumulty, 1978). These include the ability of the physicians to instill trust and confidence; the provision of hope and the concurrent removal of fear and doubt; a close personal relationship associated with concern and empathy; and effective communication. Each of these important qualities will be discussed individually.

Trust and Confidence. The capacity of the physician to enlist the patient's trust and confidence in his/her abilities is regarded as a basic tenet in the practice of medicine. To doubt one's automobile mechanic is not unusual, but to question the physician into whose hands a life has been placed is almost unthinkable. Such doubt would represent an example of cognitive dissonance. Most doctor–patient relationships begin with an assumed (and taken for granted) trust. It is incumbent for the physician to build upon this inherent good will, and the primary task can be phrased as a negative imperative. Do nothing to lose trust and confidence! Patients have been proven to be remarkably tolerant of their physician's mistakes when the patients remain convinced that the physician has been honest with them, has the patients' best interests at heart, and does not abandon them. Trust and confidence can be facilitated by effective two-way communication, a genuine personal concern shown for the patient and an empathetic relationship.

Hope and the Removal of Fear and Doubt. The instillation of hope and optimism (the components of faith) within the bounds of reality is an important therapeutic endeavor. The lay literature contains testimonials demonstrating the power of faith as an important adjuvant to healing. These reports should not be regarded as fictitious or merely rare or isolated events. The account of his illness by Cousins (1976) is a dramatic example of how one's attitudes and emotions may influence a disease process. The converse side, the loss of faith (or the giving up–given up complex) is known to be associated with medical complications, often leading to death (Engel, 1967). The physician may at times feel that it is his duty to falsely encourage a patient or to lie about a prognosis. In my opinion, such a tactic does not instill hope, but instead distrust, and thereby undermines the cornerstone of the doctor–patient relationship. The patient does not demand a cure, but rather he wishes an assurance that the physician will be there when needed, that all reasonable efforts will be made to effect cure or palliation, that he will not be allowed to suffer needlessly, and that he will not be abandoned. Within this context the majority of patients can maintain an optimistic stance that their lives will continue to have meaning.

Empathy. Empathy is the capacity of the clinician to share the feelings of his patient as if they were his own. It differs from sympathy in that sympathy has the quality of feeling sorry for or pitying the patient. The patient does not need pity from his physician, that emotion is usually adequately provided for by family and friends, but instead needs to know that his physician understands his feelings and his needs. Empathy is a difficult emotional state for physicians to handle. It must be measured and limited to some degree, for if a physician were to constantly feel the full emotional range of each patient with whom he comes in contact he would soon become exhausted, nonobjective, and ineffective. Yet unfortunately many physicians, in order to protect themselves from the anxiety-generating emotions of their patients, utilize defenses to such a degree that they are unable to comprehend their patients as people. These defense mechanisms include compartmentalization (only the diseased organ system is seen), the use of technology (ordering diagnostic studies in place of taking a history), dealing with patients only in groups rather than personally ("going on rounds"), and dehumanizing of patients by the use of slang terms such as "gomer" or "turkey" (Reiser, 1973).

A Personal Relationship Associated with Concern. Peabody has stated that the patient wants a *personal* relationship with his physician (1927). The "personal" quality can be most easily understood when considering the "parent–child" aspects of medical care. A child wants a *personal* relationship with his parents. He wants to be known, loved, and respected as an individual. The provision of material goods, food, shelter, and other basic needs are not adequate, no matter how luxurious, unless accompanied by *personal* concern. The sick patient is no different in his wish for this concern from his physician, and it is that quality which serves a vital supportive role. The famous words of Peabody, written when he knew himself to be ill with terminal carcinoma (Williams, 1950), succinctly summarizes this aspect of the doctor–patient relationship: " . . . the secret of the care of the patient is in caring for the patient" (Peabody, 1927).

Concern for a patient does not mean the expression of a continuously solicitious attitude. It has been observed that becoming angry with a patient may, at times, reflect care and concern (Flexner and Abram, 1978).

Communication. Something so simple as the communication of information from doctor to patient and patient to doctor appears to represent a major area of dissatisfaction of the general public with the medical profession (Tumulty, 1978; Waitzkin and Stoeckle, 1972). Physicians are accused of both not providing adequate information and of not listening to patients. "Confusion, negativism, anxiety, lack of compliance and lawsuits are born of failures in communication" (Tumulty, 1978). Pickering (1978) has expressed the opinion that the single greatest defect in young doctors of the United States and Great Britain is their inability to take a good history and their inability to sit down and to listen to their patients in such a manner that they really learn what problems most deeply trouble the patient.

Why communication between physician and patient should exist as a major problem is unclear. It has been hypothesized that an underlying reason is that by maintaining uncertainty in the patient the balance of power in the relationship remains on the side of the physician (Waitzkin and Stoeckle, 1972). Although this cynical theory may be difficult to refute, I would offer an alternative theory which is not mutually exclusive. The young modern physician is immersed in science and technology. This knowledge has been obtained at the high cost of years of study, and this "value" (scientific thinking) has been reinforced by the general values of society. In contrast, there is little confidence in personal abilities, it is only what is known that matters, not who one is! Words are regarded as cheap—for salesmen—the "true scientist" operates with hard data and numbers. Thus the physician may devalue himself/herself and in the process obsessively hold on to precious scientific knowledge with the unconscious fear that if it were shared with the patient the physician would lose that value which is possessed.

Whatever the reasons behind the failure to communicate effectively, an extremely valuable tool has been lost or underused. But, whether or not a physician talks to his patient, communication continues. "Everything the doctor does, says, or doesn't say is a communication on one level or another to his patient" (Joyce, 1972). Therefore the failure to talk, to listen or to commiserate is in effect saying that the physician is not interested, does not care, or feels that the patient is not important.

Communication with a patient is an intellectually challenging task. In the medical setting all messages are supercharged with emotion, and the patient frequently hears only portions of that which is told him. Distortions of understanding abound, and the nonverbal gestures of the physician are attentively scanned in order to attribute nuances of meaning onto the messages (Henderson, 1935).

The patient may have difficulty in making a direct communication of his thoughts and feelings. Henderson (1935) has advised that when one talks to a patient one must listen first, for that which the patient wishes to tell; second, for that which he does not want to tell; and third, for that which he cannot tell. Information which is shameful or painful will not be divulged easily and certain attitudes or assumptions which are of an unconscious nature cannot be verbalized. Yet, all is essential to the understanding of the patient's life, of which the illness is a part.

SPECIAL ASPECTS OF THE DOCTOR–PATIENT RELATIONSHIP

Changes in societal attitudes, particularly related to such issues as "accountability" and the "right to know" have led to the development of several new aspects of the doctor–patient relationship. Another different type of doctor–patient relationship is that of the doctor–doctor/patient relationship. An examination of these special aspects increases our overall knowledge of the complexity of interactions between doctors and patients.

Informed Consent

The major thrust of the recent emphasis upon informed consent has come through medicolegal concerns of medical practice. Informed consent can be defined as the right of the patient to make choices as to his/her medical treatment after having been advised, not only of the potential gain from the procedure, but also as to any potential adverse reactions. This doctrine that the patient has inherent rights in determining the nature of his medical care carries with it implied modifications of the paternalistic model of the doctor–patient relationship (Johnson and James, 1979). It is probably this challenge to the physician's traditional authority, more than any other factor, which has engendered the heat which emanates from discussions of informed consent. In one article in a state medical association journal a physician blamed informed consent as "causing" the patient's death (Patten and Stump, 1978)!

Not surprisingly, many patients are not too eager to assume the responsibility for the decision-making which physicians are loath to relinquish. Research which has been reported to date indicate that different investigations have found varying proportions of patients who desire an informed consent. In regard to proposed use of an experimental medication Bergler and coworkers (1980) found that most patients (95%) wanted to be informed about the drug trial, but 75% were willing to accept their physician's recommendation without an explanation. In contrast, in reference to radiologic procedures, Alfidi (1975) found that 60% did not wish to be informed. Lankton et al. (1977) found differing responses among their patients; half of their patients stated (after the fact) that they would not like to again have a complete disclosure of the risks of anesthesia. However, the latter authors noted a wide range of responses from their patients varying from gratitude to anger and resentment for the detailed risk disclosure.

What patients understand (or at least remember) concerning information offered in an informed consent does not appear to be related to the patient's level of education (Bergler et al., 1980). Patients appear to selectively remember certain parts of the information that they are given and repress other parts. There is a tendency to remember more of the indications for a proposed procedure and the benefits likely to occur from it, than to remember potential adverse effects or complications (Bergler et al., 1980; Priluck et al., 1979; Robinson and Merav, 1976). The extent to which patients can "forget" or distort information given to them in an informed consent is remarkable. Robinson and Merav (1976) tape-recorded informed consent interviews prior to surgery and 4–6 months later recontacted the patients to determine what they remembered about their interviews. Their patients remembered surprisingly little and, on occasion, severely distorted even the length of the interview. For example, one 24-minute recorded interview was recalled as follows, "All he did was lift up my shirt, put a stethoscope on my heart and that was it."

We can conclude that patients show a wide variation in their wishes concerning an informed consent. Some patients do not wish to accept any responsibility and request that their physicians make their decisions for them. Other patients are grateful for the information received. It is important to note that information concerning procedures may prove to have utilitarian value; postoperative complications have been shown to be reduced in renal transplant patients who had preoperatively been educated as to what to expect in terms of the operation, recovery room and postoperative techniques (Brock et al., 1973).

It is also clear that in some highly anxious patients an informed consent is not actually "informed"; the patient's emotional status precluded the registration of the information offered. This observation is consistent with opinions that it is the emotional quality of the doctor–patient relationship which is of the greatest importance.

Further research to determine those characteristics which influence informed consent will also lead to greater understanding of the doctor–patient relationship.

Patients Who Want to Read Their Charts

A no less heated debate than the question of informed consent is the issue of a patient's rights in regard to his medical records. Is the information contained therein the property of the physician or the patient? There appears to be a fairly well-accepted consensus that the actual physical chart is the property of the physician or the hospital. However, what right does a patient have to the facts contained within it or does he have the right to reproduce the chart through some mechanical means?

The suggestion that a patient might have a right to review his physician's records has met with outright rejection from at least one quarter (Halberstam, 1976). The passage of legislation providing residents of Massachusetts with a Bill of Rights (Curran, 1979) which includes access to their medical records has received mixed reviews. One way of interpreting the situation is to identify patients who make a request to look at their records as deviant in some way. A report by Altman and colleagues (1980), who studied patients who requested to read their hospital records, concluded that the requests were the outgrowth of mistrust directed toward the health care team and that some requests were expressions of adversarial patient–doctor relations. Most of these patients were psychologically described as hysterical, and a smaller group were described as paranoid personalities. Lipsitt (1980) has assumed a different stance on this issue and states that patients often express their emotional needs in a spectrum of behaviors. He expressed the belief that the wish to read a chart may represent a breakdown in communication and suggests that such a request can be turned into a collaborative healing transaction rather than an adverserial encounter.

My personal experience with having patients read their charts began with duty as a military physician. Military personnel usually carry their records (including medical records) with them from duty station to duty station and also carry them to medical consultations. It is a common sight to see servicemen read their records while waiting for a medical appointment. My initial reaction of being somewhat taken back by this behavior was soon changed to accepting it as a mechanism which allowed communication of information concerning health issues. I concurrently learned, and have continued the policy since leaving the military, that medical records should be written clearly with the view in mind that they may be read by the patient (and/or his attorney). On occasion I offer access to the medical record to the patients or read the contents to them. The result is an almost inevitable increase in both communication and trust.

The Doctor–Doctor/Patient Relationship

"The patient–physician relation is complex and difficult at best; but when the patient is a physician, the complexity takes on new aspects" (Pinner, 1952). This quotation is from a book chapter written by Dr. Max Pinner during his last years of suffering with chronic heart disease.

What happens when a physician becomes a patient is a fascinating study of a complex interpersonal relationship. Unfortunately, most of the information available in regard to the doctor–doctor/patient relationship is of an anecdotal nature, mostly accounts written by physicians of their own illnesses. One attempt at a systematic study of this topic was undertaken by White and Lindt (1963) who, after extensive interviews with 12 surgeons and internists, concluded (and in support of the anecdotal book of Pinner and Miller, 1952) that (1) both the patient and his physician are more likely to behave in ways that are contrary to, or deviant from, their usual traditional roles when the patient is a physician or a member of a physician's family; and (2) if the physician and/or the patient behave in a manner that deviates too much from the usual roles prescribed by tradition then the probability of a therapeutically undesirable result is increased. A review of hospital records by these investigators indicated that when a physician (or family member) was a patient then a statistically documented difference in some aspects of medical care related to hospitalization could be demonstrated when a comparison was made to the other "nonmedical-family" patients. For example, both antibiotics and narcotics were utilized less for physicians and members of their families (Franklin et al., 1965).

When the patient is a physician or a member of a physician's family there are certain advantages, such as the ability to seek out the best physician for the particular problem. However, despite this apparent advantage physicians often seek out a physician who is not necessarily the most competent but one with whom they are comfortable or with whom they do not fear a loss of "equality" in the relationship (Lipsitt, 1975). Disadvantages for the physician-patient include that he may be reluctant to seek help for fear of imposing upon a colleague's time or of appearing to be a hypochondriac (White and Lindt 1963). Even if the physician-patient is willing to surrender his automony to the treating physician and enter the sick role, the treating physician may be reluctant to treat the colleague as a patient but instead expect him to write his own history and manage his own medications (Pinner, 1952). The treating physician may be ambivalent and anxious in taking care of a colleague because, despite the flattery of having been chosen, there may be fear of criticism concerning professional competence. The response to this anxiety may be insufficient or less aggressive treatment than would be otherwise provided and the net result less than optimal.

Professional courtesy is a custom which may also interfere with optimal care (Pinner, 1952). The treating physician, because of courtesy, may be resentful of the time expenditure without remuneration, but more often it is the physician who receives courtesy who is placed in a bind. The physician-patient may be reluctant to ask for more time or visits because of the fear that he is exploiting his colleague. It is also hard to change doctors and in essence tell a physician, who has been providing free services, that his efforts are not appreciated. Because of these problems there is an increasing acceptance of the idea that professional courtesy is an anachronism and many physicians are abandoning the custom (Bass and Wolfson, 1980).

It is often suggested that the physician who becomes sick should turn the responsibility for his medical care over to another physician and that physician should treat the physician-patient the same as he would any other patient. This suggestion represents an ideal, but an ideal which is most probably never achieved. The treating physician can never really forget that his patient is also a physician, and in the interests of good care should not (Grotjahn, 1964). There are few occupations where one's job and one's personal identity are so closely woven together as in *being a doctor*. One does not stop being a physician at 5 PM or on weekends. To strip a person of one of the basic components of his identity is to depersonalize him; this is certainly *not* the way to establish a working doctor–patient relationship. Because *being a doctor* is so central a psychological issue the physician-patient cannot discard the role and maintain self-esteem. As a consequence the treating physician must remember that it is a physician whom he is treating, no matter how hard each tries to deny this special circumstance of the doctor–patient relationship. Because communication consists of not only what is said but also of what is *not* said, the need for effective communication in view of the physician-patient's medical knowledge becomes *more*, rather than less, important.

What must remain as an acknowledged aspect of this special doctor–patient relationship is that the patient, despite being a doctor, also assumes the psychological characteristics of a patient. As a patient the doctor-patient's view of the illness is from an emotional and subjective viewpoint and behavior is characterized by regression as would be the reaction of any patient. The treating physician's therapeutic tactic must be to remain aware of patient's emotional needs, including the special requirements presented by the patient's status as a doctor, but he must approach the medical care from an objective stance.

The following case vignette illustrates the effective and humane management of one physician's life-threatening disease. These particular techniques would by no means be appropriate for all physician-patients any more than there is one way to manage non-physician patients.

A 34-year-old physician and father of two children developed acute myelogenous leukemia not long after completing training and starting medical practice. Multiple outpatient and hospital admissions for chemotherapy and attendant complications were necessary. During this time, and until his ultimate death, the young physician with the help of his wife maintained a detailed personal medical record, which included all of the laboratory test results. He was assisted in this by his attending physician who provided him with all of the pertinent laboratory data. Decisions for medical management were made by the treatment team and then communicated to the patient for his concurrence. He essentially always agreed but would occasionally ask, "Have you thought of . . . ?"

The result of this treatment technique was to support the psysician-patient's effective use of intellectualization and isolation as a way to bind anxiety. In addition, his self-esteem was supported by the acknowledgment of his identity as a physician: an identity only recently won at high cost and about to be taken away from him.

THE DOCTOR–PATIENT RELATIONSHIP—A CONCEPT IN FLUX

The traditional concept of the doctor–patient relationship—the paternalistic model—is under attack from a large number of dissatisfied medical care users. The monopoly on medical care is being challenged not only by groups such as chiropractors but also by persons who want to assume responsibility for as much of their health care as is possible. This increased interest in personal responsibility for health is seen in a large number of books published for, and purchased by the lay public dealing with areas such as diet and physical fitness. The political ramifications of such an interest are demonstrated by the establishment of governmental regulatory agencies which by law have substantial representation from nonmedical segments of the society. These developments undermining the traditional authority of the physician in matters regarding health and illness are often derided by members of the medical profession, who use terms such as "consumerism" or "governmental interference" as catchwords to voice their dissatisfactions.

If one looks beneath the surface conflicts it is not unreasonable to propose that the real issue is patients' dissatisfaction with the medical model, as prevalently employed. More specifically, this dissatisfaction is focused upon frustration with the doctor–patient relationship. There are nostalgic wistful longings for the good old days of the "country doctor," "house calls," "someone who knew you and your family," and "who took time to talk with you." But if this romanticized view of medical practice ever existed, it is probable that it did not occur during the lifetimes of the overwhelming majority of living Americans. Complaints concerning the "scientific" nature of medicine were already common in the decades of the 1920s and 1930s (Henderson, 1935; Peabody, 1927). In my view a "return" to the type of medical practice which has been idealized and romanticized would be atavistic. Modern technical medicine requires specialization in order to learn highly technical procedures, and "house calls" are an extremely inefficient use of physicians' time (consider travel time). Also, once in the patient's home there is little (besides, of course, the very valuable doctor–patient relationship) that can be offered because of a lack of diagnostic and treatment agents and equipment.

To reject scientific medicine would be absurd; but we are not in an "either/or" dilemma because it is possible to maintain the advantages of modern technology and expand one's therapeutic/diagnostic potency by effective use of interpersonal skills. Engel (1981) has observed that a failure to acknowledge and utilize an important factor which has been statistically demonstrated to affect illness outcome is in itself unscientific.

To return to considerations of what changes are occurring in the expectations of the doctor–patient relationship we can observe that "consumers" (patients) are demanding change. They have difficulty in articulating exactly what they want, but are increasingly accepting responsibility for their own health maintenance. A personal acceptance of responsibility for health may be the single greatest advance in medicine in the next several decades because the next major increments in longevity are likely to be due to changes in life habits rather than technical innovations (Knowles, 1977). It is not then unreasonable for one to extrapolate that, if a person accepts responsibility for his health management, then he/she will expect some degree of control and responsibility for disease management.

From the other side of the doctor–patient relationship, physicians complain about dependent clinging patients, yet place patients in a double bind by expecting them to give up all autonomy in their relationships with the physician. If as noted above, the major advances in health will come from changes in life habits, it would appear medically prudent to transfer responsibility for these life habits to the patient. A reformulation of a relationship between a physician and his patient would emphasize that a physician must assume the role of teacher. The physician becomes a source of expert knowledge and, as appropriate, this knowledge is imparted to the patient. It is of interest to note that in Indo-European languages the words for doctor and teacher derive from similar roots (Balint, 1957).

However, when a patient becomes seriously ill there is an almost inevitable psychological regression. It is the patient who demands that the physician assume responsibility and authority. Because of this regression the patient's judgment may be impaired, and it becomes incumbent upon the physician to make medical decisions which are in the best interest of the patient. Because of this very human characteristic, it would be unreasonable to assume that a teacher–student model of the doctor–patient relationship would always be appropriate.

It follows, from the above discussion of the type of relationship that a patient may require at given times, that flexibility is required on the part of the physician. During periods of health or minor illness the physician is a teacher, a source of knowledge and a collaborator in health maintenance. At times of serious illness the physician responds to the patient's voluntary relinquishment of the partnership relationship and assumes increasing responsibility and authority as is indicated. Responsibility is returned to the patient as soon as is feasible in order to facilitate recovery and discourage undue dependency. The patient's relinquishment of authority is usually an unconscious action and may be communicated in subtle ways. For example, I have observed that patients who usually talk to me on a first name basis will, upon becoming sick, change and start addressing me by "Dr. Ford."

If it is assumed that the management of health and disease is a collaborative venture, then the conflict over medical records and informed consent suddenly becomes a nonconflict. The withholding of information is antithetical to a mutually assumed responsibility.

THE PROBLEM PATIENT

Difficulty in the doctor–patient relationship generally leads to identifying the patient as a "problem patient." Lipsitt, during a symposium devoted to dysfunctional doctor–patient relationships (Lipsitt et al., 1981), aptly noted that, while we often talk of the problem patient in reference to dysfunctional doctor–patient relationships, we rarely speak of the "problem physician." The following discussion will strive to keep in perspective that a dysfunctional doctor–patient relationship may result from difficulties on either or both sides of this emotionally intense relationship.

There are several types of patients which are recurrently identified as troublesome to physicians (Drossman, 1978; Goodwin et al., 1979; Groves, 1978; Lorber, 1975). These problem patients include those who have physical complaints but little evidence of organic disease; the somatizers (the subject to which this book is primarily addressed); patients who are covertly suicidal or are in other ways self-destructive, e.g., alcoholism; those who are demanding and clinging or uncooperative in their behavior; and those whose emotional responses are considered excessive for the degree of physical disease which they are believed to have.

It is readily apparent that a patient who does not fit a mode of the physician's expectations is soon regarded as a problem. Those expectations can be summarized as follows: a good patient presents with objective signs and symptoms of a treatable disease process, makes no emotional demands upon the physician (e.g., makes no discomforting displays of excessive emotion), cooperates in the treatment process (e.g., obeys the physician's orders) and upon getting well displays gratitude for the help received. Difficulty occurs when the above conditions are not fulfilled, and with the development of a problem the culpability is assigned to the patient. That the problem may reflect stress or strain in the social system, defined as the doctor–patient relationship, a failure of communication of mutual needs and expectations, or that the patient was unable to articulate the actual nature of his symptoms is rarely considered. Several of these issues will be considered individually.

Covertly Self-Destructive Patients

Goodwin and colleagues (1979) have observed that patients who were liked the least by their physicians were actually covertly suicidal. This observation is consistent with the opinion of Groves (1978) that one of the groups of patients found "hateful" by physicians is one which he labels "self-destructive deniers." Groves describes these patients as appearing to derive their main pleasure in defeating the physician's attempts to preserve their lives. Examples of self-destructive deniers include such patients as those who continue to drink alcohol after being warned of liver damage or patients with severe emphysema who persist in smoking cigarettes. The patient's self-destructive behavior (which may be covertly suicidal) repetitively returns them to medical care, which will transiently improve their situation but engenders a sense of futility in their caretakers. Not infrequently, the physician will react to them with overt anger or malice and perhaps will harbor a secret wish that the patient would die and get it over with. Such an emotional response or malevolent fantasy results in guilt feelings of impotence and rejection of the patient, or via reaction formation may result in overly solicitous or gratuitously heroic rescue efforts. It must be kept in mind that some of these patients may be seriously depressed and must be evaluated for potential antidepressant treatment, and that others cannot or will not accept genuine treatment of any nature. There are some patients whose need for illness, and/or self-destruction, is greater than any physician's capacity to treat them. When physicians encounter such patients, humane care must be offered but its refusal should not be equated with a sense of personal failure.

The Uncooperative Patient

The "uncooperative patient" is frequently labeled by the physician as deviant or in other ways is regarded as less than ideal. That patients should be cooperative and unquestionly accept their physician's "orders" is a concept endorsed by many patients as well as by their caretakers. In few other human situations is there such a blind and passive acceptance of authority. Because of this general expectation of obeisance the patient who questions his treatment, refuses to accept procedures, or who demands that the hospital make concessions to his needs (rather than subjugate personal needs to the idiosyncrasies of hospital rules) is frequently labeled as troublesome, bad, psychiatrically disturbed, or as having "conflicts with authority." The physician's response to the uncooperative patient is one of defensiveness, anger, or rejection. Rarely is the lack of cooperation regarded as prudent or the product of enlightened self-interest. The following clinical vignette reported by a 38-year-old woman to her psychotherapist illustrates the type of conflict over control which is common between physicians and patients.

An internist, the patient's personal physician for the preceding 15 years, recommended a new treatment for the patient's annoying but not life-threatening chronic disease. The patient demurred stating that she wanted more information and a second opinion because she had heard that the treatment was potentially dangerous. The internist's response was to become furious and he demanded to know whom she thought the doctor was: her or him? He threatened to discharge her from his practice but relented when he had calmed down. The patient observed to the psychotherapist that she had always done what the physician had prescribed in the past, just as she had always followed her mother's requests. Insightfully, she observed that her physician was very similar in personality to her controlling, domineering, obsessive-compulsive mother whom she had always obeyed. Interestingly, following a consultation with another physician, she accepted the recommended treatment and planned to continue her relationship with the original internist, commenting that "he *is* a good doctor." She regarded the confrontation as a growth experience but it is easy to imagine that with another less insightful patient the scenario may have played to a less benign conclusion.

Although conflicts over whether or not to accept therapeutic recommendations can be directly seen as an issue of cooperation, a patient's failure to get well may also be irrationally (and perhaps unconsciously) viewed as poor cooperation. I have seen multiple situations where the physician's therapeutic efforts have failed or have resulted in less than hoped for results with blame subsequently projected to the patient for failure to "cooperate." Statements such as "he got postoperative pneumonia because he wouldn't do his breathing exercises properly" are commonly heard in any hospital. The unconscious statement being made is that after treatment has been offered it is the patient's obligation to get well; a failure to do so is interpreted as a lack of cooperation.

The explanations of issues concerning struggles for control (cooperation vs rebellion) within the doctor–patient relationship are found on both sides of the dyad. Many patients struggle repetitively with any form of authority, or imagined authority, be it school, employment or the military. Psychiatric illness may also result in poor cooperation because of such factors as decreased cognitive abilities, delusions, or self-destructive attitudes associated with depression. On the other side of the dyad is the physician and the attitudes and personality characteristics, which were brought to medicine and which have been reinforced through the process of socialization into the medical profession. As noted elsewhere (Chapter 12) physicians have a high frequency of obsessive-compulsive characteristics. Persons with these personality traits have a need to control their environments and feelings of weakness or vulnerability are defended against by efforts to become omnipotent and omniscient. Power over patients is one way of reversing the sense of impotency which was experienced with parents, and the cure of a patient's disease is a way of denying one's own vulnerability to disease. Patients who fail to surrender their autonomy or who fail to respond by getting well are not well regarded because they frustrate important psychological needs of the physician. This threat to omnipotence can be handled by labeling the patient as "uncooperative" and thereby denying one's own lack of power.

The Clinging Patient

The patient who later becomes recognized as a clinging patient, and a problem, is often initially regarded as a "good patient." He or she is usually on time for appointments, cooperative with proposed treatments or procedures, and is grateful. With the passage of time the patient becomes increasingly regarded as clinging and demanding. Therapeutic efforts are unsuccessful or are followed by the development of new symptoms. The problem of the clinging patient is not unique to the medical/surgical physician. Psychotherapists may also find themselves confronted with these patients whose covert aim is not to get well but rather to perpetuate the relationship with the doctor (Safirstein, 1972). Giovacchini (1970) has noted that these patients' behavior, which becomes more angry and demanding with the passage of time in the relationship with the physician, is the result of deficient mothering in crucial periods of psychic development. In seeking medical treatment the patient is looking for something which is perceived as missing, but neither the patient nor the physician comprehend the nature of what is being sought. The patient feels deprived, makes increasing demands, and becomes angry when expectations are not fulfilled. The physician frustrated in his efforts to find a cure, feels alternately resentful of the patient's unfair and unreasonable demands and guilty because of a failure to help the patient. Ultimately the physician withdraws or attempts to avoid the patient (Groves, 1978). The hurt and angry patient leaves the relationship and repeats the cycle with another physician (Giovacchini, 1970).

One management technique is to encourage the patient's relationship with the overall clinic or hospital situation ("institutional transference") and thereby reduce the interpersonal demands upon any one person (Safirstein, 1972). Encouragement of the patient's clinging demands may be counter-therapeutic because of the impossibility of ever effectively meeting such demands and the potential for acting-out behavior by the patient when he/she inevitably feels rejected.

The Overemotional and/or Suffering Patient

Among surgical patients, those who were found to be most disliked by the medical care staff were those who were as not seriously ill in the eyes of the staff but who nonetheless acted as if they were, by their behavior of complaining, crying, and refusal to cooperate with medical procedures (Lorber, 1975). Those patients who were seriously ill and engaged in similar behavior were regarded as problem patients but were "forgiven" because of the nature of their illnesses. These reactions of the health care team to these patients, who responded to illness with exaggerated emotions, can be understood in light of Hollender's (1958b) observations concerning the seeking of sympathy or pity. He has noted that because suffering usually evokes a response of sympathy some persons may use illness as a means of extracting sympathy or pity from another. This sympathy serves to maintain an affective (emotional) quality in their interpersonal relationships. However, since sympathy or pity places a demand upon another person, it is more likely to evoke hostile reactions than are other forms of behavior such as seeking of admiration. It is these demands for increased dependent care elicited by excessive emotional expression, or a display of suffering, that evoke the negative responses in physicians and result in inappropriate clinical decisions such as early discharge (Lorber, 1975).

Another aspect of the discomfort experienced by the physician in response to emotional displays by a patient is that of the physician's characteristic rejection of emotional (affective) modes of relating to others in favor of "logical" modes of communication. The typical physician uses the logical, fact-oriented cognitive style of the obsessive-compulsive personality and is to some degree emotionally constricted.

Somatizing Behavior

A recurrent theme in this book is that physicians are repetitively consulted for somatic complaints which do not fit the bioscientific model of medicine. The patient cannot in any verbal method communicate his need. The often desperate and agonizing pleas for help are couched in symptomatic complaints of a somatic nature which demand cure. However, what may be actually underlying these physical complaints is a psychic pain which is feared even more than physical illness. This pain may be due to depression, anxiety, or the fear of completely losing one's sense of self (psychosis). The pain may also represent an unfilled hunger or sense of emptiness which reflects back to defective and inadequate parenting at a time of crucial psychosocial development (Giovacchini, 1970). The repetitive efforts to establish a therapeutic relationship with a physician are attempts to fulfill a need which can be comprehended consciously only as a defect in one's physical sense of being.

The somatizing patient is a very difficult problem for many physicians. The reason for this is the similarities between the somatizing patient and the physician. The physician through the use of reaction formation is often defending against the very issues presented by the somatizing patient. Physicians have a higher than average incidence of psychiatric problems (usually depression), use hypochondriacal ego defense mechanisms themselves, and frequently come from childhood homes where dependent needs were not adequately gratified (see Chapter 12). Because somatizing behavior in patients threatens defenses, if often elicits anxiety in the physician and is dealt with through anger, rejection or aversion. By the mechanism of projection the problem, which is both that of physician and patient, is assigned exclusively to the patient.

Because of its importance to the major theme of this book, the management of somatizing disorders, through use of the doctor–patient relationship, is discussed in a separate section below.

USING THE DOCTOR–PATIENT RELATIONSHIP WITH SOMATIZING PATIENTS

Peabody (1927) stated that the doctor–patient relationship is important in all illnesses but doubly so with the "functional disorders." Yet despite the obvious truth, Peabody's observation is too infrequently translated into the practical day-to-day clinical care of the somatizing patient. The reason for this difficulty would appear to be the frustration engendered by confusing communications and expectations on both sides of the relationship.

The patient with a somatizing disorder presents himself/herself at the physician's office with a "ticket of admission" which consists of a somatic complaint. What is really being said in form of a metaphor is, "I am in pain, I hurt and I need a good parent to relieve my distress. Moreover, because of past injustices and poor care in the past I am entitled to loving care from you." Of course, because this message is determined by unconscious factors, the patient cannot articulate it more clearly than by a demand of treatment for the somatic distress. The patient unconsciously longs for an idealized relationship with the physician and is more than willing to surrender authority and responsibility to the physician.

On the other hand, the physician responds to the somatizing patient with scientific interest in the somatic complaint, which has been accepted on face value. Employing a paternalistic model of medical care, diagnostic and treatment procedures are "ordered." The almost inevitable result of this approach is (1) The patient responds to the authority of the physician with regression (becoming more childlike); (2) The physician responds to the patient's failure to get well and to the regression with frustration and anger.

The patient, who has experienced inadequate parenting during childhood, is often remarkably tolerant of an unsatisfying doctor–patient relationship (Lipsett et al., 1981). The physician, perhaps because of defenses against emotional factors similar to those of the patient, becomes anxious and is less accepting of the relationship. The physician may seek to terminate the relationship by seeing the patient as infrequently as possible or by referral to another physician or clinic. Eventually, the relationship does end, an unsatisfactory encounter for both the patient and physician. The patient then seeks the services of another physician and the scenario is replayed, too often with exactly the same conclusion.

The initiative for changing the recurrent nontherapeutic encounters between doctors and somatizing patients must come from physicians; the patients are unaware of the origins of their behavior. One of the best brief explanations of the process of treating the somatizing patient is by Reusch (1948) who states that treatment of these patients is employing the technique of child psychiatry to adult patients. The patient cannot immediately come to grips with the fact that somatizing behavior serves as an infantile means of communicating feelings and needs. Rather, he must learn new more mature methods of relating to others. Such a process requires time and patience. The physician cannot expect rapid change, but instead must first attempt to save the patient from further somatic injury consequent to unnecessary diagnostic treatment procedures. Second, the physician can employ treatment techniques which will ultimately alter the patient's somatizing behavior. Through the relationship with the physician, the patient learns that it is permissible (and desirable) to express emotions and that there is a need to assume responsibility for oneself. For change to occur it is essential that the physician makes alterations in the paternalistic doctor–patient relationship. The patient will find such changes in the relationship initially uncomfortable, because a dependent relationship is unconsciously sought. However, similar to the situation of the good parent who with time progressively turns over responsibility to the growing child, the physician must turn over increasing responsibility for health and disease management to the somatizing patient.

It is a paradox that the model of the doctor–patient relationship preferred by physicians (the paternalistic model by which the physician maintains authority) is the mechanism which may prevent "bad patients" (somatizing patients) from becoming "good patients." The physician, in order to alter this "double bind" placed upon patients, must learn to identify personal psychological characteristics (the need for omnipotence) in order that these are not played out contrary to patients' therapeutic needs.

SUMMARY

Until the 20th century, the doctor–patient relationship presented the primary therapeutic modality available to physicians. The efficacy of the relationship to influence physiologic changes has been concretely demonstrated by the placebo effect.

The doctor–patient relationship is strongly influenced by emotional factors. The physician, through trust, confidence, and concern, helps to provide hope and to alleviate fear and doubt. In return, the relationship with the patient provides emotional and intellectual gratification for the physician.

Traditionally, the doctor–patient relationship has been paternalistic in nature, the patient surrendering autonomy to the physician. Recently, there have been societal shifts in attitudes to make the practice of medicine less authoritarian.

Several types of patients have been identified as troublesome to physicians. Prominent among these are somatizing patients who are often concurrently clinging and dependent. A proposed technique for the management of the somatizing patient is to effect changes in the doctor–patient relationship, which will increase the patient's personal responsibility for health and disease management.

With all due respect to the triumphs of bioscientific medicine, the doctor–patient relationship remains a potent therapeutic force for all illnesses; for the somatizing disorders, it is the primary means of treatment.

REFERENCES

Adler, H.M., and Hammett, V.B.O. 1973. The doctor–patient relationship revisited: An analysis of the placebo effect. Ann Int Med 78:595–598.

Alfidi, R.J. 1975. Controversy, alternatives, and decisions in complying with the legal doctrine of informed consent. Radiology 114:231–234.

Altman, J.H., Reich, P., Kelly, M.J., and Rogers, M.P. 1980. Patients who read their hospital charts. N Engl J Med 302:169–171.

Balint, M. 1957. *The Doctor, His Patient and the Illness.* New York: International Universities Press.

Bass, L.W., and Wolfson, J.H. 1980. Professional courtesv. Pediatrics 65:751–757.

Beecher, H.K. 1955. The powerful placebo. JAMA 159:1602–1606.

Bergler, J.H., Pennington, A.C., Metcalfe, M., and Freis, E.D. 1980. Informed consent: how much does the patient understand? Clin Pharmacol Ther 27:435–440.

Brock, D., Lawson, R.K., Bennett, W.M. 1973. Preoperative workshops with patients waiting for kidney transplants. Transplant Proc 5:1059–1060.

Carson, R.A. 1977. What are physicians for? JAMA 238:1029–1031.

Comfort, A. 1978. On healing Americans. J Operational Psychiatry 1:25–36.

Cousins, N. 1976. Anatomy of an illness (as perceived by the patient). New Engl J Med 295:1458–1463.

Curran, W.J. 1979. Massachusetts patients' bill of rights: Cabbages, kings, sausages and laws. N Engl J Med 301:1433–1435.

Drossman, D.A. 1978. The problem patient: Evaluation and care of medical patients with psychosocial disturbances. Ann Int Med 88:366–372.

Engel, G.L. 1967. A psychological setting of somatic disease: The 'giving-up—given up' complex. Proc Roy Soc Med 60:533–535.

Engel, G.L. 1981. The care of the patient, art or science? Rhode Island Med J 64:95–103.

Evans, F.J. 1981. The placebo response in pain control. Carrier Foundation Letter #71, pp 1–4, Belle Mead, New Jersey.

Findley, T. 1953. The placebo and the physician. Med Clin N A 37:1821–1826.

Flexner, J.M., and Abram, H.S. 1978. A hostile patient—Fighting ire with ire. Hastings Center Rep 18–20.

Franklin, R.W., Goolishian, H.A., and White, R.B. 1965. Psychological hazards involved in treatment of medical colleagues (a further report). Dis Nerv Syst 26:731–734.

Gee, H.H. 1960. Learning the doctor–patient relationship. JAMA 173–1301–1304.

Giovacchini, P.L. 1970. Characterological problems: The need to be helped. Arch Gen Psychiat 22:245–251.

Goodwin, J.M., Goodwin, J.S., and Kellner, R. 1979. Psychiatric symptoms in disliked medical patients. JAMA 241:1117–1120.

Grotjahn, M. 1964. On being a sick physician. In *New Dimensions in Psychosomatic Medicine.* Wahl, C.W., ed. Boston: Little Brown.

Groves, J.E. 1978. Taking care of the hateful patient. New Engl J Med 298:883–887.

Halberstam, M.J. 1976. The patient's chart is none of the patient's business. Mod Med 44(19):85–88.

Henderson, L.J. 1935. Physician and patient as a social system. New Engl J Med 212:819–823.

Hollender, M.H. 1958a. *The Psychology of Medical Practice.* Philadelphia: W.B. Saunders Company, pp 5–13.

Hollender, M.H. 1958b. The seeking of sympathy or pity. J Nerv Ment Dis 126:579–584.

Houston, W.R. 1938. The doctor himself as a therapeutic agent. Ann Int Med 11:1416–1425.

Johnson, B.A., and James, A.E. 1979. The radiologist and informed consent: A review comments and proposals. Current Prob in Diag Radiol 7(6):1–19.

Joyce, C.R.B. 1972. The issue of communication within medicine. Psychiatry Med 3:357–363.

Knowles, J.H. 1977. The responsibility of the individual. In *Doing Better and Feeling Worse: Health in the United States*. Knowles, J.H., ed. New York: Norton, pp 57–80.

Lankton, J.W., Batchelder, B.M., and Ominsky, A.J. 1977. Emotional responses to detailed risk disclosure for anesthesia, a prospective, randomized study. Anesthesiology 46:294–296.

Levine, J.D., Gordon, N.C., and Fields, H.L. 1978. The mechanism of placebo analgesia. Lancet 2:654–657.

Lewin, B.D. 1946. Counter-transference in the technique of medical practice. Psychosomatic Med 8:195–199.

Lipsitt, D.R. 1975. The doctor as patient. Psychiatric Opinion 12(5):20–25.

Lipsitt, D.R. 1980. The patient and the record. (editorial) N Engl J Med 302:167–168.

Lipsitt, D.R., Block, S., Drossman, D.A., and Gerson, S. 1981. Dysfunctional doctor–patient relationships: A study of 200 dyads and clinical comment. Workshop presented at the annual meeting of the American Psychosomatic Society, Boston, Mass., March 26.

Lorber, J. 1975. Good patients and problem patients: Conformity and deviance in a general hospital. J Health Soc Behav 16:213–225.

Nunberg, H. 1938. Psychological interrelations between physician and patient. Psychoanal Rev 25:297–308.

Ort, R.S., Ford, A.B., and Liske, R.E. 1964. The doctor–patient relationship as described by physicians and medical students. J Health Human Behav 5:25–34.

Patten, B.M., and Stump, W. 1978. Death related to informed consent. Texas Med 74(12):49–50.

Peabody, F.W. 1927. The care of the patient. JAMA 88:877–882.

Pickering, G. 1978. Doctor–patient relationship: The impact of recent changes in medicine and society. Acta Med Scand 204:339–343.

Pinner, M. 1952. Chronic heart disease. In *When Doctors are Patients*. Pinner, M., and Miller, B.F., eds. New York: Norton, pp 18–30.

Pinner, M., and Miller, B.F., eds. 1952. *When Doctors are Patients*. New York, Norton.

Priluck, I.A., Robertson, D.M., and Buettner, H. 1979. What patients recall of the preoperative discussion after retinal detachment surgery. Am J Ophthal 87:620–623.

Reiser, D.E. 1973. Struggling to stay human in medicine. New Physician (May), 295–299.

Reusch, J. 1948. The infantile personality: The core problem of psychosomatic medicine. Psychosom Med 10:134–144.

Robinson, G., and Merav, A. 1976. Informed consent: Recall by patients tested post-operatively. Ann Thoracic Surg 22:209–212.

Safirstein, S.L. 1972. The clinging patient—A serious management problem. Canad Psychiat Asso J 17(Supl):ss221–ss225.

Shapiro, A.K. 1959. The placebo effect in the history of medical treatment: Implications for psychiatry. Am J Psychiatry 116:298–304.

Shapiro, A.K. 1964. Factors contributing to the placebo effect. Amer J Psychotherapy 18:73–88.

Shapiro, A.K. 1970. Placebo effects in psychotherapy and psychoanalysis. J Clin Pharmacology 10:73–78.

Stein, M., Schiavi, R.C., and Camerino, M. 1976. Influence of brain and behavior on the immune system. Science 191:435–440.

Szasz, T.S., and Hollender, M.H. 1956. A contribution to the philosophy of medicine: The basic models of the doctor–patient relationship. Arch Intern Med 97:585–592.

Tumulty, P.A. 1978. The art of healing. Johns Hopkins Med J 143:140–143.

Wahl, C.W. 1964. Psychodynamics of the hypochondriacal patient. In *New Dimensions in Psychosomatic Medicine*. Wahl, C.W., ed. Boston: Little Brown.

Waitzkin, H., and Stoeckle, J.D. 1972. The communication of information about illness. In *Advances in Psychosomatic Medicine, vol. 8, Psychosocial Aspects of Physical Illness*. Lipowski, Z.J., ed. Basel: Karger, pp 180–215.

White, R.B., and Lindt, H. 1963. Psychological hazards in treating physical disorders in medical colleagues. Dis Nerv Syst 24:304–309.

Williams, T.F. 1950. Cabot, Peabody, and the care of the patient. Bull Hist Med 24:462–481.

14

SUMMARY AND CONCLUSIONS

Health, disease, and illness are processes which are determined by multiple factors: social, intrapsychic, and pathophysiologic. The services of a physician are sought because of *illness*, a personal sense of suffering, and disability. Once under the care of the physician, a person becomes a "patient." The patient's illness may, or may not, be associated with *disease*, as defined as objective evidence of pathophysiologic or anatomic deformations. Somatization is the term used to describe physical symptoms or abnormal bodily sensations which are not directly related to a disease process.

Somatization includes the use of the body as a coping mechanism for personal gain or as a means of expression of an emotional state. It is a common phenomenon, probably employed to some degree by everyone at one time or another. However, some people repetitively use somatization; for them, illness is a way of life.

Repetitive somatizers become chronic patients. Various studies have demonstrated that, depending upon the type of medical practice, up to 40% of patients seen in physicians' offices have no evidence of disease. In addition, epidemiologic studies have demonstrated that a small proportion of people account for a disproportionately large portion of all medical services rendered. Similarly, a small proportion of people account for a disproportionately large portion of work disability days. It is likely that somatizing patients comprise a significant percentage of those persons who are high utilizers of medical services and who frequently miss work because of illness.

Sick people behave in characteristic ways. Regression almost always accompanies serious disease or injury. Also very common are responses of anxiety and grief. The latter is manifested by its various components of denial, anger, depressed mood, and preoccupation with the lost object, health. Because these reactions to illness are so common and are accepted as normal, social and cultural values make provisions for the ill person. The *sick role* relieves the ill person of blame for the illness and provides relief from usual personal responsibilities. The sick role, although sanctioned by society, is considered deviant and temporary. The sick person is expected to seek medical help and to abandon the role as soon as is possible. Most people with acute illnesses do recover and leave the sick role within a socially acceptable period of time. Most people with chronic disease make necessary emotional and reality-based adjustments in their lives in order that they can reaccept responsibility for themselves and reenter the main flow of society as productive persons.

Unlike the normal person, who develops an acute disease process and abandons the deviant sick role with recovery, the somatizer persistently remains in the sick role and continues to behave as if acutely ill. Consistent with this sick-role behavior are continuing expectations by the somatizing patient that others will do something for him/her. Among these expectations are responses of pity, sympathy, and concern from others; provision of addicting medications; relief from usual responsibilities; and monetary compensation. At times the process of somatization also provides solutions to intrapsychic conflicts. For example, "pain" may be a result of a need to suffer, and "disabling" physical symptoms may serve to rationalize real or perceived inadequacies.

A major subgroup of patients who somatize are those who have limited capacities to articulate their needs and emotions. Such patients may be alexithymic and, through developmental and/or neurophysiologic defects, be unable to express their emotional distress. Cultural factors may also have an important function in inhibiting or blocking emotional expression. An open display or communication of emotional states may not be sanctioned by the person's cultural milieu. Because of sociopolitical reasons, a person may not be able to express a psychiatric disability as such. Insurance companies, governmental agencies, employers, military superiors, and family members may reject any claim for social or vocational disability on the basis of psychological impairment. A translation of a psychological disability to a somatic disorder may then make acceptable the occupancy of the sick role.

It is essential to recognize that some persons who have genuine organic disease may use their disease for personal reasons. Therefore, the presence of genuine underlying disease does not rule out somatizing behavior. Somatization may become superimposed upon the disease process for persons who have a propensity to use somatic symptoms as a form of communication or who find aspects of the sick role to be solutions to life problems. For these individuals there may be little difference between the phenomenology of their illnesses and those of people who have more pure somatizing disorders. Thus, from a clinical viewpoint, the boundary between somatizing disorders and organic disease is often very indistinct. Somatizing patients do develop organic diseases, and patients with organic disease may engage in somatizing behavior.

Somatization has been used as a unifying concept in this book to bring together a variety of disorders characterized by abnormal illness behavior. As is apparent from a review of the various somatizing disorders, there are multiple overlaps among the various diagnostic terms. There are also some important differences among these patients which may call for specific therapeutic interventions.

SIMILARITIES AND DIFFERENCES AMONG SOMATIZING DISORDERS

The remarkable number of similarities among the various somatizing disorders suggests that many of the differences among these disorders are quantitative rather than qualitative. That is not to say that all somatizing behavior is equivalent, but rather that there is less specificity to the various disorders than implied by the diagnostic terminology.

Irrespective of the specific type of somatizing behavior studies, a common finding is a history of a disturbed childhood. There are two major patterns of childhood described. The first, which is typical of patients with Briquet's syndrome, factitious disease, and Munchausen syndrome, is that of inconsistency. These childhoods are chaotic and result in overstimulation. Multiple changes in the parents' marital partners, alcoholism, physical abuse, and dealings with various social agencies have all been frequently reported. The second major type of childhood described, more typical of the hypochondriacal patient and certain types of pain patients, is one of stability but without warmth. Parents are frequently described as hypochondriacal themselves and worried. One parent was often domineering and the other, passive. In both of these types of childhood, there was a failure to have experienced close, constant and/or affectionate relationships with parents.

Frequently the somatizing patient has had personal experience during childhood with illness or chronic disease. At times it was the patient who as a child had a serious illness; in other situations, a parent or sibling was sick. The illness is remembered by the patient as altering the family relationships and may have been a means for obtaining something not otherwise available. A period of hospitalization may have been seen as a pleasant experience. Health care staff may have been warm and shown concern, and there was relief from the tension at home. For other patients, illness was seen as a means of obtaining attention from otherwise emotionally uninvolved parents. In these cases, there is often an aspect of sibling rivalry; the sick brother or sister was perceived as getting more from the parents in both attention and material goods.

There are varying manifestations of the general difficulty that most somatizing patients experience in expressing or communicating emotions.

The hypochondriacal patient usually has difficulty in expressing or verbalizing emotional feelings. The patient may look angry or depressed, but when questioned these feelings are most frequently denied. These patients are best described as emotionally constricted or inhibited, traits consistent with the obsessive-compulsive personality and the description of alexithymia. In contrast, patients with Briquet's syndrome, factitious illness, or Munchausen syndrome frequently have emotional outbursts. Emotions seem to be poorly controlled, even if not deeply felt. Despite this emotionality, the patients often have difficulty in directly expressing some feelings or ideas which are blocked from consciousness, and they must resort to somatic means of communication such as conversion phenomena.

The adult somatizing patient rarely has close, mature relationships with others. Those relationships which do exist are often neurotic in nature and/or characterized by a high degree of instability. A mature, active sexuality is not frequently seen in these patients, irrespective of the type of somatizing disorder. Patients, as adults, tend to reenact the types of childhood which they have experienced. Those patients with chaotic childhoods, marred by having an alcoholic parent, often marry an alcoholic. Many somatizing patients never marry or remain married for relatively brief periods of time. The demands of a close, mature sexual relationship with someone else are frightening or overwhelming to them. Other marriages which are more stable may involve a spouse who has a need to nurse someone or be characterized by a bland, emotionless quality.

The foregoing discussion has pointed out similarities among many somatizing patients irrespective of their diagnostic "labels." Some differences have also been alluded to. It would appear that there are some disorders which are more closely related to each other in terms of the phenomenology. I propose that a major differentiating characteristic in somatizing patients is that of cognitive style. One group of patients is typified by a hysterical cognitive style and the other, by an obsessive style. This proposal has its origins in the opinion of Briquet who, in the mid-19th century, suggested marked differences between hypochondriacs, whom he described as obsessive, and hysterics, whose symptoms he regarded as manifestations of emotions (Mai and Mersky, 1981).

Briquet's syndrome, factitious illness, Munchausen syndrome (and at times, malingering) are syndromes which have in common certain phenomenological features. These features include a dramatic presentation of symptoms and a poorly described but positive medical history. Patients with Briquet's syndrome are usually histrionic, with a gift for mimicry, and often prevaricate. The symptoms of patients with factitious disease and Munchausen syndrome are more elaborate dramatic productions, complete with simulated disease; role playing; and pseudologia fantastica. Diagnostic terms frequently applied to this group of patients include hysterical, sociopathic, and borderline personality disorders. Previous research has shown that Briquet's syndrome, hysterical personality, and sociopathy are often closely related. This proposed grouping of the disorders suggests that factitious disease and Munchausen syndrome may be similar to Briquet's syndrome but represent syndromes with more extreme symptom presentation. Patients with less-extreme symptomatic presentations (Briquet's syndrome) are usually hysterical personalities, and patients with factitious illness and Munchausen syndrome are characterized by a more severe personality disorder: borderline personality with hysterical features. Malingering is not a specific syndrome but rather a description of behavior. It is often closely associated with hysteria and sociopathy but has been described as associated with all psychiatric disorders and normal persons.

In contrast, hypochondriacs and many chronic pain patients are typified by an obsessive cognitive style. They are preoccupied with the details of their symptoms. They are superb, accurate historians often boring the physician with the minutiae of past symptoms and treatment. In addition, they are worried and fearful about the nature and any implication of diseases.

Chronic pain syndromes and disability syndromes which have been presented in this book as general categories of somatizing behavior are actually defined by the nature of the syndrome or secondary effect of the symptom rather than any basic etiologic factor. In fact, these disturbances are actually special manifestations of other disorders including Briquet's syndrome, hypochondriasis, and underlying psychiatric disorders such as depression, psychosis or posttraumatic stress syndrome.

Psychiatric illness is frequently masked by somatization. Atypical facial pain, persistent low back pain, and dermatitis artefacta are frequently symptomatic of a "masked" depression. The monosymptomatic hypochondriacal disorders appear to be closely related to underlying psychosis. In a less specific manner, some forms of somatizing behavior may be symptomatic expression of, or a defense against, psychiatric illness. For example, it has been proposed that Munchausen syndrome represents a defense against psychotic decompensation.

In conclusion, it is proposed that somatization is a nonspecific behavior pattern which most frequently has its origins in early life. There is a significant component of learned behavior. The somatizer has learned that there are advantages to being sick or that somatic illness is more socially acceptable than psychological disability. The symptomatic expression of somatizing behavior is closely related to the individual's personality and cognitive style. Briquet's syndrome, factitious disease, and Munchausen syndrome are related to each other and are on a continuum representing the severity of the underlying personality disorder. Hypochondriasis and some forms of chronic pain disorders appear to be somewhat qualitatively different and are more closely related to the obsessive cognitive style. Severe psychiatric illness may underlie any of the somatizing disorders. In at least some situations the somatizing behavior can be interpreted as a defense against further psychological decompensation.

PHYSICIANS AND SOMATIZING PATIENTS

In the introduction to this book it was stated that for patients with somatoform disorders illness is a way of life, and that in their devotion to the treatment of illness, physicians have also made illness a way of life. The two situations are two sides of the same coin!

A comparison of the characteristics of physicians and somatizers yields many similarities (see Table 1). A review of their psychological characteristics indicates that physicians have a higher-than-expected incidence of psychiatric disorders, primarily depression and drug abuse. Physicians frequently come from childhoods which were not supportive and which were often associated with illness, either in the individual or members of the family. Underlying conflicts with dependency are commonly described. Marital problems and difficulties with close interpersonal relationships are also frequently noted in physicians. All of the above characteristics are commonly seen in patients with somatizing behavior. In addition, physicians are frequently obsessive and emotionally constricted, characteristics frequently found in depressed patients who somatize and in hypochondriacs.

Physicians are *not* the same as somatizing patients. Despite the similarities, there are also some important differences. Physicians utilize reaction formation and counterphobic mechanisms to a great extent. Instead of being

TABLE I. Comparison of Characteristics of Somatizers and Physicians

Common Features of Somatizing Patients	Common Features of Physicians
Childhood homes with unmet dependency needs	Childhood homes with unmet dependency needs
Experience with illness and/or death as a child	Experience with illness and/or death as a child
Depression, often masked or denied	Depression, often masked or denied
Excessive use of medications	Increased incidence of addictions
Repressed sexuality	Increased incidence of sexual problems
Difficulty with overt expression of anger	Emotional constriction in general
Blatant dependency	Reaction formation as a means to defend against dependency wishes
Hypochondriacal preoccupation	Counterphobic in regard to disease and death
Wish for protection	Fantasies of omnipotence and omniscience

obsessed with the fear of disease and death, the physician defends against this fear by conquering disease. Rather than feeling weak and helpless, the physician maintains fantasies of omniscience and omnipotence.

Because of the psychological similarities shared with physicians, somatizing patients have the capacity to tap into the physicians' own intrapsychic conflicts. In an effort to defend against anxiety, the physician may not want to hear of depressive symptoms, dependent needs, marital problems and so forth. Because physicians may need to deny these issues, patients with similar characteristics may be subtly rejected. To the contrary, as a way of denying uncomfortable feelings, the physician may overcompensate and become solicitous and unwittingly reinforce somatizing behavior. Schildkrout (1980) lists four types of behavior that young physicians may utilize as a means of avoiding direct confrontation with emotional aspects of the doctor–patient relationship. These include (1) focusing upon an organic problem rather than confronting emotional issues, (2) using premature assurance when patients express concern about prognosis, (3) being "overprotective" (see above) when dealing with disliked patients, and (4) making a premature referral to another specialist before it is necessary. These forms of behavior may be directed toward any patient who elicits uncomfortable emotional responses in a physician. As suggested, such a response is especially likely to occur with a somatizing patient.

Because of the primacy of the doctor–patient relationship in the effective management of the somatizing disorders, it is important, perhaps essential, that the physician is aware of his/her emotional responses to certain types of patients and/or symptoms. With this awareness, the probability of unintentional antitherapeutic actions is substantially reduced.

THE MANAGEMENT OF SOMATOFORM DISORDERS

The initial step in managing somatization must be recognition. Identification of abnormal illness behavior is not always easy. There may be unconscious collusion between both patient and physician to avoid confronting the psychosocial issues which are influencing the patient's illness. It must also be kept in mind that somatizing patients cannot easily articulate their underlying psychological distress. If they could, somatization would not be necessary! Therefore it is not unusual for somatoform disorders to remain undiagnosed until considerable time has passed, medical expenses compiled and, perhaps, iatrogenic morbidity has occurred.

No single symptom or sign is indicative of a somatoform disorder, and abnormal illness behavior may be superimposed upon organic disease. There are, however, several features which may suggest the possibility that the patient's symptoms represent somatization. These include a lengthy past history of poorly defined illnesses; multiple surgical procedures; difficulty in discussing emotional feelings; a vague, dramatically presented medical history or, on the contrary, an obsessively detailed history. Other features which suggest the possibility of somatization are concurrent symptoms characteristic of depression. These symptoms include sleep disturbance, appetite disturbance, gastrointestinal changes, impaired concentration, and a loss of interest in usual activities.

When somatization has been identified, it is important, to the degree possible, to establish a more exact diagnosis. Does the patient have Briquet's syndrome? Is the symptom a signal of an acute psychosocial crisis? Are the symptoms an effort to establish a relationship with the physician? Is the patient suffering from an underlying depression or defending against a psychosis? Is the symptom indicative of a strain in the doctor–patient relationship?

In spite of the recognition that the patient's symptoms are not due to a disease process, it is still necessary to maintain the relationship. Referral to a psychiatrist is frequently not well-accepted and not necessarily of benefit. Most patients with somatization disorders do best with one physician who knows them, their histories and social situation, and who is able to interpret new symptoms which could represent the development of disease. With this type of ongoing relationship, there is a reduced probability of potentially dangerous, but unindicated, invasive diagnostic and therapeutic interventions. Regularly scheduled appointments will reduce the patient's need to develop a symptom in order to have an excuse to see the physician.

Underlying psychiatric disease (usually depression) must be treated. Often the primary care physician can effectively treat depression with pharmacological agents and in the context of the ongoing doctor–patient relationship. If the depression is of psychotic proportions (e.g., somatic delusions), a referral to a psychiatrist is indicated because of the risk of suicide.

The doctor–patient relationship is potentially the single most important treatment modality for somatizing patients. As the doctor becomes better acquainted with the patient, there can be increased recognition of the patient's use of physical symptoms as a metaphor. Symptoms are often attempts to convey feelings of hurt, needs for affection, anger, and a wish for help in an ongoing psychosocial crisis. The physician's ability to communicate that these feelings have been recognized, without ever directly confronting the patient concerning the symptom, may alleviate the need for the symptom. With receptive encouragement extending over time, the patient may gradually learn to express emotions and needs more directly, thereby making somatization unnecessary. Thus education becomes an important therapeutic technique as the somatizer learns new forms of illness behavior.

A doctor–patient relationship which emphasizes mutual participation (instead of the paternalistic model) will tend to undermine the patient's use of physical symptoms as a way to obtain gratification of dependency wishes. The patient's fantasies of the physician as an omnipotent, omniscient good parent tend to encourage regression and dependency. The physician, by refusing to play the "god-doctor" role and by co-opting the patient into responsibility for his/her health and disease management, encourages the patient to become more mature.

There are differences of management techniques among the various somatoform disorders. The "crock" may benefit from support of existing strengths and the encouragement to be more expressive of emotions. The hysteric (Briquet's syndrome) may need encouragement to be less volatile and emotionally labile and to express needs more directly with less manipulation through somatic symptoms. A family treatment approach is often indicated for patients with Briquet's syndrome because of the high frequency of these patients' chaotic life circumstances. Patients with factitious illness and Munchausen syndrome require patience, understanding and support. Patients with these disorders have severe characterological disorders, and their behavior often serves as a defense against a more severe psychological decompensation. However, despite the severity of the underlying psychopathology, these patients may do better with a primary care physician, with whom they can have a long-term relationship, than with a psychiatrist.

In response to the above suggestions concerning the management of somatization, the practicing physician might well respond with claims of insufficient time. This excuse is actually a straw man. A good history which documents Briquet's syndrome is obviously more cost- and time-effective than a continuing pattern of multiple hospitalizations! What is proposed above is basically a change in attitude and strategy toward patients. It has been demonstrated that physicians often know more about their patients than they had realized (Pittenger, 1962). Learning alternative ways of interpreting information and a willingness to confront psychosocial issues broadens therapeutic usefulness. This comes from an understanding that whatever the physician does or says has an immediate effect upon the patient, and that the doctor is really practicing medicine when sitting and listening to the patient (Pittenger, 1962). Physicians who have more interest in psychotherapy per se can incorporate this mode of treatment into their medical practices by the use of brief, time-limited therapy techniques (Castelnuovo-Tedesco, 1965).

Efficacy of Psychotherapeutic Interventions in Somatoform Disorders

The effectiveness of alternative treatment techniques of somatoform disorders remains for further investigation. Although not proven, it would seem reasonable that psychotherapeutic approaches to psychosocial crises would be more effective and humane than repetitive surgical operations. Similarly, the "treatment" of hypochondriacal suffering by repetitive diagnostic tests would appear to be a poor substitute for effective antidepressant therapy.

A few studies do suggest that somatizing behavior can be altered with a resultant decreased utilization of medical services. It has been proposed that group psychotherapy for chronic somatizing patients can reduce their utilization of medical services (Ford and Long, 1977; Friedman et al., 1979; Mally and Ogston, 1964; Roskin et al., 1980; Schoenberg and Senescu, 1966; Valko, 1976). This favorable response is presumably secondary to meeting the patient's affiliative needs through relationships within the group and the learning by group members to utilize new mechanisms to communicate and to alter their relationships with others.

Most investigations indicate that psychiatric consultation and/or psychotherapy subsequently decrease patients' medical utilization (Follette and Cummings, 1967; Goldberg et al., 1970; Jameson et al., 1978; Longobardi, 1981; Schlesinger and Mumford, 1982). The mechanism of this effect is not known. Possibilities include a specific therapeutic effect by the psychiatrist and/or a communication of relevant information and treatment recommendations back to the primary care physician.

Even modest interventions involving emotional support and/or the provision of information significantly reduce morbidity, length of hospitalization and the period of convalescence in surgery and heart attack patients (Mumford et al., 1982). If patients with demonstrated organic disease respond well to emotional support, it would seem reasonable that patients who somatize would also do well with support from primary physicians.

A long-term follow-up study indicated that behavior modification treatment of chronic pain in selected patients was highly effective (Roberts and Reinhardt, 1980). However, differentiation of specific therapeutic effects in pain control is often difficult because patients have received multiple simultaneous treatment modalities.

In summary, there is reason to believe that psychological interventions are effective in some forms of somatizing behavior. Further investigation will help elucidate the best therapeutic modality for each type of patient which has been discussed.

CONCLUSIONS

The use of somatic symptoms to cope with stress and to communicate with others is facilitated by a culture which emphasizes the disease model to interpret illness. Such somatization may occur in the presence or absence of a disease process.

Health, illness, and disease are all fluid states of being, the boundaries of which are determined by the interactions of environmental, physiologic, intrapsychic, and interpersonal factors. As with illnesses of all etiologies, the treatment of the somatizing patient must take into account all of the above factors. Primary among the therapeutic modalities available for the somatoform disorders is the physician, administered via the doctor–patient relationship. To be effective the physician must be aware not only of those qualities of the patient which determined the somatization but also of his/her own intrapsychic factors which influence this emotionally intense relationship.

Some persons appear to prefer a lifestyle characterized by illness, and they are resistant to all efforts to modify their patterns of somatization. Other patients who have previously made illness a way of life will, with treatment, develop new methods of coping and communicating and are able to discard their symptoms.

Helping to restore a patient to health, irrespective of the etiology of the illness, is one of the most personally satisfying aspects of being a physician; healing the patient is what it is all about.

REFERENCES

Castelnuovo-Tedesco, P. 1965. *The Twenty Minute Hour: A Guide to Brief Psychotherapy for the Physician*. Boston: Little Brown.

Follette, W., and Cummings, N.A. 1967. Psychiatric services and medical utilization in a prepaid health plan setting. Med Care 5:25–35.

Ford, C.V., and Long, K.D. 1977. Group psychotherapy of somatizing patients. Psychother Psychosom 28:294–304.

Friedman, W.H., Jelly, E., and Jelly, P. 1979. Group therapy for psychosomatic patients at a family practice center. Psychosomatics 20:671–675.

Goldberg, I.D., Krantz, G., and Locke, B.Z. 1970. Effect of a short-term outpatient psychiatric therapy benefit on the utilization of medical services in a prepaid group practice medical program. Med Care 8:419–428.

Jameson, J., Shuman, L.J., and Young, W.W. 1978. The effects of outpatient psychiatric utilization on the costs of providing third-party coverage. Med Care 16:383–399.

Longobardi, P.G. 1981. The impact of a brief psychological intervention on medical care utilization in an army health care setting. Med Care 19:665–671.

Mai, F.M., and Merskey, H. 1981. Briquet's concept of hysteria: An historical perspective. Can J Psychiatry 26:57–63.

Mally, M.A., and Ogston, W.D. 1964. Treatment of the 'untreatables'. Int J Group Psychother 15:369–374.

Mumford, E., Schlesinger, H.J., and Glass, G.V. 1982. The effects of psychological intervention on recovery from surgery and heart attacks: An analysis of the literature. Am J Public Health 72:141–151.

Pittenger, R.A. 1962. Training physicians in the psychologic aspects of medical practice. Penn Med J 65:1472–1474.

Roberts, A.H., and Reinhardt, L. 1980. The behavioral management of chronic pain: Long-term follow-up with comparison groups. Pain 8:151–162.

Roskin, G., Mehr, A., Rabiner, C.J., and Rosenberg, C. 1980. Psychiatric treatment of chronic somatizing patients: A pilot study. Int J Psychiatry Med 10:181–187.

Schildkrout, E. 1980. Medical residents' difficulty in learning and utilizing a psychosocial perspective. J Med Educ 55:962–964.

Schlesinger, H.J., and Mumford, E. 1982. The effects of psychotherapy on the utilization of medical care services. Presented at the Annual Meeting of the American Psychosomatic Society, Denver, Colorado, March 25.

Schoenberg, B., and Senescu, R. 1966. Group psychotherapy for patients with chronic multiple somatic complaints. J Chronic Dis 19:649–657.

Valko, R.J. 1976. Group therapy for patients with hysteria (Briquet's disorder). Dis Nerv Syst 37:484–487.

INDEX